Handbook of Neurc
Techniques

Dear Dr Lopez,

Ovr most esteemed Clleague

Respectfully,

Shuvanes Heyt.

.2/6/17

Shah-Naz H. Khan
Andrew J. Ringer

Handbook
of Neuroendovascular
Techniques

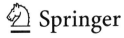 Springer

Shah-Naz H. Khan
Institute of General and Endovascular
 Neurosurgery (IGEN)
Flint, MI
USA

and

Department of Surgery
College of Human Medicine
Michigan State University
Flint, MI
USA

Andrew J. Ringer
Mayfield Clinic
Chief of Neurosciences, TriHealth System
Cincinnati, OH
USA

ISBN 978-3-319-52934-9   ISBN 978-3-319-52936-3   (eBook)
DOI 10.1007/978-3-319-52936-3

Library of Congress Control Number: 2017933849

Printed on acid-free paper

This Springer imprint is published by Springer Nature
The registered company is Springer International Publishing AG
The registered company address is: Gewerbestrasse 11, 6330 Cham, Switzerland

Preface

The necessity of a neuroendovascular handbook was recognized during the authors' fellowships. While numerous endovascular texts are available, none of them specifically address 'techniques' exclusively. We undertook this project initially from the perspective of someone just starting out in the specialty. All the mainstream procedures are described and step-by-step instructions provided such that the operator will know precisely what to do even if performing the procedures for the very first time. For the same reason, the text is written as if in points and any discussion that detracts from performance has been intentionally avoided. Our objective is that the reader should be able to open the book at any technique and find complete stepwise instructions in that particular chapter, without having to flip back and forth between various chapters or refer to multiple books. Therefore, this book can also be likened to an 'operative atlas.' The format and descriptions make this a useful manual not only for beginners, but also for more advanced practitioners who may not have performed a particular technique previously or may have done so infrequently. We have included practical tips that usually are not found in books and are gleaned by word of mouth, or learnt through performing the procedure repeatedly.

We recognize that there are many ways to skin a cat. The techniques described herein are mainstream and as practiced at our endovascular laboratories. Where indicated, alternatives have been described.

This is the first edition and first step in our project. While the standard handbook by itself will enable the reader to undertake any technique, we also intend to exploit the electronic version to its full potential. In this vein, video clips and other enhancing material will be available in the near future.

Finally, we deeply appreciate and welcome feedback from our readers and will use the comments and suggestions to make future editions even better.

Shah-Naz H. Khan
Flint, MI, USA

Andrew J. Ringer
Cincinnati, OH, USA

Acknowledgements

The authors wish to acknowledge the contribution of Ms. Farrah Garno (R)(VI) (ARRT), Radiology Supervisor/Clinical Instructor, Hurley Medical Center, Flint, MI, and Ms. Melanie Ashley RT(R)(VI), Hurley Medical Center, Flint, MI, for their invaluable assistance with obtaining most of the photographic images used in the handbook.

We would be remiss if we were not to recognize Ms. Stephanie Frost of Springer. Her professionalism as well as, her even-keeled, diplomatic and friendly temperament, went a long way in bringing this project to fruition.

Contents

Preparing for Angiography

Preparing the Angiography Equipment Table

- The sterile angiography equipment table is positioned behind the operator who faces the angiography operating table (Fig. 1.1).
- The equipment table should be kept clean and uncluttered. The length of the table should be long enough that catheters and wires may be stretched out over it during preparation. If needed, two tables may be placed end to end for adequate space.
- The table and the contents upon it are part of the operating field, and sterile precautions are maintained.
- Sterile drapes for the patient and angiography operating table and sterile gowns and gloves for the operators may be opened on this table according to operator preference.
- The table bears a round basin with sterile heparinized saline. The basin should be large and deep enough to hold wires and catheters when they are not in use. To ensure that the various catheters and wires don't get entangled, each one is looped to fit the basin and may be wrapped at one point in a moist Telfa® or gauze piece. It is ensured that the heparinized saline in the bowl is clean and devoid of any clots or other foreign bodies. If a clot is detected, discard the saline for a clean supply.
- A moist piece of Telfa or particle-free sponge should be available to wipe the wires when they are retracted from the catheter, and it should be replaced when any clot or debris is noted upon it.
- A foam-bedded container for sharps is provided, and the micropuncture needle, scalpel, suture needle, etc., are stuck into it after use. Do not attempt to recap needles.
- A manifold with a one-way valve may be used to dispense sterile heparinized saline, contrast, and waste fluids from syringes into a closed system. The manifold may be clipped to the equipment table or the angio table depending upon the preference of the surgeon.
- Sterile cotton gauzes (4 × 4) and towels are also provided.

© Springer International Publishing AG 2017
S.H. Khan and A.J. Ringer, *Handbook of Neuroendovascular Techniques*,
DOI 10.1007/978-3-319-52936-3_1

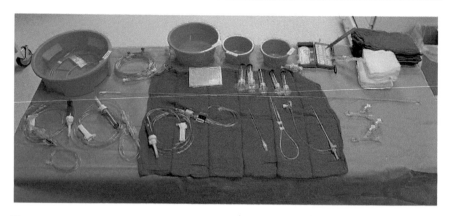

Fig. 1.1 A sterile angiography table is usually positioned behind the surgeon for easy access to equipment. The setup shown is prior to the patient being prepped and draped. The tubing in the *left* lower corner of the figure will be used for heparinized flushes of sheath and catheters and will come to lie on the sterile drape of the operating table, rather than the angiography table. A guide wire in its sheath can be seen in the *large blue bowl*. Heparinized saline will be added to the bowl, and once the hydrophilic coating of the guidewire is activated, it is kept wet at all times. Same is the case for catheters. A micropuncture kit and access sheath lie next to the tubing on the surgical towel. A Guide catheter can be seen lying across the table. The red foam container for sharps with scalpel, syringe with local anesthesia, micropuncture needle, and 2-0 silk suture can be seen

Instruments

- The following basic equipment would be required for any procedure, diagnostic or interventional: micropuncture kit: 21G needle with 0.018 guidewire and 4 Fr dilator OR single wall needle: 18G.

Medications (with Typical Doses)

- *Fentanyl* (e.g., 50–100 μgm IV) and *Versed* (0.5–1 mg) for sedation prior to arterial puncture. Administer additional doses through the procedure to maintain mild to moderate sedation, alleviating any anxiety while the patient is still able to follow instructions. These medications are not necessary if the procedure is done under general anesthesia.
- *Heparin* is present in the flush systems (see below) and is also administered IV to maintain the desired ACT during interventional procedures. For flush systems, 6000 IU of heparin in 1000 ml of normal saline (6 IU/ml) is continuously administered at a rate of 30 ml/hr through each indwelling catheter or sheath used. During interventional procedures, a 5000 IU (or 70 IU/kg) of heparin bolus is usually administered after arterial access or once the Guide catheter has

been secured in its position. In case of ruptured aneurysm, the heparin bolus may be deferred until the first coil has been placed. The ACT is measured 20 min after the bolus and then hourly. Additional heparin is administered as needed to maintain desired ACT. For goal ACTs, refer to specific procedure.

- Consult a hematologist first, in case of heparin-induced thrombocytopenia.
- *2% Lidocaine* for local anesthesia. Infiltrate skin with lidocaine prior to stab incision. Initially, raise a skin wheel and then advance the needle deeper into soft tissue. Before injecting, aspirate to ensure the needle tip is not in a vessel. Aspirate and inject as the needle is withdrawn.

Guidewires

- We typically use 0.035″ or 0.038″ to support 5 Fr and larger catheters, e.g., Glidewire® (Terumo Interventional Systems, Somerset, NJ) for diagnostic catheters and Guide catheters.

Shape

- Curved tip (30–60°) is useful for most selective catheterization.
- Straight tips are useful when navigating the abdominal aorta to avoid renal or splanchnic vessel selection.

Coating

- Hydrophilic coating, e.g., Glidewire®, may minimize friction and clot formation.
- Coated wires should NOT be used with arterial access needles as the coating may be stripped if the wire is withdrawn through the needle, resulting in embolic complications. For certain procedures where a sheath is not inserted and repeated angiographies via the same artery are anticipated (e.g., intra-arterial chemotherapy for brain tumors), we use a Bentson wire (Cook Medical, Bloomington, IN). It can be inserted and slid back through the arteriotomy needle without sheering off any coating.
- Table 1.1 shows common wires for diagnostic angiography. Refer to Chap. 5 for greater details.

Table 1.1 Common wires for diagnostic angiography

Wire type	Caliber	Length (cm)	Tip shape
Glidewires (Terumo) **Standard**, long taper, stiff shaft, stiff shaft long taper, long taper, 1 cm taper	0.032, 0.035, 0.038	120, **150**, 180, 260 cm	**Angled**, Shapeable tip, J-tip, Bolia curve
Bentson (Cook medical)	0.025, 0.032, 0.035, 0.038	145, 180, 200, 260 cm	1.5, 3 mm J

Refer to Chap. 5 for greater details

Sheaths

- Placed to enable exchange of wires, catheters, etc., without losing arterial access or causing repeated trauma to the vessel (Fig. 1.2a, b). The sheath is connected to a continuously running flush of heparinized saline.
- 5 Fr for diagnostic procedures; 6 Fr or larger for interventional procedures, e.g., coiling.
- 10–11 cm length is used for normal vasculature, 14 cm or longer for tortuous vasculature. May need to use an 80-cm or longer sheath, e.g., shuttle® sheath (Cook Medical, Bloomington, IN) in case intervention is required in tortuous vasculature.
- 2-0 silk suture or Tegaderm patch to secure the sheath, so that it is not displaced during procedure.
- In children, a 4-Fr sheath should be used for diagnostic purposes.
- Table 1.2 shows commonly used sheaths. The more commonly used specifications are indicated in bold. Refer to Chap. 5 for greater details.

Catheters

- One typically selects one or two catheters as standard workhorses for diagnostic angiography. Familiarize yourself thoroughly with one or two diagnostic and guide catheters. Then, a few for situations like tortuous vasculature that is not amenable to navigation with the usual diagnostic or guide catheters. We typically use a 5-Fr glidecath® (Terumo Bloomington, IN) as our diagnostic catheter (Fig. 1.3a, b) and a 6-Fr or larger (depending upon the intervention) Envoy® guide catheter (Fig. 1.4a, b; Codman & Shurtleff Inc, Raynham, MA) for interventional procedures. If we anticipate that the diagnostic angiography will be immediately followed by intervention and the patient's vasculature is not tortuous, we may use the Envoy guide catheter as the diagnostic catheter as well. This saves time and equipment, as switching from diagnostic to guide catheter is eliminated.

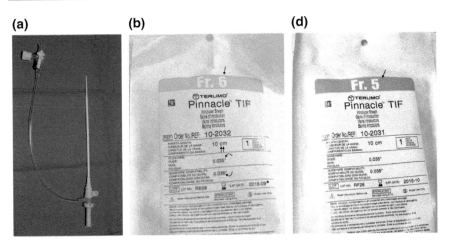

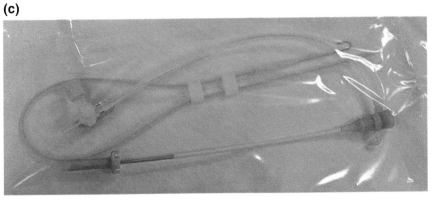

Fig. 1.2 a Terumo Pinnacle sheath. Typically, 5 Fr is used for diagnostic purposes, while 6 Fr and larger are used for intervention. The sheaths are frequently color coded for size. In this picture, the dilator (tapered *blue* end extending beyond the *white* sheath tip) has been inserted into the sheath and is ready to be inserted over the wire into the vessel. The short tubing enables attachment of the sheath to continuous flush. The additional port on the side can be used to draw blood or for injections. The labeling at the back of the package enables rapid access to information for sheath election **b**. The size of the sheath (*arrow*) and its length (*double arrows*) and the size of compatible wires (*curved arrows*) are shown. The number in a *rectangle* (in the first row with *double arrows*) indicates the number of sheaths in the package. The expiry date (*asterisk*) can be seen. The package contents can be easily visualized from the front **c**. The color of the sheath and dilator cap readily indicates that it is 6 Fr. The packaging of a 5-Fr sheath can be discerned from the 6 Fr label shown above by the number as well as the different color (**d**, *arrow*). Similarly, the sheath itself and the dilator cap are also colored *gray*

- In case of difficult vasculature, alternative catheters such as H-1 (Terumo) or Simmons 2 (Terumo) are used, instead of the usual diagnostic catheters (Fig. 1.5a, b). In the same vein, instead of an Envoy guide catheter, a shuttle sheath may be used, which is advanced to its intended position over an H1 slip catheter (Cook Medical) and 0.035 glidewire. The slip catheter and wire are

Table 1.2 Commonly used sheaths are indicated below

Type	Inner diameter (Fr)	Length (cm)	Length of protruding dilator (cm)	Guidewire
Pinnacle (terumo)	4, **5**, **6**, 7, 8, 9, 10, 11	10, 25	2.5	0.035[a]
Super arrow Flex (arrow)	**5**, **6**, 7, 8	11, 24, 35, 45, 65, 80		

The more commonly used specifications are indicated in bold. Refer to Chap. 5 for greater details
[a]Available with and without prepackaged 0.035 stainless steel mini-guidewire

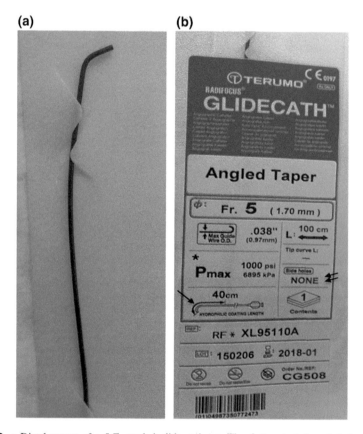

Fig. 1.3 **a** Distal aspect of a 5-Fr angled glide catheter. The demonstrated angled tip shape is commonly used for angiography in normal vasculature. **b** Similar to the sheath, pertinent information is on a label and follows the same arrangement. The distal 40 cm of the catheter (*arrow*) is hydrophilic. The maximum pressure (P max) that this catheter can tolerate is 1000 psi (*asterisk*). Pressures greater than this will cause the catheter to burst. The label also indicates that the catheter has no side holes (*double arrows*)

(b)

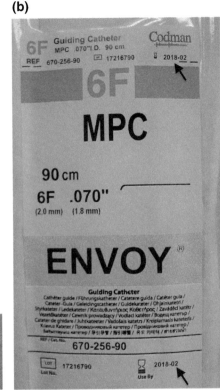

(a)

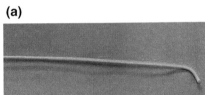

Fig. 1.4 Envoy guide catheter. A conduit for other devices to be readily advanced and retracted during endovascular interventions. It also provides stability, decreasing the likelihood of microcatheter collapsing during intervention. **a** The distal aspect of MPC (multi-purpose catheter) with the angled tip that aids in vessel selection. **b** The label demonstrates the size (6 Fr), inner diameter (0.070″ or 1.8 mm), length (90 cm), and the type of catheter (guide catheter). The expiry date is also readily seen (*arrow*)

removed once the shuttle sheath is suitably positioned. Refer to Chap. 5 for selection of appropriate catheters, sheaths, and wires.

Difference Between Sheaths and Catheters

- The size of the sheath describes the internal (luminal) diameter, while in case of catheters it alludes to the outer diameter. Therefore, a 6-Fr sheath has a larger lumen than a 6-Fr catheter. Practically, this means that a catheter can be inserted into a sheath of same size, but not vice versa.

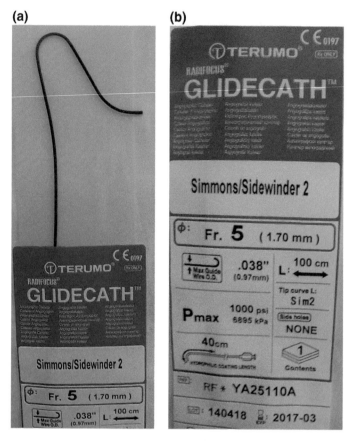

Fig. 1.5 Example of alternative diagnostic catheter. **a** Simmon's 2 catheter. The tip is available in multiple modifications with larger of tighter loop. **b** The label demonstrates its name, size (5 Fr), caliber of compatible guidewire (up to 0.038″), length (100 cm), P max (1000 psi), curve tip type (Sim 2), etc. The arrangement of the label enables access to relevant information at a glance

Setting up Flushes for Sheaths and Catheters

- Heparinized saline in concentration of 6000 IU of heparin in 1000 ml of normal saline (6 IU/ml) is used for flush systems. The heparin is injected into the saline bag, maintaining sterile precautions. Run the heparinized saline through the tubing until it is completely free of any air bubbles. For neurointervention, no air bubbles or foreign bodies are acceptable in the tubing or catheters as they may result in embolic strokes.
- To achieve a bubble-free system, priming is performed as follows:
- Add 6000 IU heparin to a liter bag and ensure the bag is free of any residual air. Pre-prepared heparinized saline bags are also available.

- Place the proximal tip of the tubing (the one closest to the drip chamber) into the provided inlet of the bag, maintaining sterile precautions.
- Clamp the distal end of the tubing (this usually lies in the sterile field).
- Pinch the line just distal to the chamber and squeeze the chamber. Then allow the inflow from the bag to fill one-third of the chamber.
- Flick away any bubbles out of the chamber.
- Do not completely fill the chamber with fluid, as monitoring of the flush rate will not be possible.
- Now gradually release the hand pinching the line distal to the chamber. The fluid will advance from the chamber distally into the tubing.
- Inflate the pressure system around the saline bag to 300 mmHg.
- The distal clamp (on the sterile field) is released. The air in the tubing will advance out of the tubing, to be replaced by the air-free flush solution.
- The flow rate of flush may be controlled using the distal clamp. We prefer using a pediatric transducer, which allows the fluid to flow at a uniform rate of 30 ml/hr. When needed, the rate of flow may be increased (e.g., when cleaning out the catheter or Touhy-Borst Y-Connector aka rotating hemostatic valve of blood) by releasing the regulator of the transducer. Depending upon the brand, this is done by action such as pressing the wings on either side of the transducer or pulling the 'tail' on the transducer (Fig. 1.6).
- When a neonatal transducer is used, the distal clamp of the tubing is kept completely loose because the flow rate is controlled by the transducer.

Attaching Flush System to the Sheath

- After a sheath has been placed in the artery, it will need to be connected to the flush system without introducing any air into the vasculature.
- The sidearm of the sheath (intended for flush systems) usually has a built-in three-way stopcock. Turn it to allow backflow of blood into the sidearm tubing. Then make a wet connection with the flush system.
- Turn the stopcock to also irrigate the side portal of the stopcock and purge any air. Then turn it again to open it to the sheath, with the blood being replaced by the clear heparinized saline.
- To prevent unnecessary blood loss, close the three-way stop to the sheath during sheath insertion.
- Connect the flush tubing to the sheath. There will be egress of saline through the open port of the stopcock. Press the wings (or alternative provided mechanism) of pediatric transducer to enhance the flow rate through the portal.
- Then, the valve/stopcock is briefly closed to the flush system by turning it clockwise, resulting in backflow of blood (and any air) through the open sideport.
- Then turn the stopcock to close it to the patient again and irrigate the side open portal clean.

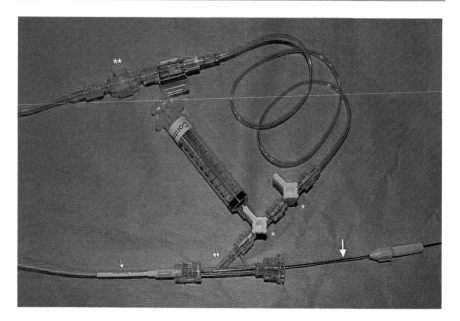

Fig. 1.6 Proximal aspect of Envoy guide catheter (*single arrow*) attached by its hub (*yellow*) to a rotating hemostatic valve (RHV, *double arrows*). The guidewire (*thick arrow*) is introduced into the catheter through the RHV. The catheter is advanced over the guidewire into the patient's vasculature. The wire is rotated back and forth as it is advanced, to prevent its tip from engaging and dissecting the vessel wall. This rotatory movement can be performed using the fingers holding the wire or a torque device (*green* and *white*) as shown attached to the wire, in a rubbing fashion against each other. It is ensured that the RHV cap is rotated clockwise to tighten around the traversing guidewire enough to prevent back bleeding, but still enable unobstructed movement of the wire. Two three-way stopcocks (*asterisk*) are attached to the side arm of the RHV, and the catheter is irrigated with continuous heparinized saline by tubing attached to the stopcock. The advantage of two stopcocks is that one can be used for manual injections while the other is used for connecting tubing from the autoinjector. The latter need not be disconnected since another port is available, and the preservation of a closed system prevents potential complications, e.g., introduction of air into the system. A neonatal transducer (*double asterisks*) is interposed between the tubing that enables continuous irrigation at 30 ml/hr. If a faster rate of irrigation is needed (e.g., to clean blood out of the catheter), the tabs/wings on either side are pressed together on this particular type of transducer

- Finally, close the stopcock to the sideport, establishing a continuous fluid column between the flush system and sheath.
- We place a piece of gauze (4 × 4) at the sideport to soak up the exiting fluid and thereby maintaining a clean operating field.
- An alternative technique is to connect the sheath to the flush tubing prior to insertion into a vessel. A continuous fluid column is ensured and then the dilator is advanced into the sheath, for insertion.
- When the sheath has been introduced into the vessel and the dilator and guidewire removed, the stopcock is transiently closed to flush system, to allow backflow of blood.

- Then the stopcock is turned anti-clockwise, so it is 'closed' to the patient. The neonatal transducer is used to quickly irrigate the vacant portal with heparinized saline.
- The stopcock is turned to close the sideport and continuous fluid column established.
- Be vigilant and ensure that the flush system continues to flow.
- Any blood backing up into the tubing must be investigated. It may have occurred consequent to the pressure on the saline bag being inadequate (which should be 300 mmHg). Or, the system may be open to air at some point.
- Do not allow blood stasis in the catheter or tubing as it can result in clot formation and emboli entering the patient's vasculature.

Attaching Flush to the Catheter

- This is usually performed while the catheter is still outside the patient.
- Attach the flush tubing via three-way stopcock to the sidearm of the rotating hemostatic valve, which in turn is attached to the proximal portal on the catheter (Fig. 1.7).
- Allow heparinized saline to run through the tubing and catheter. For a short period, there may be an interruption in fluid emanating from distal the tip of the catheter, as the air is evicted (Fig. 1.8). Subsequently, continuous fluid flow will resume.
- Ensure the entire system including the rotating hemostatic valve is free of air.
- When introducing a wire into the catheter, hold the rotating hemostatic valve upright and then close it down just enough to ensure air does not enter the system. The RHV should be tight enough to prevent back bleeding or air entry, but still have some room so that the wire can be freely manipulated (Fig. 1.6).

Preparation of Patient

- Position the patient supine on the neuroangiography table (Fig. 1.9a, b).
- A pillow or support under the knees may improve comfort for cases done under conscious sedation.
- When the patient arrives in the suite, introduce the personnel and explain the procedure in simple terms (in elective cases, this should also have been done earlier). Explain what the patient might experience, e.g., a warm sensation on

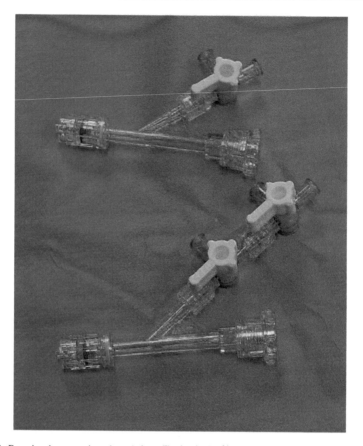

Fig. 1.7 Rotating hemostatic valves (a.k.a., Touhy-Borst Y-Connector or 'Touhy') with attached three-way stopcocks. For a diagnostic or guide catheter, we attach two stopcocks inline. This enables dedicating one stopcock outlet to the autoinjector, while the second can be used for manual injections or aspiration of blood. For microcatheters, a single three-way usually suffices, as we do not use autoinjectors with microcatheters

either side or back of face or neck when contrast is injected. Also warn about possible discomfort or pain when contrast is injected into branches of the external carotid artery. Explain the importance of remaining still when required and review the anticipated instructions such as holding of breath during angiography. During the procedure, periodically inform the patient about the progress and reassure that everything is going as anticipated.

- Ensure good intravenous access with at least two large bore angiocaths.
- Attach patient to monitors, such that heart rate, blood pressure, and respiratory rate are visible to the surgeon on the overhead monitor.
- Ensure all pressure points are padded.
- In case of interventions like carotid stenting where arrhythmias may be common, some operators prefer that the patient be attached to a pacemaker, so that

(a)

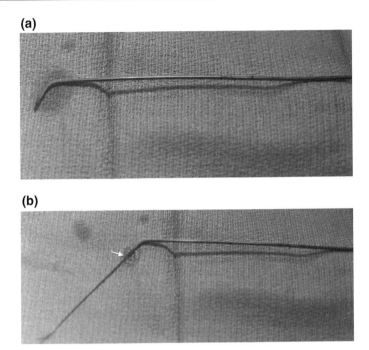

(b)

Fig. 1.8 a Distal aspect of a front angled glidecath. The proximal aspect of the catheter is connected to a continuously running flush of heparinized saline, as shown in earlier figures. Prior to insertion into patient's vasculature, ensure the catheter is air-free. Saline droplets should be noted to emanate continuously, without any interruption due to air bubbles. The hydrophilic catheter coating is activated by wiping it with moist Telfa and then not allowed to dry. **b** Once continuous column of heparinized saline running through the catheter is ensured, a moist guidewire is introduced into it, without allowing in any air bubbles. To achieve the same, the RHV is held upright when the distal softer end of the wire tip is introduced into it. The saline flush is accelerated by using the mechanism on neonatal transducer, to expel out any air that may have inadvertently entered during this process. The figure shows the distal tip of wire exiting out of the catheter tip (*arrow*). Prior to introduction of catheter into the sheath, the wire is completely retracted into the catheter. Once the catheter is within the patient's vasculature, the wire is advanced such that it leads the catheter. A vessel is selected with the wire, and then the catheter advanced over it. When retracting the system, the wire should be entirely within the catheter

in case of significant bradycardia pacemaking can be performed. Alternatively, atropine may be administered IV.

- A headrest may be used, but sometimes may need to be eliminated if difficulties are encountered with the lateral view (B plane).
- An adhesive tape may be placed across the patients' head and around the table to encourage them to remain still. It should not be too tight to cause discomfort.
- Shave both femoral regions and then prep using Chloroprep or Betadine. Maintain same sterile precautions as in the operating room.
- The patient's hands are kept at his/her side. If necessary, they may be gently restrained.

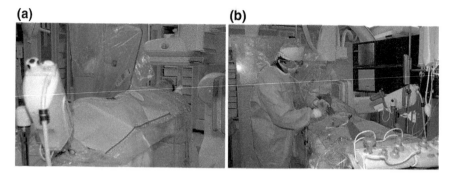

Fig. 1.9 **a** A neuroangiography suite with the patient lying on the table prepped and draped. The autoinjector is prominent in the foreground, to the *left*. **b** Procedure underway. The Biplane angio with its prominent gantry at the head end of the patient is obvious. The monitor for visualizing fluoroscopic images is positioned such that the surgeon can view the images without any difficulty. Note the remote control within sterile pouch that the surgeon may use to perform tasks such as scrolling through images or angiography runs. The equipment table (not in view) is positioned behind the surgeon

- The patient is then draped with both femoral regions available for arteriotomy.
- Administer anesthesia (local vs general) per operator's preference and patient characteristics. We perform most procedures under local anesthesia with conscious sedation.
- Conscious sedation is performed with 0.5–1 mg versed and 50–100 μgm fentanyl intravenously, prior to arterial access and periodically as needed throughout the procedure.
- General anesthesia is induced by anesthetist.
- Refrain from exclamations or remarks that may cause the patient anxiety or offense.
- When performing arteriotomy closure at the end of procedure, forewarn the patient about possible transient discomfort. Administer additional dose of fentanyl and versed. Instruct the patient to take slow deep breaths, rather than holding breath and bearing down in response to pain.
- Briefly review the results of procedure with the patient and whether further treatment is/is not anticipated. Advise the patient that you will be looking at the imaging in great detail later, and so the preliminary impressions may alter.

Suggested Readings

1. Osborne AG. Diagnostic cerebral angiography. Philadelphia: Lippincott Williams & Wilkins; 1999. p. 421–45.
2. Pearce M. Practical neuroangiography. Philadelphia: Lippincott Williams & Wilkins; 2007. p. 36–85.

Femoral Access Using Modified Seldinger Technique

- Prepare the micropuncture equipment by inserting the dilator into the 4 Fr sheath (Fig. 2.1).
- Partially pull out the 0.018″ guidewire provided in the kit from its sheath, to ensure no difficulties will be encountered in introducing it into the needle.
- Keep these items on a towel spread close to the draped groin, so that they can be retrieved readily during access, without having to stretch out, or having to let go of the needle in the vessel.
- After the groin region is appropriately prepped and draped, palpate the pulse for femoral artery.

  – Span from the anterior, superior iliac crest to the pubic symphysis with left hand to approximate the ilioinguinal ligament. Bisect the span with right hand, which indicates the location of femoral artery. Palpate for the pulsations of the femoral artery at this spot (Fig. 2.2a).
  – One may also confirm the planned puncture site by placing tip of hemostat or scissors over the pulse and visualizing its relationship to the femoral head fluoroscopically. The femoral artery should be punctured at the inferomedial aspect of the femoral head.

- Immobilize a segment of the artery between the index and middle fingers of left hand.
- Infiltrate the skin overlying the immobilized segment with local anesthesia, using 1% lidocaine with epinephrine.
- Also infiltrate the tissues overlying the artery, aspirating prior to injecting, to ensure the lidocaine is not administered into the arterial lumen. If the artery lumen is entered, blood will be aspirated into the syringe, indicating that the needle needs to be withdrawn.
- Make a small, superficial stab incision in the skin overlying the immobilized segment.

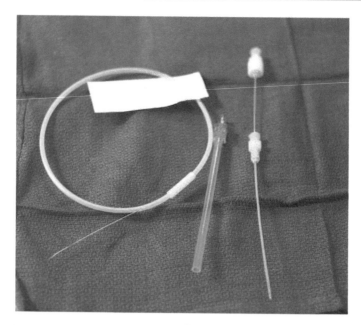

Fig. 2.1 Components of a micropuncture set. The 7 cm 21G needle (*green hub*) is still in a protective sheath that will be discarded when the needle is ready for use. The 40 cm 0.018″ wire is seen exiting its sheath. Once the needle is introduced into the blood vessel, the wire is advanced into the vessel through the needle hub. The needle is then retracted and removed. The micropuncture sheath (*gray*) is seen on the *right side*. The introducer can be seen extending out of its hub. The introducer is advanced fully into the sheath such that its cap securely clips on to sheath hub. The tip of introducer then extends beyond the tip of sheath. This unit is threaded over the wire into the blood vessel. Once the sheath is appropriately positioned, the introducer and wire are simultaneously removed, leaving the sheath in place

- The needle used for puncturing the artery may be from 21 to 23G.
- Using the free right hand, hold the needle with the thumb, index, and middle fingers, with the bevel leading and the opening pointing upwards. Enter through the stab at 45° over the site where arterial pulsations are felt. An indentation in the hub (aligned with the bevel, which should be positioned superiorly) of the needle also assists in correct positioning of the needle tip.
- When the artery is punctured and needle is in its lumen, blood will emanate from the needle hub.
- Stop advancing the needle once within the lumen and avoid going through the facing arterial wall, resulting in a double wall puncture.
- Without moving the needle any further, gently cover the hub with your thumb.
- Use your free hand to pick the provided wire and advance it into the needle hub, introducing it into the arterial lumen (Fig. 2.2b, c, d).
- If any resistance is sensed, fluoroscopically confirm the location and correct intravascular trajectory of the wire (Fig. 2.2e).
- Make sure to have control of some segment of the wire at all times, a part of which should always extend out of the needle hub.

- Once the wire is 5–10 cm into the arterial lumen, retract the needle over the wire (Fig. 2.2f). Make sure to have control of some segment of the wire at all times.
- Introduce the pre-assembled micropuncture sheath with dilator over the wire into the artery (Fig. 2.2g, h). Again, ensure a hold of some segment of the wire at all times and advance the microsheath completely (Fig. 2.2i).
- Withdraw the wire and introducer, leaving the sheath in the artery (Fig. 2.2j, k).
- Cover the hub of the sheath with your thumb to prevent unnecessary blood loss (Fig. 2.2l).
- Introduce a J wire (60–70 cm) into the sheath, until it is in the artery well beyond the sheath (Fig. 2.2m, n). Again, ensure that access is available to some segment of the wire at all times (Fig. 2.2o).
- Maintaining control of wire at all times, retract, and completely withdraw the small sheath over the wire.
- Compress the artery with the same (left) hand which is holding onto the wire to prevent bleeding from the enlarged entrance wound.
- Introduce the 5 Fr or larger sheath over the wire into the arterial lumen (Fig. 2.2p, q, r).
- Retract and remove the wire and sheath introducer, when the sheath has been positioned in the artery (Fig. 2.2s, t).
- Connect the sheath to previously prepared tubing with a neonatal transducer to ensure the continuously running heparinized saline solution is at a rate of 30 ml/hr (Fig. 2.2u).
- Prior to even beginning the procedure, the heparinized saline flush systems for the sheath and at least one catheter should be prepared. It should be ensured that the entire tubing system is free of air bubbles, or any other foreign material (see Chap. 1).
- Make a wet connection so that no air bubbles enter the vascular system (Fig. 2.2v, w, x; also see Chap. 1).
- Secure the sheath by suturing it to the skin using 2-0 silk, or covering it with Tegaderm adhesive to the skin (Fig. 2.2y, z).

Micropuncture Technique

- Use a 21G needle and the 4 Fr micropuncture kit that includes a sheath, dilator, and wire.
- We prefer using micropuncture technique for all elective cases as the arteriotomy puncture is small, with less likelihood of significant blood loss in cases of loss of access during sheath insertion.

Using Single-Wall 18G Needle

- In emergent cases, e.g., stroke where time is of the essence, a larger bore single-wall needle with a J wire or a 0.035 Bentson wire is used to gain a quicker access and place the sheath directly, eliminating the use of the 4 Fr micropuncture set and the involved additional steps.

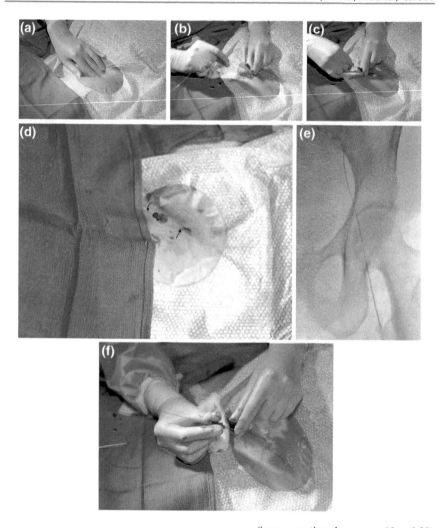

(images continued on pages 19 and 20)

Fig. 2.2 a The pulsations of femoral artery are palpated at the point midway between anterior superior iliac spine and symphysis pubis. **b** The needle is stabilized with one hand as the microwire is introduced into the needle hub with the other and then advanced into the artery (**c**). **d** The microwire (*curved arrow*) has been introduced into the femoral artery through the micropuncture needle (*arrow*). **e** In case of any resistance, fluoroscopy can be performed to verify that the microwire is indeed intravascular. **f** Once the microwire has secured access to femoral artery, the needle is removed over wire. **g, h, i** The microsheath unit is then threaded over the wire, taking care that the wire is not inadvertently pulled out of the artery. **j** Following complete insertion of micropuncture sheath, the introducer hub is detached from that of the sheath. As can be seen in the figure, one hand maintains the micropuncture sheath securely in place, while the other withdraws the introducer and wire (obstructed from view by hand) simultaneously. **k** The introducer is almost completely out of the sheath hub, which is maintained in place. The retracting hand is holding on to the introducer hub and wire concurrently. **l** As soon as the wire and introducer are withdrawn, cover the hub of micropuncture sheath with thumb, to prevent unnecessary blood loss.

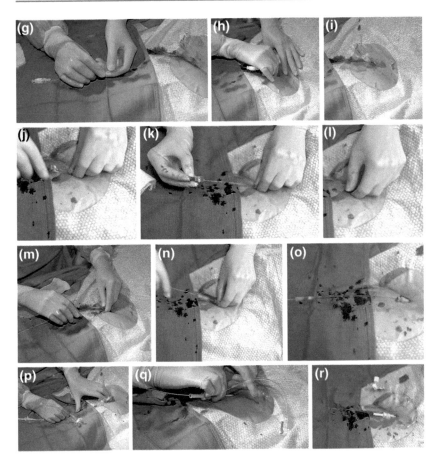

(images continued on next page)

Fig. 2.2 m The J wire is inserted into the microsheath. The white introducer, obvious between the hands, enables easy insertion of the wire into microsheath by straightening out the 'J' shape of the tip. The same can also be done by holding the wire between index finger and thumb and then sliding the thumb back. This movement straightens out the J shape. **n** Advance additional wire further into the sheath, to ensure it extends into the vessel beyond sheath tip. **o** After insertion of the wire into the sheath, adequate length still remains outside, to ensure against inadvertent loss of wire into patient's vasculature. **p, q** After removal of the smaller sheath, the sheath to be used for procedure is introduced over the wire and advanced over it into the accessed vessel (**q**). The sheath has its introducer in place, to enable smooth insertion. **r** The sheath is completely advanced into the vessel, such that its hub is right next to the skin. **s, t** The wire and introducer are removed from the sheath simultaneously, leaving the sheath in place (**t**). **u** The sheath is connected to a continuously running flush of heparinized saline. **v** It must be ensured the flush system is bubble free. To this end, the three-way stopcock at site of connection has been turned toward the saline flush. This results in back bleeding that exits through the free port. A gauze is used to soak up most of the exiting fluid, in an effort to keep the operative site clean. **w** The three-way stopcock is then turned toward the sheath. This results in occlusion of back bleeding while the saline flush flows out of the free port, cleaning it. The sequence of occluding the flush and then the sheath, washes out any air bubbles, clots or other particles through the free port.

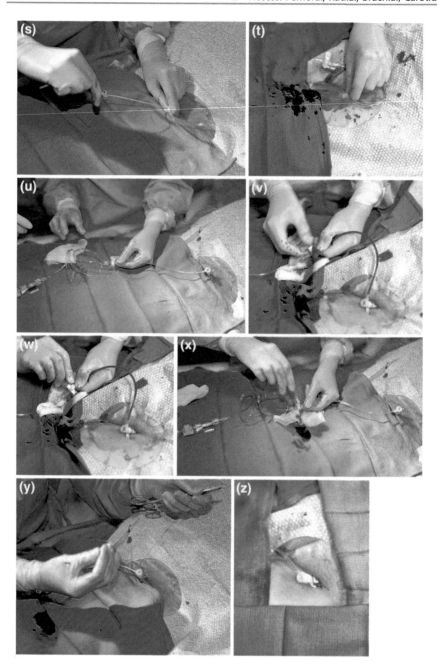

Fig. 2.2 x The three-way stopcock is finally turned to freeport, resulting in establishment of continuous heparinized saline flow to the sheath. y The sheath is secured by suturing to the patient's skin using the eyelet on the sheath provided for this purpose, to avoid inadvertent dislodgement. z Following completion of suturing, the operative site is cleansed. The operator should also ensure her/his gloves are clean, free of blood. Meticulous hygiene is practiced at all times to ensure there is no introduction of clots or foreign bodies into patient's vasculature

- This may also be helpful when the arterial pulse is not palpable with the smaller access needle.

- Care should be observed to avoid a double puncture of the arterial wall. A punctured bleeding site, unsecured by angioseal or similar means, may be a cause of significant bleeding, especially in patients who have received heparin, TPA, or similar blood thinners for the intervention.

Using Image Guidance in Difficult Access

- If difficulty is because of inability to palpate the femoral artery pulse, use the anatomic landmarks, e.g., if the thumb of your hand is on the patient's anterior superior iliac spine and the hand spans across such that the little finger is on the symphysis pubis, the location of the artery is demarcated by using the index finger of the other hand to bisect the hand span.
- If the femoral vein is entered, retract and clean the needle. Apply manual pressure on the vein for a minute, or so. Then, direct the needle slightly lateral to the previous course, as the femoral artery lies lateral to the vein.
- Ultrasound may be used to access a difficult artery (Fig. 2.3).
- A 5–10 MHz linear probe is used for femoral artery with a depth setting of 2–3 cm.
- It is placed in a sterile sheath with transmission gel applied to it (Fig. 2.3a, arrow).

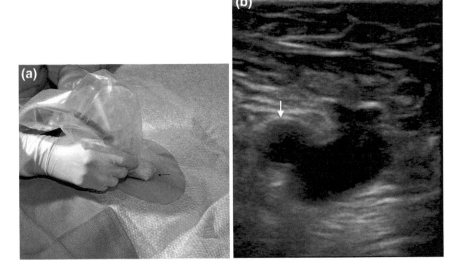

Fig. 2.3 a, b An ultrasound probe in a sterile sheath may be used to locate the femoral artery and access it, in case of difficulty feeling arterial pulse. Ultrasound gel is used (*arrow*) to enable satisfactory conduction. **b** Femoral artery (*arrow*) and vein can be seen side by side. The artery is recognizable by its more circumferential shape and pulsations. The needle can be advanced into the artery by visualizing its shadow as it is advanced and guided into the vessel

- Apply the probe at the level estimated to be superior to femoral bifurcation.
- The probe is applied transverse to the course of the artery, resulting in visualization of axial plain.
- The artery will be superficial to the vein, and more circumferential.
- The vein is more readily compressible by application of pressure using the probe.
- If the site interrogated is at or inferior to femoral bifurcation, two arterial circumferences will be seen.
- Introduce the needle into the skin inferior/caudal to the probe and advance it toward the artery at about 40° angle.
- The anterior wall of the artery is kept under the central target line (markers visualized as dots/circles), which indicates the path of the needle.
- Blood will emanate from the needle hub, once vessel has been entered.
- If difficulty is encountered during insertion of sheath over the J wire or, during exchange to a larger sheath over a wire:

  - Use fluoroscopy to ensure the J wire is in appropriate position.
  - Use a mosquito forceps to dilate the stab incision/subcutaneous tissue that may be providing resistance to the advancing sheath. This may happen due to scarring from previous procedures or tension in the deep fascia.
  - If a smaller size sheath is already in place, e.g., the 4 Fr sheath from the micropuncture kit, perform angiography through it to assess for stenosis or dissection.
  - In case of difficulty upsizing to a larger sheath, e.g., from 5 to 6 Fr, use a 5 Fr dilator over the wire, followed by 6 Fr dilator, if needed, and then reattempt insertion of the 6 Fr sheath.
  - A stiff 5 Fr micropuncture sheath can also usefully function as a dilator when resistance from scar tissue is encountered.

Radial Access

- Radial access is usually elected when vascular anatomy makes intervention difficult by the femoral route (i.e., aortic coarctation or, subclavian stenosis). Other situations that may require opting for radial access include skin infection in the femoral region or, unusual obesity rendering femoral access very difficult, if not impossible.
- Prior to performing arteriotomy, perform Allen's test with pulse oximetry to ensure the hand has satisfactory vascular supply, just in case the procedure results in radial artery occlusion.

Allen Test

- Palpate the radial and ulnar arteries.
- Place a pulse oximeter on the thumb or index finger.
- Make the patient flex and extend their fingers repeatedly.

- With digital pressure, compress both the radial and ulnar arteries during finger extension and maintain the compression until the oximetry pulse is lost.

  - Ensure the wrist is maintained in approximately 20° flexion, in order to avoid false positive tests which may happen with wrist hyperextension.
  - Release the pressure on the ulnar artery. Measure the time taken to achieve visual capillary refill in finger pads and at least 92% oxygen saturation.
  - Normal capillary refill time is <5 s, refill times of 5–15 s are considered equivocal. A refill time longer than 15 s is abnormal.
  - Allen's test can also be performed using ultrasonography.

Reverse Allen Test

- This should be performed when the radial artery is being subjected to a repeat procedure.
- With digital pressure, compress both the radial and ulnar arteries during finger extension and maintain the compression.
- Ensure the wrist is maintained in approximately 20° flexion, in order to avoid false positive tests that may happen with wrist hyperextension.
- Release the pressure on the *radial* artery. Measure the time taken to achieve visual capillary refill in finger pads and at least 92% oxygen saturation.
- Normal capillary refill time is <5 s, refill times of 5–15 s are considered equivocal. A refill time longer than 15 s is abnormal.
- An abnormal filling time indicates proximal radial artery disease. Therefore, repeat procedure on the artery should be avoided.

Access Technique

- Maintain the forearm in supine position.
- If required, use towels under the wrist to support it.
- The hand and or forearm may also be taped down to maintain supine position.
- Anesthetize the skin overlying the radial artery using 0.5 or 1% lidocaine.
- Take care not to puncture the artery, or cause it to go into spasm.
- Use two fingers to immobilize the arterial segment to be catheterized.
- As described above for femoral artery catheterization, use modified Seldinger technique and perform arteriotomy with a micropuncture set to secure arterial access.

  - Do not attempt arterial access with a larger bore single-wall needle.
  - Avoid entering the needle into artery at a steep angle, as this may cause difficulties in threading the wire through the artery. Remember, the radial artery is much smaller than femoral.

- Advance the 0.018″ wire through the needle hub into the radial artery and remove the needle.

- Use the tip of the scalpel blade to make a nick in the skin over the wire, to aid in smoother insertion of larger sheaths. This nick can also be made prior to arteriotomy with needle, provided it is done carefully and not going too deep.
- Advance the 4 Fr micropuncture sheath (with dilator) over the wire.
- Remove the wire and dilator.
- Advance 0.035″ wire through the sheath and then remove the sheath over the wire.
- A 5 Fr or 6 Fr sheath may be placed in radial artery, provided upsizing is performed after placing a 4 Fr catheter.
- Prior to upsizing, administer a cocktail of heparin (5000 IU/ml), verapamil (2.5 mg), lidocaine (2%, 1.0 ml), and nitroglycerin (0.1 mg) through the introducer sheath to relieve and/or prevent vasospasm.

  - Forewarn the patient about an uncomfortable but transient sensation of severe burning as the cocktail is injected into the artery. Usually analgesic administration prior to cocktail injection in unnecessary because of the very transient nature of the sensation.

- Following completion of procedure, _Do Not_ use angioseal or similar device for arteriotomy closure.
- Use manual compression only and apply pressure for 15–20 min, until hemostasis is achieved.
- In order to decrease the likelihood of radial artery occlusion, use the smallest size of sheath through which the procedure can be performed. We usually use a 4 Fr or 5 Fr sheath.

Brachial Access

- If possible, avoid the use of brachial artery. However, sometimes its use may become necessary, e.g., unavailable femoral and radial arteries.
- The access method is the same as for femoral artery, using modified Seldinger technique.
- Preferably start with a 4 Fr micropuncture kit, unless the situation is urgent and access with the larger single-wall needle appears reasonably assured.
- The use a closure device in the brachial artery is not presently FDA approved.
- Apply manual compression for approximately 15 min after the sheath is removed.

Carotid Access

- Carotid Access is best avoided because of the high risk of potential emboli going directly to the cerebral circulation during the puncture and the risk of ante grade dissection. This embolic risk is mitigated the farther the access arteriotomy is from the cerebral circulation. Furthermore, dissection in a vessel such as femoral artery would be retrograde, amenable to self-repair.

- If necessary, access is obtained by using modified Seldinger technique as described above for femoral artery.
- It may be advantageous, especially for the interventionists with neurosurgical background to make an incision and dissect to perform a direct exposure of the carotid artery.
- Arterial access should be performed at the Common carotid artery rather than the internal carotid.
- Usually the vessel is of sufficient caliber and superficial enough that access may be commenced with an 18G single-wall needle.
- Be very careful not to advance the J wire beyond the cervical carotid.
- Confirm the location of the tip of the J wire using fluoroscopy.
- Do not use a closure device for closure. Instead, apply manual compression.
- Ensure that the contralateral carotid is not being compressed concurrently.
- Conversely, if a cut down to the carotid was performed, then a purse string suture using 4-0 prolene is applied for closure.

Choice of Sheath or Access Device

- When performing a procedure electively, we gain access with a single-wall 21G needle 7 cm in length, using it with a 4 Fr micropuncture set. This results in less trauma to the femoral artery, and the lack of double puncture eliminates the risk of persistent bleeding in a heparinized patient.
- In emergency cases, e.g., when performing an intervention in stroke patients a larger 18G needle with 0.035 glidewire may be used, instead of the 21G needle with micropuncture set.
- Usually a 5 Fr Short sheath suffices for diagnostic procedures (e.g., an 11 cm length sheath).
- At least a 6 Fr sheath will be needed for most interventional procedures.
- In case of stroke where use of larger caliber devices is anticipated, we usually insert at least a 7 or 8 Fr sheath from the very outset.
- Use a longer sheath when the patient has a tortuous vasculature, e.g., elderly patients. In such situations use at least a 22 cm sheath, instead of the usual 11. A longer sheath will eliminate the tortuosity of segment traversed by it, making the navigation and manipulation of a catheter further distally, easier.
- When the vasculature is particularly tortuous or, in procedures such as stenting where the stability of catheters and devices is imperative, use a 60 cm shuttle sheath (see Chap. 5 for further details and examples of different types and sizes of sheaths).

Problems Encountered and Solutions

- Table 2.1.

Table 2.1 Problems and maneuvers

Problem	Maneuver
Resistance is felt on advancing the Microguidewire (0.018") through the needle	• Stop, as soon as any resistance is felt. Perform fluoroscopy to ascertain the location of the wire (Fig. 2.2e). If the guidewire appears crumpled up, retract and discard. If blood is no longer emanating from the needle hub, it indicates that arterial access has been lost. Retract the needle and apply pressure for a couple of minutes on the puncture site. Clean the needle and reattempt arteriotomy
	• If blood is still emanating from the hub after the microwire is removed, it is indicative of the needle still being in the artery. Ensure that bevel of the needle is directed superiorly (by checking that the divot of the hub is pointing up). Drop your hand slightly if the angle appears too steep. If angle was appropriate and divot was pointing superior, rotate the needle slightly to change the direction of bevel. After confirming blood is still emanating from the hub, advance a fresh microwire through the needle into the vessel
The wire initially advanced through the sheath, but then resistance was encountered	• This may happen with the microwire or the J wire. A common reason could be the wire advancing laterally into a branch such as circumflex iliac artery, instead of medially into the external iliac artery. Retract the wire partially so that it is out of the selected branch and back in the femoral artery. Attempt to advance the wire medially under direct fluoroscopy while rotating it back and forth at its distal end, to select the correct direction. The sheath may need to be retracted back slightly and then advancement of the wire attempted. If this is unsuccessful, retract and remove the wire and perform angiography to assess the cause of resistance. The angiogram can be used as a roadmap (e.g., 'smartmask' feature on the Phillips system). Do not give up access, unless it is inevitable based on site or arteriotomy. If the resistance is because of significant stenosis in the femoral or iliac artery, consider using access through the contralateral vessel
Previously palpable pulse is lost	• Inspect the skin distal to arteriotomy on the affected extremity. If it appears well perfused and with good capillary refill, observe
	• Obtain a peripheral vascular consult
	• If punctate mottling of digital skin alone is seen, close observation alone may suffice and no further action may be necessary
	• If the extremity appears compromised, perform angiography to inspect the cause of vascular compromise. Consider the following options:
	(continued)

Table 2.1 (continued)

Problem	Maneuver
	– For femoral artery compromise, perform arteriotomy on the contralateral femoral artery and navigate the catheter into the affected vessel staying proximal to the site of suspected injury and perform angiography
	– For radial artery, consider retrograde angiography via the brachial or subclavian artery
	– If angiography demonstrates a thrombus, local intra-arterial TPA may be administered
	– If angiographic appearance is consistent with a dissection, stenting with or without angioplasty is an option. Since neurointerventionists usually have limited experience of peripheral vasculature, requesting consultation from a peripheral interventionist may be prudent
Persistent bleeding despite adequate Angioseal deployment	• Ensure the appropriate size closure device is selected. The size should be the same or larger than the sheath placed in the vessel. Sometimes, due to use of Heparin or thrombolytics, persistent oozing is encountered. This is usually innocuous and is addressed by applying a few minutes of manual compression followed by pressure dressing. Such oozing will abate after the anticoagulant/thrombolytics are stopped. In case of overnight heparinization to prevent embolic complications, it is usually unnecessary to stop the medication for a mild continuous ooze
Plug pulls out of arteriotomy during deployment	• Ensure the appropriate size closure device is selected. When this occurs, arterial access has already been lost. Therefore, manual compression is applied for at least 20 min. If necessary, manual compression may be followed by usage of Femostop esp. if therapeutic dose of blood thinners have been used during intervention
	• In case a Femostop is used, ensure that proper positioning over arteriotomy site is maintained. To achieve this, the see-through inner circle of the Femostop dome should be positioned 1 cm superior and 1 cm medial to the actual puncture site. Inflate the Femostop to 20–30 mm Hg above the patient's systolic pressure. If this does not result in hemostasis, inflate to higher pressures until distal pulses are occluded. Maintain distal pulse occlusion for 5–7 min, then readjust the manometer pressure until good pedal pulse and good color of extremities is achieved. Once hemostasis occurs, reduce manometer pressure to half the number and observe the site for 2–3 min
	• Additionally, continue to check the pressure applied, as the device may have a tendency to deflate spontaneously. Continue to progressively decrease the applied pressure over the course of several hours, until the device can be discontinued entirely

(continued)

Table 2.1 (continued)

Problem	Maneuver
Patient complaining of weakness, nausea, dizziness or rapid pulse with/without hypotension	• Usually, a Femostop is maintained for 6–12 h • First and foremost ensure the patient is not continuing to lose blood from the arterial puncture site causing a retroperitoneal hematoma. This problem is more likely to be encountered following an interventional procedure, rather than a diagnostic one. These symptoms may occur within hours to several days following the procedure. The symptoms may be no more than a vasovagal response. However, the possibility of persistent blood loss needs to be ruled out. Do the following: – Monitor pulse, BP continuously, until condition diagnosed or ruled out – Send labs including CBC, electrolytes, aPTT, INR and if need be cardiac enzymes and troponins – Perform EKG – Insert foley catheter – Monitor intake and output – Administer 1 litre bolus of 0.9% normal saline and then a continuous running infusion at 125–150 ml/h – A smaller or larger bolus may be administered depending on the patients' clinical condition, e.g., a smaller bolus may be prudent in a hemodynamically stable patient with CHF. Similarly, the infusion rate may be titrated depending on the individual patient. However, it is better to aggressively overhydrate rather than under resuscitate the patient, which may compound the initial problem further, e.g., onset of ARF – Perform ultrasonography to rule out femoral pseudoaneurysm. The ultrasonography may also prove therapeutic as the USG probe may be used to compress and occlude the femoral artery pseudoaneurysm – If the ultrasound is negative and the suspicion of pseudoaneurysm remains, obtain an abdominal-pelvic CT scan – Usually the presence of pseudoaneurysm or retroperitoneal hematoma only requires supportive care including, IV fluids with/out PRBC – However, obtain a vascular consult in case surgical/endovascular intervention for treating the pseudoaneurysm is required

Suggested Reading

Levy EI, Boulos AS, Fessler RD, Bendok BR, Ringer AJ, Kim SH, et al. Transradial cerebral angiography: an alternative route. Neurosurgery. 2002;51:335–42.

Closure Techniques

3

Manual Compression

- Ensure ACT is <150.
- Ensure BP is under control.
- Patient should be in supine position with the accessed extremity kept straight.
- Prior to removal of sheath, palpate the artery proximal to arteriotomy location.
- Compress the proximal segment of the artery as the sheath is removed.
- Once the sheath is completely removed, increase the compression so that the pulse is completely or near completely obliterated.
- The site of compression is proximal to the skin puncture site, not at the puncture site since the arteriotomy is usually proximal to the puncture.
- Apply manual compression for at least 15–20 min.
- The duration of manual pressure also depends on the size of sheath. Use the following approximate durations in Table 3.1.
- Gradually decrease the applied pressure (every 5 min or so) while maintaining hemostasis.
- Following 15–20 min, when the pressure has been completely relieved, the puncture site should not be bleeding. If visible bleeding or soft tissue swelling is noted after releasing pressure, reapply occlusive pressure for another 5 min, then check again.

Compression Devices

Femostop®

- Ensure BP is under control.
- Patient should be in supine position.

© Springer International Publishing AG 2017
S.H. Khan and A.J. Ringer, *Handbook of Neuroendovascular Techniques*,
DOI 10.1007/978-3-319-52936-3_3

Table 3.1 Size of sheath and manual compression

Size of sheath (Fr)	Duration of manual compression (min)
4–5	15
6–7	20–25
7–10	30

- We prefer applying manual compression for 15–20 min prior to the application of Femostop, but a shorter duration is acceptable if the ACT is low (<150).
- Place the Femostop belt under the patient's hips, in line with the puncture site.
- Ensure that Femostop is properly positioned over the arteriotomy site.
- To achieve this, the see-through inner circle of the Femostop dome should be positioned 1 cm superior and 1 cm medial to the actual puncture site and over the femoral artery.
- Fully compress sidearm levers on compression arch to allow belt to be threaded. Adjust the belt to a snug fit. The arch should be level and sit squarely across groin area.
- Inflate the Femostop to 20–30 mmHg above the patient's systolic pressure. If this does not result in hemostasis, inflate to higher pressures until distal pulses are occluded. If the Femostop is positioned properly, the distal pulses will attenuate with device inflation.
- The properly positioned device will push straight downward upon the artery and not be tilted, or at an angle other than 90° to the underlying artery.
- Maintain distal pulse occlusion for 5–7 min and then readjust the manometer pressure until good pedal pulse and good color of extremities are achieved.
- Once hemostasis occurs, reduce manometer pressure to half the number and observe the site for 2–3 min. Additionally, continue to check the pressure applied, as the device may have a tendency to deflate spontaneously.
- Continue to progressively decrease the applied pressure over the course of several hours, until the device can be discontinued entirely.
- Usually, a Femostop is maintained for 6–12 h in anticoagulated patients.
- While the Femostop is applied, continue neurochecks, vital signs, O_2 sats; pedal pulses, limb color, sensation of warmth; puncture site for bleeding, hematoma on a flowchart. The following frequency of observations may be considered:

  - Every 15 min for 1 h.
  - Every 30 min for 2 h.
  - Every hour until Femostop is discontinued.

- Instruct the patient to inform the nurse immediately of any obvious bleeding, sensation of wetness, burning or tearing at the puncture site.
- After the Femostop is removed. Continue monitoring for signs of vascular complications, e.g., tenderness; groin mass, pulsatility; bruit, signs of leg ischemia.
- The following frequency of monitoring may be considered:

  - Every 15 min for 1 h.
  - Every 30 min for 2 h.
  - Every hour for 4 h.

Percutaneous Closure Devices

Angioseal (St. Jude Medical, Minnetonka, MN)

- This is our device of choice for closure due to its simplicity of use and reliability. Additionally, unlike most other percutaneous devices, it does not cause attenuation of vessel lumen.
- Available in 6 Fr and 8 Fr sizes.
- Angioseal device consists of 3 components: (i) arteriotomy locator, (ii) insertion sheath, and (iii) carrier tube (Fig. 3.1). The arteriotomy locator is advanced into the insertion sheath until it locks in place. The single unit so formed is then advanced over the wire into the artery, after the sheath used for procedure is removed over the wire, leaving the wire in place. The arteriotomy locator and the wire are withdrawn concurrently, leaving the insertion sheath in the artery. The carrier tube is advanced into the insertion sheath for completion of the closure. The details are as follows:

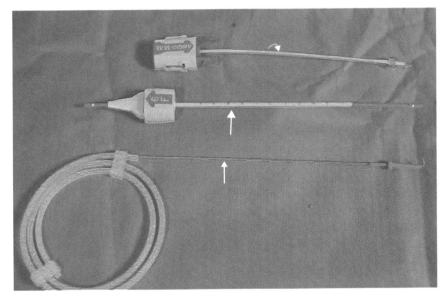

Fig. 3.1 Components of Angioseal. The J wire (*arrow*) is introduced into the vessel through the access sheath, and the sheath is then removed, taking care that wire remains within the vessel. The arteriotomy locator (with * on either end) has been inserted into the 6 Fr sheath (*thick arrow*), ready to be advanced over the wire into the artery. Once in the artery, the locator is removed and the sheath left in place. The carrier tube (*curved arrow*) is then inserted into the sheath, until it snaps in place

- Perform femoral angiography to ensure the arteriotomy is proximal to femoral bifurcation and that vessel diameter ≥ 4 mm.
- Remove any catheter traversing the femoral sheath.
- Cut the suture securing the sheath to the skin (if an anchoring suture was used).
- Continue to maintain sterile field.
- Remove the Angioseal device contents from the foil package. Pull the foil apart completely, before removing the Angioseal device to ensure none of the contents get kinked.
- Insert the arteriotomy locator into the insertion sheath, until the two pieces snap securely in place (Fig. 3.2).
- When inserted correctly, the arrow mark on the arteriotomy locator is aligned with a similar mark on the insertion sheath.
- Insert the J wire provided in the Angioseal kit, or longer exchange wire as required for longer access sheaths, into the femoral sheath and advance it into the artery.
- Remove the femoral sheath over the J wire and discard it. Ensure that the J wire maintains its position so that arterial access is not lost.
- Thread the arteriotomy locator-insertion sheath unit onto the J wire. Advance it over the wire into the artery, until blood is noted to pulsate out of the drip hole located at the outer (proximal) aspect of the arteriotomy locator (Fig. 3.3).
- Disengage the arteriotomy locator from the insertion sheath, by gently rocking the locator side to side at its junction with the insertion sheath (Fig. 3.4).
- Remove the locator and J wire concurrently, while maintaining the sheath in place
- Ensure the arrow marker on the sheath is facing upward. If not, rotate the sheath until it does (Fig. 3.5).
- Now pick the carrier tube by grasping it at the flared (distal) end, with only a small part of the bypass tube extending beyond the finger tips (Fig. 3.6).
- Ensure the reference arrow on the (proximal) tab of carrier tube is facing upward.
- Carefully thread the distal tip (a.k.a. bypass tube) of the carrier tube into the insertion sheath.
- The arrows on the insertion sheath and carrier tubes must face up and align with each other, for the two components to snap together (Fig. 3.7).
- Hold the insertion sheath stationary with one hand such that it does not move further into or out of the artery.
- With the other hand, pull back the tab/cap at the outer end of the carrier tube, until a slight resistance is felt (Fig. 3.8).
- Rock the cap/tab of the carrier tube from side to side. A snap/click will be heard every time this is done.
- Place your right thumb and index finger on either side, in the space created between the tabs of insertion sheath and carrier tube.

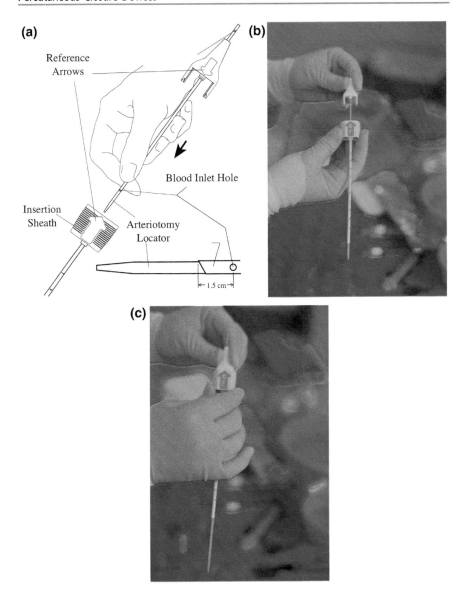

Fig. 3.2 Diagrammatic representation of Angioseal **a** The arteriotomy locator is about to be inserted into the insertion sheath. The *arrows* on the sheath and arteriotomy locator are appropriately facing the same side. The same is demonstrated in the photograph **b** where the arteriotomy locator is being inserted into sheath. The markings on the sheath indicate that it is 6 Fr in size. The arteriotomy locator has been completely inserted and snapped into position in the sheath **c** (Figure 3.2a courtesy St. Jude Medical, Minnetonka, MN. Angioseal™ is a trademark ofSt. Jude Medical, Inc. or its related companies. Reprinted with permission from St. JudeMedical™, © 2012. All rights reserved)

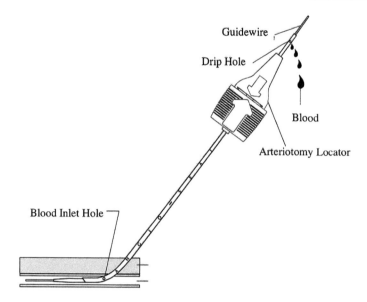

Fig. 3.3 When the sheath is at least 1.5 cm within the artery, blood is seen to spurt out of the drip hole at the proximal aspect of the arteriotomy locator (Figure courtesy St. Jude Medical, Minnetonka, MN. Angioseal™ is a trademark of St. Jude Medical, Inc. or its related companies. Reprinted with permission from St. Jude Medical™, © 2012. All rights reserved)

- With the fingers wedged between the tabs pull back at an angle of 45° to the incision (Fig. 3.9), until resistance is felt because the collagen plug is apposed against the arteriotomy site. Provide counter traction with your other hand by gently pressing in around the incision site.
- Continue to maintain tension with the right hand and advance (toward the patient's incision) the 'tamper tube' with the left, until the black 'compaction' mark on suture is visualized (Fig. 3.10). To do so, you may need to push the 'tamper tube' component on the suture down with left index finger and thumb, while pulling back with right hand. A black mark will be revealed at the superior end of tamper tube.
- If the mark is not visualized, additional upward tension on the suture while pushing down the tamper tube usually reveals it. Once visualized, there is no need to continue pulling to see the entire mark. This will cause over tightening and the risk of tearing off the collagen plug.
- Let go of the Angioseal device to confirm hemostasis. If some bleeding is noted, you may tamp down with the tamper tube while pulling the suture, again.
- After hemostasis is achieved, cut the suture below the lower end of tamp tube such that the remaining suture retracts under the skin (Fig. 3.11).
- Clean the puncture site and apply dressing.

Fig. 3.4 Once entry of the sheath into the artery is confirmed, disengage the arteriotomy locator from the sheath by rocking it from side to side while holding the sheath in place (Figure courtesy St. Jude Medical, Minnetonka, MN. Angioseal™ is a trademark of St. Jude Medical, Inc. or its related companies. Reprinted with permission from St. Jude Medical™, © 2012. All rights reserved)

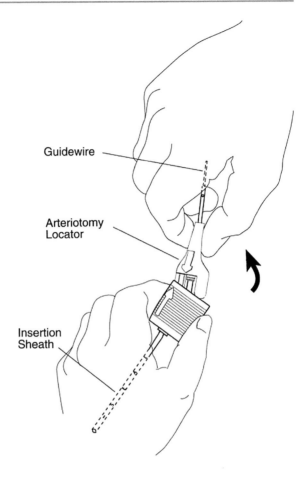

Guidewire

Arteriotomy Locator

Insertion Sheath

- Have the patient lie for 2 h with the leg on the side of Angioseal deployment kept straight.
- Perform periodic neurochecks and distal pedal pulses.
- Usually, the patient can be mobilized after 2 h. For outpatient procedures, we recommend observation while ambulatory for 1 h prior to discharge to minimize the risk of delayed closure failure.

Cautions

- Angioseal should not be used in an artery <4 mm in diameter. The small arterial size may prevent the Angioseal from deploying properly.

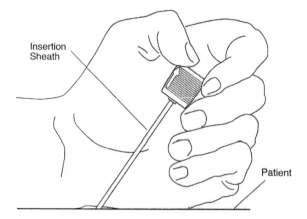

Fig. 3.5 Arteriotomy locator and the J wire have been removed concurrently, while the sheath is carefully maintained in position (Figure courtesy St. Jude Medical, Minnetonka, MN. Angioseal™ is a trademark of St. Jude Medical, Inc. or its related companies. Reprinted with permission from St. Jude Medical™, © 2012. All rights reserved)

Fig. 3.6 Carrier tube about to be inserted into the sheath. The *arrows* on the sheath and carrier tube, both face upward (Figure courtesy St. Jude Medical, Minnetonka, MN. Angioseal™ is a trademark of St. Jude Medical, Inc. or its related companies. Reprinted with permission from St. Jude Medical™, © 2012. All rights reserved)

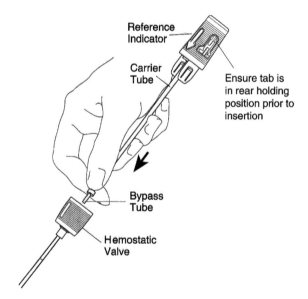

- Open the device foil pouch, just prior to actually using it. The device should be used within an hour of removal from its foil pouch because its biodegradable components begin to deteriorate upon exposure to ambient conditions.

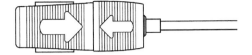

Fig. 3.7 When the carrier tube is correctly inserted and clipped into the sheath, the arrow on one aligns with the other (Figure courtesy St. Jude Medical, Minnetonka, MN. Angioseal™ is a trademark of St. Jude Medical, Inc. or its related companies. Reprinted with permission from St. Jude Medical™, © 2012. All rights reserved)

Fig. 3.8 Tab/cap of the carrier tube has been pulled back, while maintaining the sheath stationary (Figure courtesy St. Jude Medical, Minnetonka, MN. Angioseal™ is a trademark of St. Jude Medical, Inc. or its related companies. Reprinted with permission from St. Jude Medical™, © 2012. All rights reserved)

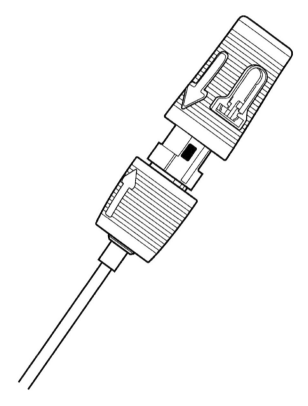

Exoseal (Codman, Miami Lakes, FL)

- This device has a similar use, deployment, and reliability to Angioseal, but may be better tolerated by conscious patients. Like the Angioseal, the Exoseal is inserted percutaneously through the arteriotomy sheath, placing an extravascular collagen plug for hemostasis, but it does not require a wire exchange and comes packaged as a single unit device. As it utilizes the deep femoral fascia to secure its plug, it does not utilize a suture at the arteriotomy, which may be a source of discomfort for some patients receiving the Angioseal. The details are as follows:
- Remove the Exoseal device from its packaging prior to anticipated sheath removal.

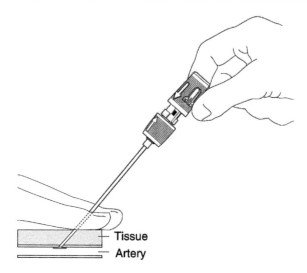

Fig. 3.9 Rather than holding the cap as shown in the figure, wedge the index finger and thumb in the space between the cap/tab of carrier tube and the cap of the sheath. As the device is pulled back at 45°, counter traction is provided with the other hand by pressing down on the patient's skin with index and middle fingers on either side of the sheath. Continue pulling back until a resistance is felt (Figure courtesy St. Jude Medical, Minnetonka, MN. Angioseal™ is a trademark of St. Jude Medical, Inc. or its related companies. Reprinted with permission from St. Jude Medical™, © 2012. All rights reserved)

- Perform femoral angiography and remove any suture securing the sheath, as described above for Angioseal.
- Insert Exoseal through sheath until blood return is observed at the indicator tube.
- While stabilizing Exoseal with the right hand, slowly withdraw the sheath with the left hand until it locks into place on Exoseal with an audible click. Blood return should continue.
- Slowly withdraw the sheath and Exoseal together as a single unit, watching the indicator window for closure of the white, arrowhead-shaped chevrons.

  - Closure is effected by tension on a wire stopper as it pulls against the inner wall of the arteriotomy, indicating ideal placement of the extravascular plug.
  - Closure followed by appearance of red chevrons indicates that the wire stopper has been overstretched and that the device should not be deployed. Slightly re-advance the sheath and Exoseal until the chevrons close again.

- Deploy the device by squeezing the trigger on the side of the device and holding for a count of 2.
- Release the trigger and remove the device with the right hand while applying manual pressure with the left hand as described in the manual closure section above. Hold subocclusive pressure for 2 min only.

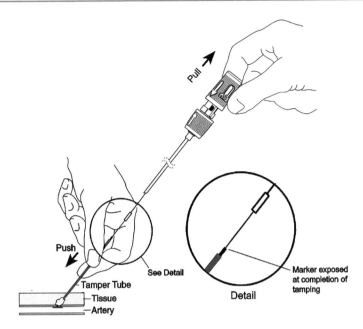

Fig. 3.10 While tension is maintained with the *right hand*, the tamper tube is pushed down with the *left*, until a black mark becomes visible on the thread. This indicates that the tamping is complete, as demonstrated in the *inset* (Figure courtesy St. Jude Medical, Minnetonka, MN. Angioseal™ is a trademark of St. Jude Medical, Inc. or its related companies. Reprinted with permission from St. Jude Medical™, © 2012. All rights reserved)

- Observation, ambulation, and discharge criteria are identical to those for Angioseal.
- Other percutaneous devices available include Starclose, Perclose, and Mynx.
- We use Angioseal and Exoseal almost exclusively because while the hemostatic plug employed in it eventually resorbs without compromising vessel lumen, devices like Starclose and Perclose use a clip or ligature, which would result in some luminal sacrifice. This is of particular concern when multiple angiographies would lead to multiple closures.
- Mynx on the other hand places the collagen plug on the outside of the arteriotomy. In our personal experience, we have found it to fail more frequently than Angioseal. However, it causes less discomfort during deployment.
- Unlike Angioseal, safe usage of Mynx is limited to 5 Fr and 6 Fr sheaths only.
- Starclose is contraindicated in patients with hypersensitivity to nickel-titanium.
- For further details on the usage of these devices, refer to the user manuals provided with these devices.

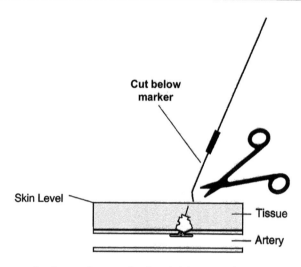

Fig. 3.11 Once tamping is complete, cut the thread right at the skin while also gently pressing down on the skin with the scissors. This will ensure the remaining thread retracts under the skin (Figure courtesy St. Jude Medical, Minnetonka, MN. Angioseal™ is a trademark of St. Jude Medical, Inc. or its related companies. Reprinted with permission from St. Jude Medical™, © 2012. All rights reserved)

Problems Encountered During Closure and Solutions

Femostop

See Table 3.2.

Table 3.2   Problems encountered during closure and solutions Femostop

Problem	Solution
Pain from Femostop compression	• Consider prescribing analgesics and some sedation prn • Ensure the Femostop is not positioned too laterally, overlying the femoral nerve instead of the artery
Extremely high inflation pressures (>200 mmHg) required to achieve hemostasis	• The belt may not be put on properly and requires adjustment
Decreased HR, BP, loss of consciousness	• This may be a vasovagal episode from pain and discomfort due to the Femostop. Ensure symptoms are not due to hypovolemia from ongoing blood loss • Administer 500–1000 ml of 0.9% NS bolus • Loosen or adjust Femostop belt • Atropine 600 μg IV once or twice, for bradycardia • Analgesics

(continued)

Table 3.2 (continued)

Problem	Solution
Bleeding or hematoma despite Femostop application	• The dome may have slipped out of position or may not have been positioned appropriately. If the bleeding site cannot be seen, or the Femostop cannot be repositioned, remove the Femostop from the belt, quickly clean area with sterile gauze, and apply manual digital pressure proximal to the puncture site to achieve hemostasis • Do not hesitate to and call for assistance if there appears to be ongoing bleeding despite manual compression

Angioseal

See Table 3.3

Table 3.3 Problems encountered during closure and solutions Angioseal

Problem	Solution
Persistent oozing despite adequately tamping down and visualizing the black marker	• Sometimes, a little oozing is noticed despite adequate closure. In such a situation, just cut the suture below the tamper tube as usual. Then, apply gentle manual pressure for a few minutes, which usually results in complete hemostasis
No place to cut the suture between the patient's skin and tamper tube	• In this case, cut above the tamper tube (Fig. 3.12). Slide the tamper tube off the suture. Now cut the suture right at the skin (Fig. 3.11), so it will retract under the skin
Loss of vascular access during exchange of sheath for Angioseal device	• If access is lost, apply manual pressure for 20–30 min, or longer if necessary. Do not attempt to continue advancing the insertion sheath or carrier tube, if vascular access is lost
Pain at access site persisting beyond several hours	• Apply a warm compress to the access site to soften any residual hematoma and administer oral NSAIDs (i.e., Ibuprofen 400–800 mg)

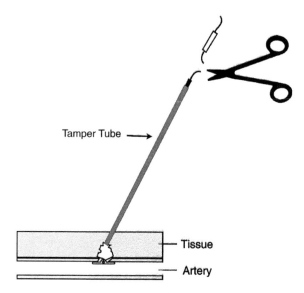

Fig. 3.12 Thread is cut at the proximal end of the tamper tube, when there is no space available between the tamper tube and patient's skin. The tamper tube can then be slid off the thread, enabling it to be cut at the patient's skin (Figure courtesy St. Jude Medical, Minnetonka, MN. Angioseal™ is a trademark of St. Jude Medical, Inc. or its related companies. Reprinted with permission from St. Jude Medical™, © 2012. All rights reserved)

Suggested Readings

1. Angioseal User Manual. St Jude Medical, Minnetonka, MN.
2. Schneider PA. Endovascular skills. Guidewire and catheter skills for endovascular surgery. New York: Marcel Dekker, Inc; 2003. p. 335–45.

Contrast Agents

4

Choices

- The following table (Table 4.1) lists the commonly used agents in endovascular neurosurgery. All agents listed are nonionic.
- While usually high-osmolality contrast media (HOCM) are safe and effective and these agents cost less, if possible these should be avoided in patients at higher risk, e.g., patients with CHF, renal insufficiency, diabetes. HOCM will typically cause more discomfort for the patient on injection. HOCM include very hypertonic monomers, e.g., 1500 mOsm/kg for 300 mgI$_2$/ml.
- Low-osmolality contrast media (LOCM) are relatively more expensive and cause less discomfort and minor (1% vs 5%) or major (0.015% vs 0.1%) adverse reactions. Most LOCM are nonionic, e.g., 300 mOsm/kg for 300 mgI$_2$/ml.
- Some centers use LOCM exclusively, while others use it in patients at high risk. High-risk patients include:

  - History of adverse reaction to iodine-containing contrast agents (sensation of warmth, flushing, or a single episode of nausea/vomiting is not considered adverse reactions).
  - History of serious allergic reaction to materials other than contrast agents.
  - Severe arrhythmia, unstable angina or, recent MI.
  - Renal insufficiency, especially in the presence of diabetes.
  - General severe debilitation, etc.

Adverse Effects

- The pathogenesis of adverse effects may be multifactorial. The etiology may include:

© Springer International Publishing AG 2017
S.H. Khan and A.J. Ringer, *Handbook of Neuroendovascular Techniques*,
DOI 10.1007/978-3-319-52936-3_4

Table 4.1 Commonly used agents in endovascular neurosurgery

Agent	Chemical structure	Anion	Cation	% Salt concentration	% Iodine concentration	Iodine mg/ml	Viscosity 25 °C	Viscosity 37 °C	Osmolality mOsm/kg H$_2$O
Visipaque™ 270 (GE Healthcare)	Iodixanol	Nonionic	Nonionic	None	27	270	12.7	6.3	290
Isovue™ 300 (Bracco)	Iopamidol 61.2%	Nonionic	Nonionic	None	30	300	8.8	4.7	616
Omnipaque ™ 300 (GE Healthcare)	Iohexol 64.7%	Nonionic	Nonionic	None	30	300	11.8	6.3	672
Optiray™ 300 (Mallinckrodt inc)	Ioversol 64%	Nonionic	Nonionic	None	30	300	8.2	5.5	651
Optiray™ 320 (Mallinckrodt inc)	Ioversol 68%	Nonionic	Nonionic	None	32	320	9.9	5.8	702

- Specific chemical formulation of the contrast (chemotoxicity).
- Hypertonicity.
- Binding of small contrast agents in the blood to activators.
- Ca-chelating substances.
- Substances leeched from rubber stoppers in bottles or syringes.
- Patient anxiety.

- A previous h/o adverse event to contrast injection is the best predictor of recurrent event. Recurrent events occur in 8–30% patients.
- Adverse events include the following (Table 4.2).

Management of Adverse Reactions

- Monitor all patients regardless of duration or complexity of procedure. Always have crash cart available.
- Assess vital signs rapidly.
- Ensure airway is protected and patent and the patient is breathing adequately. Intubate and ventilate if needed.
- If needed, call a code.
- Identify the cause of reaction and address it, e.g.,

Table 4.2 Adverse events

Adverse event	Comment
Urticaria	Due to histamine release, usually urticaria and other allergic reactions are more likely to occur in patients with a h/o allergic reactions
Bronchospasm	More likely in patients with h/o asthma
Acute pulmonary edema	Prone to occur in patients with left HF who are less able to compensate for negative chronotropic events associated with contrast agents. Use LOCM in such patients
Hemodynamic changes	More likely in patients with severe cardiovascular disease, e.g., aortic stenosis or, severe CHF
Hypotension/tachycardia	May be consequent to the hypertonicity of the agent
Vasovagal reaction	Due to increased vagal tone, which causes decreased SA and AV nodal activity, decreased AV conduction and peripheral vasodilatation. The result is hypotension and bradycardia. The vasovagal reaction may be consequent to anxiety and therefore may occur during taking consent, or placing needle, or injecting contrast. It is usually mild and self-limiting. However, if it is not monitored or treated, it may progress to hemodynamic collapse
PEA/cardiac arrest	May be consequent to sudden drop in serum ionized Ca caused by specific contrast formulation or additive
Seizure	Like CVS, CNS is a key target of these agents

- Hypotension and tachycardia may be indicative of hypovolemia because of blood loss; anaphylactic reaction to contrast agent, or other drug administered; or, consequent to hypertonicity from contrast administered.
- Arrhythmia may be because of the tip of the catheter being in the atrium, causing irritation.
- Sudden hemodynamic instability during intervention may be due to aneurysmal rupture, e.g., posterior circulation aneurysms may cause profound hypotension. The rupture may occur due to the force of contrast expulsion from an autoinjector, esp. in case of an already ruptured aneurysm. In such a situation, rapid ventriculostomy (if an EVD is not already in place) may make the difference between life and death.

- Based on symptoms, assess whether adverse reaction is mild, moderate, severe, and whether it is organ specific, in order to respond appropriately.

Mild Reactions: e.g., Nausea, Vomiting, Sensation of Warmth, Urticaria

- The incidence of above increases with high-osmolality ionic contrast agents.
- Pain on injection may be due to hypertonicity of contrast agents.
- Mild reactions usually do not require treatment.
- However, these must be monitored for at least 20–30 min as they may progress to more severe reactions.

Moderate Reactions: e.g., Symptomatic Urticaria, Vasovagal Reactions, Bronchospasm, Tachycardia, Mild Laryngeal Edema

- Not immediately life threatening, but may progress to be so.
- Monitor closely until completely resolved.
- Treat as needed for specific symptoms, e.g.,

  - Hives: diphenhydramine, hypotension: raise legs/volume resuscitation /Vasopressors.
  - Bronchospasm: ß-agonist inhaler.
  - Laryngeal edema: epinephrine.

Severe Reactions: e.g., anxiety, diffuse erythema, sudden cardiac arrest, vasovagal reactions; moderate to severe bronchospasm, severe laryngeal edema, loss of consciousness

- These are Potentially or Immediately Life Threatening.
- In severe reactions, time is of the essence. Act immediately.
- Institute ACLS protocols including, ensuring ABC's.

Organ-Specific Adverse Reactions: These Include

- Pulseless electrical activity, pulmonary edema, seizures.
- Venous thrombosis: Contrast agents are known to have effect on endothelial function.
- Disorders of hemostasis.
- Renal damage: The risk is low with normal serum creatinine, even in elderly with decreased body mass and decreased GFR.
- Elevated creatinine: Effects primarily related to dose. When contrast agents cause elevated creatinine, in most patients the elevation is transient and levels return to baseline in 2–3 weeks.

Special Considerations

Diabetes

- Pre-disposes to contrast media induced renal dysfunction.

  - Ensure that patient is well hydrated.
  - In diabetics with renal dysfunction: limit the volume of contrast used or, if possible consider an alternate exam.
  - Avoid Metformin when contrast agent has been administered in patients with renal/hepatic dysfunction, ETOH abuse, S. CHF, as all these conditions limit Metformin excretion, increase lactate production, increase likelihood irreversible/fatal lactic acidosis (50% mortality).
  - Do not resume until 48 h post-procedure, only after renal function checked and found to be normal.

Diabetes and Renal Insufficiency

- Use LOCM or nonionic iso-osmolal contrast media (IOCM) that are less nephrotoxic.

Renal Insufficiency
Salivary gland swelling ('iodide' mumps) and syndrome of acute polyarthropathy are more frequent in renal dysfunction and may also occur with HOCM/LOCM.

- Delayed symptoms, e.g., rash and itching, may occur as late as 1–7 days after contrast injection.

- Paraproteinemias esp. multiple myeloma pre-dispose to irreversible renal failure after contrast injection due to protein precipitation in renal tubules.
- Obtain baseline BUN and Cr.
- Ensure patients are well hydrated before, during and after study.
- Limit the volume of contrast used.
- Consider if there is an alternate study, which would result in avoidance of use of contrast.

Contrast Nephrotoxicity

It is a sudden change in renal status after contrast administration, where no other etiology appears likely.

- It is the third most common cause of in-hospital renal failure, (after hypotension and surgery).
- Defined as:

  - Serum Cr. rise >25% if baseline Cr <1.5 mg/dl.
  - Serum Cr. rise >1 mg/dl if baseline Cr >1.5 mg/dl.

- It occurs within 72 h of contrast administration.
- It occurs consequent to renal hemodynamic changes, direct tubular toxicity of contrast agents. Both osmotic and chemotoxic mechanisms may be involved.
- Risk factors for contrast nephrotoxicity include renal insufficiency (S. cr. >1.5 mg/dl), diabetes, dehydration, CV disease, diuretics, age ≥ 70, myeloma, hypertension, hyperuricemia. Patients with pre-existing renal insufficiency and diabetes are at the greatest risk of contrast-induced ARF.
- The outcome of contrast nephrotoxicity depends on baseline renal status, coexisting risk factors, degree of hydration and contrast dose.
- The serum Cr rises within 24 h, peaks in 96 h (4 days) and returns to baseline in 7–10 days. Temporary or permanent dialysis is rarely needed.

Prevention/Treatment of Contrast Nephrotoxicity

- Hydration: Pre-angiographic volume expansion with normal saline or sodium bicarbonate has been demonstrated to reduce the risk of nephrotoxicity.
- N-acetylcysteine: antioxidant. 600 mg p.o. bid, a day before and on day of contrast administration, or half an hour prior to contrast administration: 150 mg/kg over 30 min and then 50 mg/kg over 4 h.
- Limit contrast use; as a rule of thumb, the volume of LOCM tolerated may be estimated as [5 ml x body weight (kg)]/serum creatinine.
- Serum Cr should be measured in:

- Adults with kidney disease including tumor and transplant.
- Family h/o renal failure.
- Diabetes.
- Paraproteinemia syndromes or diseases, e.g., myelomas.
- Collagen vascular diseases.
- Medications including Metformin or Metformin combinations, NSAIDs, use of nephrotoxic antibiotics, e.g., aminoglycosides.

- BUN may indicate state of hydration, but is not a reliable indicator of renal dysfunction.
- Other patients undergoing a routine contrast study do not need a S. Cr measurement.

Renal Dialysis Patients
Contrast agents (CA) are not protein-bound, have low molecular weight and are readily cleared by dialysis.

- Osmotic load of CA is a primary concern.
- At least theoretically, CA may cause direct chemotoxicity of heart and bundle branch block.
- Urgent dialysis is only needed if there is severe cardiac dysfunction or, a very large volume of CA is used.
- In such patients, limit the dose of CA. Use a nonionic LOCM.

Prep/Pre-medication for Iodine Allergy

- Pre-medication is usually performed for patients with history of moderate or severe (not mild reactions).
- In addition to pre-medication, use a different contrast agent than the one that caused a reaction in the past.
- In case of a history of severe contrast reaction, avoid administering contrast agent at all unless the potential benefits outweigh the risks.

Elective Cases

- Prednisone 50 mg orally at 13 h and 1 h before contrast injection, plus
- Diphenhydramine (Benadryl) 50 mg IV, IM or PO 1 h before contrast injection or.
- Methylprednisolone 32 mg PO 12 h and 2 h before contrast injection. Antihistamine can also be added to the regimen as indicated above.
- If patient is unable to take oral medications, then substitute hydrocortisone 200 mg IV for oral Prednisone.

Emergency Cases

- Methylprednisolone sodium succinate (Solu-Medrol) 40 mg or hydrocortisone sodium acetate (Solu-Cortef) 200 mg IV every 4 h (q4 h) until contrast study required, plus diphenhydramine (Benadryl) 50 mg IV 1 h before contrast injection, or
- Dexamethasone sodium (Decadron) 7.5 mg or betamethasone 6 mg IV q4 h until contrast study. Plus, diphenhydramine (Benadryl) 50 mg IV 1 h before contrast injection. Also diphenhydramine (Benadryl) 50 mg IV 1 h before contrast injection, or
- Omit steroids entirely and give diphenhydramine (Benadryl) 50 mg IV.

Suggested Readings

1. ACR Committee on Drugs and Contrast Media. Media, A.C.o.D.a.C., ACR Manual on Contrast Media Version 9, 2013.
2. ACR Committee on Drugs and Contrast Media. Media, A.C.o.D.a.C., ACR Manual on Contrast Media Version 10.1, 2015.
3. Lasser EC, Berry CC, Talner LB, et al. Pretreatment with corticosteroids to alleviate reactions to intravenous contrast material. New Engl J Med. 1987;317(14):845–9.
4. Greenberger PA, Patterson R. The prevention of immediate generalized reactions to radiocontrast media in high-risk patients. J Allergy Clin Immunol. 1991;87(4):867–72.
5. Greenberger PA, Halwig JM, Patterson R, Wallemark CB. Emergency administration of radiocontrast media in high-risk patients. J Allergy Clin Immunol. 1986;77(4):630–4.

Choice of Sheaths, Wires, and Catheters

5

Sheaths

- These are required for maintaining vascular access, enabling catheter exchanges without traumatizing the blood vessel and minimizing blood loss.

Short Sheaths (10–45 cm)

- Use a 5 Fr 10-cm sheath (e.g., Terumo®, Pinnacle) for diagnostic angiography. Change to a 6 Fr (sometimes will need 7 Fr or larger) for interventional procedures (Fig. 5.1a, b).
- If anticipating intervention, use at least a 6 Fr sheath from the very outset. It is time-saving and often the same closure device (6 Fr) will be used if the sheath used is 5 Fr or 6 Fr.
- In case of stroke, start off with a 7 or 8 Fr sheath.
- In case the femoral artery is tortuous, using a longer sheath, e.g., 25 cm (Terumo®, Pinnacle) instead of 10 cm, may help straighten out the artery.

Long Sheaths (90–100 cm)

- Also called 'Guiding sheaths,' these may be needed for supporting the catheter in a tortuous vasculature where the catheter would otherwise drop out of, or cannot be placed in the target vessel, e.g., in older patients.

Shuttle® Sheath: One option is placement of shuttle® sheath (Cook Medical Inc, Bloomington, IN). To do this:

S.H. Khan and A.J. Ringer, *Handbook of Neuroendovascular Techniques*, DOI 10.1007/978-3-319-52936-3_5

(a)   **(b)**

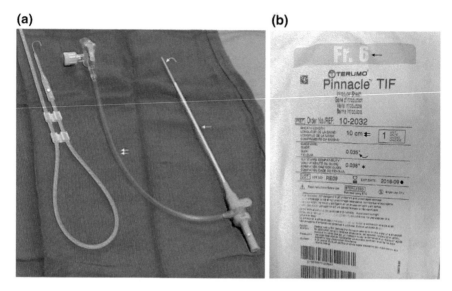

Fig. 5.1 Components of a sheath (**a**): The sheath (*straight arrow*) is introduced into the blood vessel using an introducer (*curved arrow*) that snaps onto the hub of the sheath when fully inserted. The introducer is threaded over the wire placed into the vessel. Once the sheath is introduced into the vessel, the introducer can be removed by detaching at its cap end (*asterisk*) from the sheath hub. The hub of the sheath has an eyelet to enable it to be sutured to the skin. The sheath is connected to a continuous flush of heparinized saline via provided tubing (*double arrow*). The guidewire used to place the sheath into the artery is lying to the left, still within its plastic container tubing. The plastic introducer (*dot*) can be used to straighten the tip of the J-tipped wire, enabling easier insertion into the needle, or sheath. The sheaths are color coded for size. Additionally, the label (**b**) is designed to provide appropriate information at a glance. The label of the pictured sheath readily demonstrates that it is 6 Fr (*arrow*) in size, the length of the sheath is 10 cm (*double arrow*), and the provided guidewire is 0.035″ in thickness (*curved arrow*). However, the sheath can take a guidewire up to 0.038″ in thickness (*asterisk*). The expiry date is also indicated (*black dot*)

- Access is obtained using modified Seldinger technique (see Chap. 1) and an exchange length 0.035 glidewire is advanced into the descending aorta.
- A shuttle sheath (e.g., 6 Fr) with its dilator inserted is threaded onto the glidewire and advanced to the descending aorta.
- Ensure that the tip of the glidewire always leads once the sheath is within vasculature.
- If the shuttle sheath needs to be positioned in a vessel other than aorta, then:

    - Remove the dilator completely and thread a slip catheter (5.5 or 6.5 Fr for 6 Fr and 7 Fr shuttles, respectively; H1, JB1 or Simmons 2 shapes) over the glidewire and into the shuttle sheath.
    - Advance the slip catheter over the glidewire and position it in the target vessel, e.g., CCA.

– Advance the shuttle sheath over the slip catheter to the target vessel.
– Remove the glidewire and slip catheter once the shuttle sheath has been appropriately positioned.

Special Considerations

- Use a braided long sheath where the patient is positioned in a manner that is inconvenient for angiography, e.g., prone or three-quarter prone positioning in the operating room. A considerable length of the sheath remains outside to assist easy access. As the sheath is braided, it is less likely to kink if the patient is lying on it.
- If the sheath needs to be left overnight, e.g., in case the patient is expected to return to the angio laboratory in a day or so, it should be completely secured, such that inadvertent accidents involving removal, disconnection, or injections into it do not occur. If a microcatheter has also been left in place, e.g., when administering tPA into a sinus, both sheath and microcatheter should be protected to prevent accidental retraction, disconnection, or accidentally pushing the microcatheter forward.
- If a long sheath was used, consider exchanging it for a short sheath, if the sheath is to be left in situ overnight.
- Table 5.1 shows examples of commonly used sheaths.

Wires

Guide wires

Terumo® Front Angled Glidewire (0.035", 150 cm): Our preferred wire in navigating the arch and neck vasculature. Compared to others, it is easier to manipulate and has a hydrophilic coating that remains lubricious within the catheter.

Table 5.1 Examples of commonly used sheaths, available sizes, lengths, and wire compatibility

Brand	Size (Fr)	Length (cm)	Wire (in.)
Pinnacle®, Terumo	4, **5**, **6**, 7, 8, 9, 10, 11	**10**, 25	0.035
Super ArrowFlex®, Arrow International	**5**, **6**, 7, 8, 9, 10, 11	**11**, 24, 45, 65, 90	0.035
Shuttle Select Sheath™, Cook Medical	5, **6**, 7	90	0.038

The most commonly used sizes and length are shown in bold

- Use of coated wires through the percutaneous access needle should be avoided, as withdrawing coated wires may shear the coating at the needle's tip.

Bentson® Wire (0.035″, 150 cm): An uncoated, braided stainless steel wire. Its straight shape may be advantageous when avoiding inadvertent selection of splanchnic or renal arteries from the aorta. However, remember to shape the tip to give it an angle (e.g., 45°) if intended for selective catheterization off the aortic arch. Otherwise, it will be difficult to manipulate. Bentson wire may be used as the primary choice in certain situations requiring frequent femoral artery access, e.g., patients receiving intra-arterial chemotherapy, where placement of sheath is avoided to minimize trauma to arteries accessed repeatedly over a short course of time. A Bentson® wire is advanced through the needle used to gain arterial access. The coating of a Glidewire® may be damaged and shorn during movement directly through the needle. This is not a problem with Bentson wires due to the lack of such coating.

Stiff Wires

- A stiff wire may be needed in situations where more support is necessary, e.g., during advancing a catheter with stent or angioplasty balloon. Options include the stiff Glidewire® or an Amplatz® wire may also be used. These less flexible wires are less prone to deformation while advancing rigid devices around vascular curves and may serve to straighten tortuous anatomy to improve navigation.
- Do not cross a severely stenosed segment with a large or stiff wire as it may injure plaque. A good strategy is to cross the lesion using a soft microwire and microcatheter [e.g., use a Prowler® 10 microcatheter (Cordis Endovascular) with a Transend Microguidewire (Stryker Neurovascular, Fremont, CA)]. Once the catheter is distal to the lesion, switch to an exchange length stiffer microwire. As an example, this situation may arise during treatment of severe carotid stenosis, in which case, if need, perform an angioplasty to enable usage of larger wires and catheters.

Exchange Length Wires

- Used to maintain access in a catheterized vessel and enable catheter exchange in a vessel that has proven difficult to catheterize. It must be roughly twice the length of the catheter being removed, usually 200–300 cm in length. This allows the operator to maintain wire access at the distal end of the catheter and to always have direct contact with the wire outside the patient as the catheter is removed.
- Table 5.2 shows examples of guidewires.

Table 5.2 Examples of guidewires, available types, lengths, diameter, and tip shape

Brand	Types	Length (cm)	Diameter (in.)	Tip shape
Glidewire®, Terumo	**Standard**	150	0.032	**Angle; straight**
		120ª, **150**, 180, 260	**0.035**	
		120ª, 150, 180, 260	0.038	
		150	0.035, 0.038	J-Tip
	Shapeable	150, 180	0.035	Shapeable
		150	0.038	
	Stiff	80ª, 150, 180, 260ᵇ	0.035, 0.038	Angle; straight
Bentson®, Cook Medical	TFE-coated stainless steel	145, 180, 200	0.035	Straight/shapeable
		145	0.025, 0.032, 0.038	
	TFE-coated stainless steel with heparin coating	80, 145, 180, 200	0.035	
		145, 260	0.038	
Amplatz®, Cook Medical	Stiff	145, 180, 260ᵇ	0.035, 0.038	Straight/shapeable

The kind most commonly used by us is highlighted in bold
ªAvailable only in angle tip
ᵇAvailable only in 0.035 diameter

Shaping a Wire

- Usually, a gentle 45° angle to the guidewire or microwire suffices. They also come pre-shaped. However, the wire may require shaping specifically to address the peculiarities of vasculature or location of the lesion. The technique is as follows:

  - Using a mandrel soaked in normal saline, hold the distal portion of the wire intended for shaping between the forefinger and thumb, pinching the wire against the mandrel (or other shaping device such as hemostat).
  - Slide the mandrel toward the wire tip maintaining the finger pinch on the wire and mandrel. This motion is similar to curling ribbon on a package wrapping.
  - The wire may be bent to create a tighter curve.
  - A second curve in the reverse direction just proximal to the first may create a shepherd's hook shape useful in access acute vascular takeoffs such as the anterior cerebral artery from the internal carotid.

Microguidewires

- These are used for placement of microcatheters in smaller vessels, e.g., the intracranial vasculature or branches of ECA.
- They also are used in larger vessels, e.g., crossing tight stenosis in ICA.
- Our workhorses are Transend® 0.014 or Synchro2 (Stryker, Fremont CA) with Excelsior SL-10 or 1018 Microcatheters (Stryker).
- Other good options include X-Pedion (Covidien, Plymouth, MN) or Agility® steerable guidewire (Cordis Neurovascular, Miami Lakes, FL). We use these in difficult vasculature where navigation with Synchro2 or Transend has proved unsuccessful. Each of these wires has a very good 1:1 torque response.
- Table 5.3 shows examples of commonly used Microguidewires.
- For venous sinus access, we prefer using Headliner wires as they are stiffer and may negotiate the sigmoid sinus better.

Table 5.3 Examples of commonly used Microguidewires, available types, sizes, lengths, and microcatheter compatibility

Brand	Type	Size (in.)	Length (cm)	Catheter (in.)
Transend®, Stryker Neurovascular	**Standard**	**0.010**	**205**	Excelsior SL10
	Standard	**0.014**	**182**	
	Soft tip; floppy; platinum	0.014	205	
	Extra support; floppy	0.014	300	
Synchro² Stryker Neurovascular	Soft; soft pre-shaped; standard; standard pre-shaped	0.014	200, 300	
[a]Agility®, Steerable Wires, Cordis Neurovascular	Standard; soft	0.010	195	
	Standard; standard XL	0.014	205, 350	
	Soft	0.014	205	
	Standard; soft	0.016	145, 175, 205	
	Standard XL	0.016	350	
X-Pedion™, Covidien		0.010	200	
		0.014	175	
Mirage™, ev3		0.008	200	Marathon™
Headliner®, Terumo	Standard: 45°, 90°, 90°/60° double angle, 1.5 mm J-Tip angle	0.012	200	
	Floppy: 45°, 90°, 90°/60° double angle, 1.5 mm J-Tip angle	0.016	200	

The most commonly used sizes and length are shown in bold
[a]The agility wire tips are straight (shapeable)

- When shaping tips, bear in mind the variance in pliability of different microwire tips, e.g., marathon tip requires to be shaped with gentler force than X-Pedion. Typically, smaller diameter and softer wires are shaped with less pressure.

Catheters

Guide catheters

- Used for interventional procedures involving neck and cerebral vasculature, where the Guide catheter supports the interventional catheter.
- We commonly use Envoy® 6 Fr for most of our interventions (Fig. 5.2a).
- In some cases, a larger size Guide catheters will be necessary e.g., during dual catheter procedures like, balloon-assisted aneurysm coiling.
- In procedures such as carotid angioplasty and stenting, a shuttle sheath may be used in lieu of Guide catheter in particularly tortuous vasculature (see 'Sheaths' above).

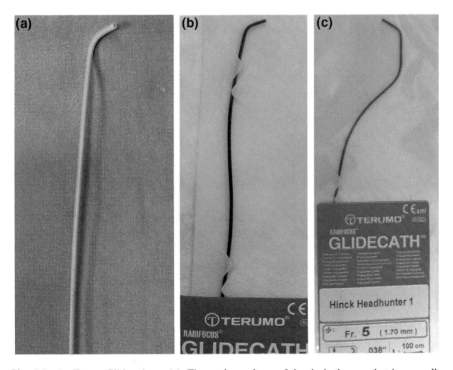

Fig. 5.2 An Envoy Glidecatheter (**a**). The angle or shape of the tip is the one that is generally used, and in this case, this product is known as 'multi-purpose catheter' (MPC). A front angled Glidecatheter (**b**). The 45° tip is commonly used. For more difficult catheterization, an H1 catheter may be used (**c**)

- Another option is a 6 Fr Neuron Delivery catheter (Penumbra Inc., Alameda, CA) that may be advanced into the intracranial carotid. However, it is not as robust in selection of supraaortic vessels. Therefore, the supraaortic vasculature may need to be selected using standard wires and catheters (e.g., 0.035 glidewire with 5 Fr Terumo glide catheter) and then an exchange made using an exchange length glidewire, to place the neuron catheter.
- Alternatively, advance a 5 Fr H1 Neuron Select™ catheter (Penumbra Inc., Alameda, CA) connected to a continuously running flush of heparinized saline through the Neuron Delivery catheter and tighten the Delivery catheter RHV around the Select catheter, so that the two act as a single unit. This is our modus operandi.
- When assembled, the coaxial system will comprise of the Select catheter (120, 130 cm length) that extends beyond the Delivery catheter (95, 105 cm length).
- Advance the 0.035 glidewire through the Select catheter and tighten the RHV around the wire just enough so that back bleeding is prevented, while the wire can be manipulated with ease.
- Introduce this system into the sheath and then advance the glidewire so that it leads the coaxial system.
- Using fluoroscopy and roadmapping, catheterize the desired vessel by advancing the Neuron Select catheter over the wire.
- Once in the desired position, loosen the Delivery catheter RHV, which is securing it to the Select catheter and then advance the delivery catheter over the positioned wire and Select catheter.
- The advantage of a neuron catheter is that it has a very soft tip and if required, may be advanced intracranially into the cavernous carotid.
- Table 5.4 shows examples of commonly used Guide catheters.

Diagnostic Catheters

Routine: A Terumo® 5 Fr front angled catheter may be used for most diagnostic procedures (Fig. 5.2b).

Challenging Vasculature, e.g., unusually tortuous and ectatic vasculature in an elderly patient, consider a Simmons 2 or a Headhunter H-1 (Fig. 5.2c).

- The Simmons 2 catheter is particularly useful for acute vascular origins, such as a steep, Type 2 or 3 aortic arch. It requires reformatting the secondary curve of the catheter after insertion. This can be performed one of two ways:

  - Lodge the distal catheter tip in a renal artery or left subclavian origin, and then advance the catheter while torqueing so that the secondary curve advances beyond the tip, ultimately dislodging it.
  - With the guidewire proximal to the secondary catheter curve, torque the catheter to form a loop in the arch and pull the catheter back so the loop is in the proximal descending aorta. Then, re-advance the wire beyond the distal

Table 5.4 Examples of commonly used Guide catheters, available types, sizes, lengths, and wire compatibility

Brand	Type	Size (Fr)	Length (cm)	Wire (in.)
Envoy®, Cordis Neurovascular	CBL, H1, **MPC**, MPD, Str	5	**90**, 100	0.035
	Mod CBL, HH1, **MPC**, MPD, Str, SIM2	6	**90**, 100	0.035
	CBL, H1, MPC, MPD, Str	0.014	205	
Shuttle Select Sheath™, Cook Medical		6, 7	80	0.035, 0.038
		5, 6, 7, 8	90	0.035, 0.038
		5, 6, 7	110	0.035, 0.038
Neuron 070 Delivery Catheter	Straight, MP	6	95, 105	0.035
Neuron Select Catheter	H1, Sim, Ber	5	120, 130	0.035
Navien™, ev3	Straight, MP 25°	5.2	105, 115, 125, 130	0.035, 0.038
		6.3	95, 105, 115, 125, 130	0.035, 0.038

The most commonly used sizes and length are shown in bold

> catheter tip until the wire stiffness opens the loop, flipping the distal catheter tip proximal to the secondary curve.
> - The wire may be removed and the catheter manipulated while on heparinized saline flush, or injected with contrast to visualize target arteries.
> - Once re-formatted, the catheter tip is advanced into a selected artery origin by gently withdrawing the catheter and is withdrawn from that artery by advancing the catheter, opposite to the movements of a single-curve catheter such as the Terumo glide or H1 catheter.

- An H1- or JB1-shaped catheter may be useful in aiding in selection of acute origins or second-order arteries where the deflection of an angled glide catheter and glidewire is insufficient and the Simmons 2 cannot be steered or advanced over the wire, such as selecting the right subclavian artery from the innominate. Typically, however, the H1 shape is more difficult to torque than the angled glide catheter.

Cerebrocervical Aortic Arch: We usually avoid performing aortic arch angiograms, as they have been associated with a higher risk of complications and the benefit of information yielded is often low. However, in cases of unusual anatomy (e.g., aberrant right subclavian origin, situs inversus) or atherosclerosis of the great vessel origins, performing an aortic arch injection will result in visualization of the entire brachiocephalic vasculature concurrently which may save time and avoid risky selective catheterization. The technique is as follows:

- Use a 5 Fr pigtail catheter for this purpose (the usual diagnostic catheters are not meant for the high-volume injections and may burst and lack the side holes for rapid opacification of a large diameter space such as the aorta).
- The catheter is positioned in the ascending aorta, proximal to the innominate artery.
- Center the image intensifier or detector over the patient's head and neck, ensuring both right and left sides are in the field.
- Inject contrast at a rate of 20 mL/s for a total of 30 mL.

Interventional Catheters/Microcatheters

Aneurysms

- Microcatheter selection depends on the size of aneurysm and the type of coils to be used for embolization.
- The microcatheters for detachable coils have 2 markers on their distal aspect, 3 cm apart.
- The most distal marker indicates the tip of the microcatheter. This marker must be within the aneurysm sac prior to coil deployment.
- The more proximal marker aligns with a marker on the coil pusher when the coil has been deployed completely in the aneurysm. Any further advancement beyond this point will result in the pusher entering the aneurysm, likely causing aneurysm rupture.
- Use Excelsior SL-10 for small aneurysms, or when planning to place 0.010″ coils, e.g., GDC-10 or Target (Stryker, Fremont, CA).
- When planning to use larger coils, e.g., GDC-18 or large diameter Target (with or without 0.010″ coils), use a larger microcatheter, e.g., Excelsior 1018 for 18 coils.
- Table 5.5 shows examples of commonly used microcatheters.
- If the aneurysm is to be treated with Pipeline™ Embolization Device (PED, eV3 Neurovascular, Irvine, CA), then a Marksman™ (eV3) microcatheter is used. To provide reliable support, in such cases we use an 8 Fr short sheath and a 6 Fr shuttle or Neuron Delivery catheter. The shuttle or neuron is advanced over a 5 Fr H1 catheter and 0.035 wire into the target vessel, e.g., the ICA. A 5 Fr Navien (ev3) catheter is prepared by connecting to a continuous flush of heparinized saline and the marksman catheter introduced into it (also connected to heparin flush). The microwire is inserted into the marksman. This system is then advanced as a unit to target location intracranially. This triaxial system (Shuttle/Neuron + Navien + Marksman) improves support and trackability during pipeline deployment. Additionally, the likelihood of catheter collapse out of cerebral vasculature is also significantly attenuated.

Table 5.5 Examples of commonly used microcatheters available, types, sizes, lengths, and microwire compatibility

Brand	Type	Size (Fr) proximal/distal OD	Size (in.) inner diameter	Length (cm) total/distal	Wire (in.)
Excelsior® SL-10, Boston Scientific	Straight, **45°, 90°, J, C, S**	2.4/1.7	0.0165	150/6	0.010, 0.014
Excelsior® 1018, Boston Scientific		2.6/2.0	0.019		0.014, 0.016
Prowler® Select® LP ES, Cordis	Straight, 45°, 90°, J	2.3/1.9	0.0165	150/5	0.010, 0.014
Prowler® Select® Plus, Cordis		2.8/2.3	0.021		0.014, 0.016

The most commonly used types are shown in bold

AVMs

- For embolization with Onyx®, we use Echelon™ and Marathon™ microcatheters (compatible with DMSO, the solvent used in conjunction with Onyx®). Echelon is reinforced to improve trackability over a wire and prevent ovalization that would interfere with coil advancement. Marathon lacks distal reinforcement making it softer and is preferred in smaller, more fragile vasculature.
- Examples of DMSO compatible catheters are indicated in Table 5.6.
- For particle embolization of tumors and epistaxis, the microcatheter chosen should have sufficient inner diameter so as not to be prematurely clogged by particles that are too large for it.
- Table 5.7 indicates the inner diameter of the microcatheters and compatible size of the particles to be used with it. For concomitant coil deposition may use Excelsior SL-10 microcatheter.

Stroke

- For administration of tPA into the cerebral artery, use Excelsior SL 10, Rapidtransit or another suitable catheter. Single-tip catheters may avoid confusion about catheter position.
- When using Merci® device, use the Merci microcatheter provided in package as these are reinforced specifically to support the device.
- May use Penumbra® as guide catheter, because the guide catheter provided with the Merci Kit frequently performs unsatisfactorily in tortuous vasculature.

Table 5.6 DMSO compatible microcatheters, types, sizes, lengths, and microwire compatibility

Brand	Tip configuration	Size (Fr) proximal/distal OD	Length (cm) usable	Catheter volume (ml)	Wire (in.)
Marathon™, EV3	Straight	2.7/1.5	165	0.23	Mirage **0.008**
Echelon 10™, EV3	Straight, 45°, 90°	2.1/1.7	150	0.34	**X-Pedion 0.010**, 0.014
Echelon 14™, EV3		2.4/1.9			
Rebar 10™, EV3	Straight, steam shapeable	2.3/1.7	153	0.27	0.010, 0.012
Rebar 14™, EV3		2.4/1.9		0.29	0.010, 0.012, 0.014
Rebar 18™, EV3		2.8/2.3	130, 153		0.014, 0.016, 0.018
UltraFlow™, EV3	Straight, steam shapeable	3.0/1.5	165	0.26	0.008, 0.010

The most commonly used types are shown in bold

Table 5.7 Table indicates the inner diameter of the microcatheters and compatible size of particles to be used with it

Brand	Size (Fr) proximal/distal OD	Catheter volume (ml)	Wire (in.)	Inner diameter (in.) distal	Compatible particle sizes (μm)
Marathon™, EV3	2.7/1.5	0.23	**Mirage 0.008**	0.013	40–120, 100–300
Echelon 10™, EV3	2.1/1.7	0.34	**X-Pedion 0.010**, 0.014	0.017	40–120, 100–300
Echelon 14™, EV3	2.4/1.9				
Rebar 10™, EV3	2.3/1.7	0.27	0.010, 0.012	0.015	
Rebar 14™, EV3	2.4/1.9	0.29	0.010, 0.012. 0.014	0.017	
Rebar 18™, EV3	2.8/2.3		0.014, 0.016, 0.018	0.021	40–120, 100–300, 300–500
Rebar 027™, EV3	2.8/2.8		0.014, 0.016, 0.018	0.027	40–120, 100–300, 300–500, 500–700, 700–900
UltraFlow™, EV3	3.0/1.5	0.26	0.008, 0.010	0.012	40–120, 100–300
Prowler Plus™ Codman	2.8/2.3	0.55	0.014, 0.016, 0.018	0.021	40–120, 100–300, 300–500
Rapid transit Codman	2.3/2.3	0.55	0.014, 0.016, 0.018	0.017	40–120, 100–300, 300–500

- When using Penumbra system® (Penumbra, Inc., Alameda, CA), choose the aspiration catheter from the available options, selecting the largest diameter appropriate for the size of the vessel to be treated, e.g., 054 (aka 5 max) catheter for ICA or M1 vessels (see Chap. 15, Stroke for further information). The large catheter may be advanced over a smaller, longer catheter to aid in tracking.
- When using the Solitaire™ (eV3) or Trevo™ (Stryker) 'stentreivers,' select the Marksman™ catheter (0.027" ID, eV3/Covidien) or Trevo™ Pro Microcatheter (0.027" ID, Stryker). In case of Trevo retrievers, Trevo™ Pro 14 is used with 3 × 20 mm retrievers, while Trevo™ Pro 18 is used with the larger 4 × 20 mm retrievers. The latter is the more commonly used retriever size. For a Trevo 6 × 25 mm retriever, an Excelsior XT-27® Microcatheter (Stryker) is used.
- When proximal flow arrest is desired, such as clot retrieval with Merci, Solitaire, or Trevo, a balloon guide catheter is recommended. These include Merci® Balloon guide catheter (Stryker Neurovascular, Fremont, CA) or Cello™ (eV3). Alternatively, we have consistently performed successful thombectomies by aspirating on a non-balloon guide catheter (e.g., Envoy or Shuttle) with a 60-ml syringe as the Trevo stentriever is retracted.

Navigation

6

General Tips

- Ensure the catheter is advanced with the guidewire leading (Fig. 6.1).
- To ensure maximal control, advance the wire or the catheter independently while stabilizing the other.
- When manipulating/rotating catheter, ensure that the catheter outside the patient is completely straight. This will prevent counter torque from developing.

Aortic Arch

- When advancing an angled catheter, ensure the tip is pointing downwards and the wire is distal to the catheter tip so that it does not inadvertently scrape the vessel wall.
- When retracting the catheter to select a vessel, turn it approx 15° counter-clockwise, so the tip is pointing upwards and withdraw slowly until the catheter 'jumps' into position indicating catheter engagement in the great vessel origin.
- The origin of a vessel is identified by the anatomical landmarks, e.g., the brachial trunk is usually at the level of right second rib head in the LAO view.
- We usually do not perform aortic angiograms except for situations such as aberrant anatomy, stenosis of the great vessel origins, or stroke (when CTA of head and neck has not been performed), where the aortic arch and the entire brachiocephalic vasculature bilaterally is visualized in a single AP run.
- In case of difficulty catheterizing the vessel arising of the aortic arch, ask the patient to take a deep breath and hold it.
- A Simmons 2 catheter may also be used, if the usual catheters are unsuccessful in catheterization. It is used as follows:

© Springer International Publishing AG 2017
S.H. Khan and A.J. Ringer, *Handbook of Neuroendovascular Techniques*,
DOI 10.1007/978-3-319-52936-3_6

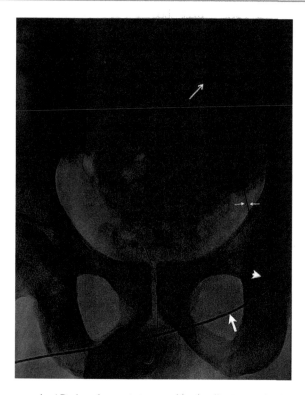

Fig. 6.1 Fluoroscopy in AP view demonstrates a guidewire (*long* arrow) advanced through the femoral and iliac arteries toward the aorta. The sheath (delineated by the opposing *small arrows*) is already in place enabling convenient advancement of wires, catheters, and other devices. The hub of the sheath is faintly visible (*arrowhead*). The diagnostic catheter (*thick arrow*) has just been introduced over the guidewire into the sheath. The tip of the catheter is just beyond the hub. Usually, catheters are advanced with the guidewire leading and retracted with the guidewire tip within the catheter

- Advance the catheter over wire into the aorta.
- When the catheter is in the ascending aorta, retract the wire well into the shaft. However, do not withdraw the wire completely out of the catheter.
- Rotate the catheter counterclockwise, which will result in the distal aspect of the catheter acquiring a ⟳ like shape.
- Maintaining this shape, gradually withdraw the catheter until it is positioned almost vertically in the descending aorta, with its tip just short of the aortic arch.
- Advance the guidewire through the catheter and continue to advance until the tip of the catheter drops into the descending aorta. The distal aspect of the

catheter will have reformed into an 'inverted U' shape with the convexity of the U leading.

– Withdraw the wire from the catheter completely.

- Advance the reformed catheter into the ascending aorta with the convexity leading and tip inferior.
- Turn the catheter clockwise so that the tip points upwards.
- Now gradually retract the catheter.
- The tip will be seen to 'catch' the origin of brachiocephalic (BCT).
- Pulling the catheter further will cause the catheter to advance further up in BCT.
- Turning the tip medially or laterally during manipulation will result in selection of common carotid arteries (CCA) or Subclavian artery (SCA).
- To retract the catheter from BCT, push/advance forward. Due to the shape of catheter, this will narrow the secondary curve resulting in the tip's retraction out of BCT.
- Keeping the tip pointing downward retracts the catheter until it is proximal to BCT origin and then rotates the catheter to point the tip up again. Further retraction will result in selection of left CCA.
- After selection of CCA, further retraction of catheter will result in its advancement further into CCA.
- As indicated above, pushing the catheter forward will result in its retraction from the CCA and then pointing the tip down, pulling it back, pointing the tip up and pulling further still result in selection of left SCA. When removing the catheter out, simply withdraw the catheter to lose the secondary curve format (taking care not to allow the tip to advance unsafely first) or reinsert the wire just short of the tip, so that it does not inadvertently reform in the descending aorta while being withdrawn, and select branches such as renal artery.
- One of the authors does not attach a Simmons 2 catheter to the flush system, to enable greater manipulation. This necessitates even greater vigilance to ensure against emboli. If the intention is to maintain the Simmons as a Guidecatheter or if the navigation is protracted, then it must be connected to a continuous flush of heparinized saline.
- During difficult catheterization, one may also do an aortic angiogram and use it as an 'image overlay'. For aortic angiography a pigtail catheter should be used, the rate of injection is 20 ml/s for a total of 30 ml ('20 for 30'). The usual diagnostic catheters may burst at this rate of injection. In such a case, exchange the pigtail catheter over exchange length catheter for the Simmons or other selected catheter because the table cannot be moved to follow the catheter up from the groin.
- In difficult navigation, using a stiffer guidewire may help.

Brachiocephalic Trunk

- Once the brachiocephalic trunk is selected with the catheter tip, advance the wire and then the catheter over it, e.g., may advance the wire well into subclavian or brachial artery so that it gives the catheter good support as it is advanced.
- Usually, the right SCA and CCA can be catheterized without angiographic visualization. However, roadmapping may be performed, if needed.
- To catheterize the SCA, the catheter tip is pointed laterally and it is advanced over the wire that has been advanced well into the SCA.
- If the catheter tip is maintained in the subclavian, proximal to the vertebral artery (VA), the VA is frequently clearly visualized on angiography without having to catheterize it. If the catheter tip is distal to the VA, or the VA is not clearly visualized, then a blood pressure cuff may be applied to that arm and inflated. This will result in contrast reflux into the VA and better visualization.
- For angiography in the brachiocephalic trunk, we use an injection rate of 6 ml/s for a total of 8 ml ('6 for 8'). The frame rate is between 2 and 4/s with a rate rise of 0.4 s.
- If the contrast injection is causing the catheter to kick out of the vessel, then the rate rise may be increased.
- If the pathology is not clearly visualized, then one remedy may be to increase the number of frames/s.

Subclavian Artery

- If difficulty is encountered in catheterizing the right SCA, the catheter is initially placed in the CCA. The wire is retracted into the shaft, and then the catheter is gradually retracted with the tip pointing laterally (to the patient's right). A slight jump will be visualized as the catheter enters the subclavian ostium. Advance the wire into the subclavian, followed by the catheter.
- The presence of wire in the shaft of the catheter diminishes the likelihood of its prolapse into the aorta.
- In case a tortuous artery makes subclavian artery catheterization difficult, try a catheter with a sharper angle at its tip, e.g., HeadHunter H1.
- The left subclavian artery is usually quite easy to catheterize. It is often in line with the descending aorta, and therefore frequently may be catheterized when the catheter is being advanced in the descending aorta. Should this happen, complete any required angiography via left SCA before retracting the catheter, in order to prevent repeat catheterizations.
- For SCA angiography, the injection rate usually remains 6 ml/s for a total of 8 ml ('6 for 8'). The frame rate is usually 4/s with a rate rise of 0.4.

Vertebral Arteries

- If VA needs to be catheterized, the catheter is advanced over wire into the SCA, the wire is retracted into the catheter, the tip of catheter pointed upwards, and then the catheter slowly retracted back until the tip catches the VA origin.
- There is no need to unnecessarily advance the catheter further into the VA beyond its origin.
- On either side, the VA is diagonally across the internal mammary artery.
- Visualization of the vertebral artery origin may be easier from a slight contralateral oblique AP view because it arises posteriorly and medially from the subclavian artery.
- The left VA is easier to catheterize than the right VA, since the latter arises off the SCA that in turn arises off the brachiocephalic trunk, creating a tortuous path from the aortic arch. On the other hand, the left SCA arises directly off the aortic arch and is almost in line with the descending aorta and therefore is far easier to catheterize.
- If VA catheterization is needed, consider catheterizing the left VA. Reflux into the RVA may result in visualization of right posterior inferior cerebellar artery (PICA), in which case the catheterization of right VA, e.g., in case of SAH, becomes unnecessary. If the contralateral PICA is not visualized, then catheterization and angiography via the right VA is needed (Fig. 6.2).
- If confusion arises whether the catheterized vessel is VA or carotid, pay attention to its course: the position of VA is medial to the projected course of the carotid; on AP projection, the VA overlies transverse process; on oblique view, the VA courses through foramina transversaria.
- The superior thyrocervical trunk may also be confused for VA, until contrast is injected for visualization. Bear in mind the origin of VA is diagonally opposite to internal mammary artery.
- If angiography is performed with the catheter tip in the SCA, then contrast is injected at 6 for 8 with the settings indicated above under 'Brachiocephalic trunk'.
- If the catheter tip is in the VA, then we use a rate of 4 ml/s for a total contrast dose of 6 ml ('4 for 6'). Usually, the rest of the settings for frame/s, rate rise, etc., can be the same as for brachiocephalic trunk.

Carotid

Right Common Carotid

- To catheterize the right CCA, the tip of the catheter in the BCT is pointed rostrally and medially.
- The guidewire is advanced to secure access and enable advancement of the catheter. If additional wire support is needed, the wire is preferably advanced into the ECA.

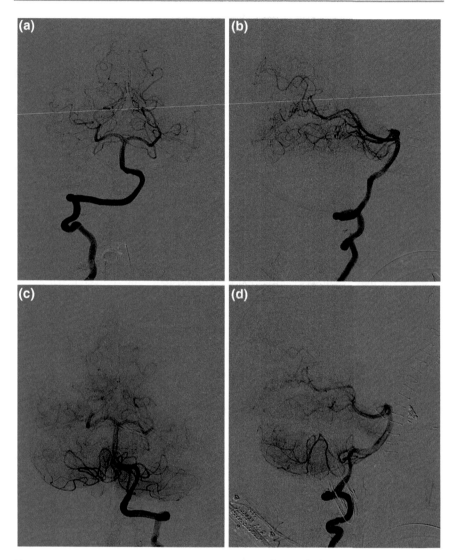

Fig. 6.2 *Right* vertebral angiography Townes **a** and lateral views **b** demonstrate obvious absence of PICAs. *Left* vertebral angiography **c** and **d** show both PICAs having common origin from LVA. There is relative avascularity in the anterior inferior cerebellar artery (AICA) distribution in all four figures, which is particularly noticeable on lateral views. The AICA territory is most likely supplied by terminal branches of SCA and PICA

Left Common Carotid

- To catheterize the left CCA, the tip of the catheter is maintained pointing up as it is gently retracted back from the BCT.

- As it is retracted out of BCT, it will then be seen to 'jump' as it pops into the origin of left CCA.

  - Frequently, the catheter needs to be torqued counterclockwise for about 15° as it is being retracted back out of BCT, to enable successful catheterization of left CCA origin.

- Once the origin of left CCA is selected with the catheter tip, advance the wire forward into the CCA and then advance the catheter over it.
- If further rostral access of wire is needed to enable catheter advancement, preferably advance the catheter into the ECA rather than ICA.
- Always be cognizant of wire and catheter tip positions.
- For angiography with catheter tip in CCA, use an injection rate of 5 ml/s for a total of 7 ml ('5 for 7'). The frame rate is 4/s with a rate rise of 0.4.
- If the contrast injection is causing the catheter to kick out of the vessel, then the rate rise may be increased.
- If the pathology is not clearly visualized, then one remedy may be to increase the number of frames/s.

Internal Carotid Artery (ICA)

- The approach to the right and left ICAs from the common carotids is identical.
- Prior to catheterization, visualize the ICA to detect any pathology, e.g., stenosis, dissection. If such pathology is present and the operator is unaware, the consequence of manipulating the wire without due care may be embolism, spasm, or dissection.
- The ICA usually lies posterolateral to the ECA.
- If difficulties are encountered, navigation can be performed by using AP and lateral carotid angiograms as 'image overlay'. Conversely, roadmapping in these projections may be performed.
- When selecting the ICA, from BCT or proximal CCA, initially advance the guidewire tip into the ECA or the distal CCA below the bifurcation. Advance the catheter just short of ICA bifurcation, then retract the wire. Point the tip of catheter laterally (on AP view) and posteriorly (on lateral view) to face the origin of ICA and advance the wire into it. Always visualize the tip of wire and catheter.
- If needed, obtain AP, lateral or oblique views to better visualize the bifurcation for catheterization.

External Carotid Artetry (ECA)

- Catheterization of the ECA is comparatively safer than ICA. However, vigilance should continue to be maintained.

- From the common carotid artery, orient the catheter tip anteriorly and medially. Advance the wire into the proximal ECA and advance the catheter over the wire.
- Be cognizant of the tendency for the catheter and wire to select the superior thyroid artery which arises anteriorly from the proximal external carotid. Catheter position distal to the superior thyroid artery may be necessary to avoid catheter kick out or contrast reflux into the internal carotid.
- Contrast injection into the ECA and its branches is usually painful. Therefore, power injections should be avoided if possible. A smooth, gentle hand injection is performed instead. When power injection is necessary, limit injection to 3 ml/s for 4 ml total volume ('3 for 4') and use a prolonged rate rise of up to 1 s.

Selective Cerebral Artery Catheterization

Anterior Cerebral Artery (ACA)

– The (ACA) is more difficult to catheterize due to its acute origin, as compared to middle cerebral artery (MCA) which is more of a continuation of the ICA. If the usual 45°–90° shaped microwire tip is unhelpful, then fashioning the tip of

the Microguidewire into a shepherd's crook may be useful (see Chap. 5) 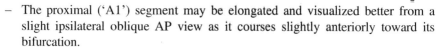 .

– The proximal ('A1') segment may be elongated and visualized better from a slight ipsilateral oblique AP view as it courses slightly anteriorly toward its bifurcation.
– When planning to coil an anterior communicating (AComm) aneurysm, perform angiography from right and left ICA to study which side is more amenable to navigation and also cross-flow across the AComm, e.g., if there is cross-flow from right to left, but not left to right, it may be better to access the aneurysm from left so that if the left A1 is inadvertently occluded, there will still be blood flow to distal ACAs. The choice of side to use will also depend upon which artery leads more directly to aneurysm.
– Additionally, the side which is easier to access is less tortuous and therefore provides better stability to the Guide catheter and/or microcatheter is also taken into consideration in deciding which artery to navigate.
– Perform angiography in two planes for navigation (Fig. 6.3).
– When angiography is needed through microcatheter, perform hand injections using 3–5 ml syringe. Using a power injector may result in disruption of the microcatheter and possible associated complications.

(a)   **(b)**

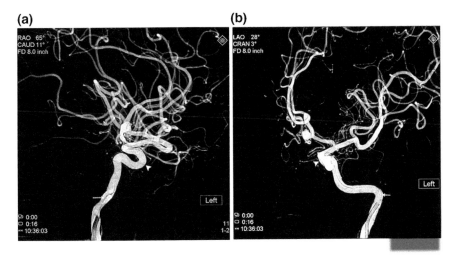

Fig. 6.3 Roadmap of anterior communicating aneurysm in lateral (**a**) and left oblique (**b**) views. The guide catheter is appreciated in *upper* cervical segment. The microcatheter and microwire can be seen (*small arrow*). The importance of two views for navigation is apparent. The carotid siphon (*arrowhead*) is best navigated using the lateral view. The oblique view is more suitable for selection of ACA and entering the aneurysm

Middle Cerebral Artery (MCA)

- Usually, this is easier to catheterize than ACA, as it is a continuation of ICA (Fig. 6.4).
- The proximal ('M1') segment may be elongated and visualized better from a slight contralateral oblique AP view as it courses slightly anteriorly toward its bifurcation.
- When angiography is needed through microcatheter, perform hand injections using 3–5 ml syringe. Using a power injector may result in disruption of the microcatheter and possible associated complications.

Vertebrobasilar System

- When possible, navigate through the non-dominant VA. In case of equidominant VAs, use the left VA, which usually has a more direct or straight approach and is usually easier to catheterize.
- When the proximal VA is tortuous, distal catheterization may straighten the artery resulting in limitation of flow. This should be avoided unless the contralateral VA provides sufficient flow to the vertebrobasilar system.
- When the Guide catheter is positioned in the proximal VA, the power injector should not be used at a rate higher than 4 for 6, unless the VA is very large.

Fig. 6.4 *Right* carotid
angiography. The MCA
(*arrow*) is obviously a
continuation of the ICA.
The ACA branches at an
acute angle (*arrowhead*) and
is more difficult to catheterize.
A microwire can be
appreciated in the MCA

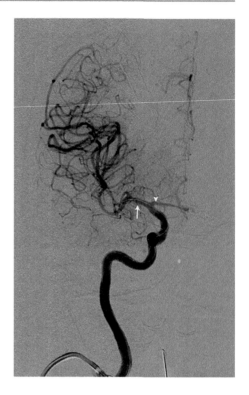

- Angiography through a microcatheter is performed using hand injections of contrast.
- For microcatheter selection of the basilar artery (BA), the BA may be elongated by using a slightly caudal, transfacial AP view as it courses slightly anteriorly toward its apex.

Techniques in Case of Difficult Navigation

- Consider using a softer or stiffer guidewire/microguidewire than the one already being used.
- Consider using a different catheter.
- Using a 'buddy wire' concurrently alongside the guidewire within the catheter being navigated up may straighten the blood vessel and provide greater catheter support to avoid prolapse during attempted catheter advancement.
- Using a longer sheath, or a shuttle sheath esp., where there is significant tortuosity of the proximal vasculature.

- If navigation via femoral artery is proving difficult, consider access through an alternate route, e.g., radial or brachial for vertebrobasilar access, or directly through carotid for MCA/ACA access.

Postoperative Management and Follow-Up

- If the procedure was diagnostic, the patient is monitored for approx. 2 h and then discharged if he/she remains asymptomatic.
- In case of an interventional procedure, we usually admit the patient to NSICU for at least 24 h. During this time, he/she is maintained on heparin for 12 h (900 IU/h for patients weighing less than 75 kg and 1300 IU/h for those weighing more than 75 kg). Alternatively, the patient may be administered 15 IU/kg/h. Any inexplicable change in neurological exam should lead to thorough investigation including CT Head and, if indicated, repeat angiography to rule out new vascular occlusion with ischemia that may not be seen on CT.
- Also monitor the access site (usually femoral artery) for pseudoaneurysm, vessel occlusion, etc.
- Site of access should be documented, so that in a future study the contralateral side is used. We recommend alternating access sites so that a single vessel is not unduly traumatized.
- Any unusual aspect encountered during navigation including difficult vasculature and how it was addressed should be documented (e.g., in dictation of procedure) for future reference.

Venography

Access

- The technique of gaining access is similar to arterial access using modified Seldinger technique. However, the stab incision and vessel puncture are made medial to the arterial pulsations.
- Take into consideration the femoral anatomy, whereby the femoral vein lies medial to the artery and the femoral nerve is lateral to the artery.
- When successfully punctured, dark blood will emanate from the needle at low pressure and without the pulsations characteristic of arterial puncture.
- Place sheath in the vein using modified Seldinger technique, in the same manner as when you catheterize the artery.
- Connect the sheath to a continuously running flush of heparinized saline and secure the sheath to adjacent skin using 2-0 silk suture.

Navigation

- Navigate the catheter connected to a continuous heparinized saline flush over wire using fluoroscopy.
- The course of inferior vena cava is usually right of aorta and will lead to right atrium.
- The catheter is then advanced over wire into the superior vena cava.

Vessel Selection

- The guidewire is then directed left (for left internal jugular vein [IJV]) or superiorly (for right IJV), depending on which IJV needs to be catheterized.
- Unlike the arteries, veins have valves and therefore resistance might be encountered as the closed valve is encountered. Do not push through forcefully. Time the advancement and manipulation with inspiration. Follow with the catheter.
- When performing roadmapping to assist with navigation, remember to wait at least 3 s after the arterial injection, before performing fluoroscopy to get the roadmap to avoid arterial contamination of the image.

Techniques in Case of Difficult Navigation

Sigmoid Sinus

- The sigmoid sinus can be very difficult to navigate across, particularly with a larger catheter, e.g., AngioJet™ or Penumbra. Consider the following strategies in case of difficulties:

    - Create a coaxial system.
    - Advance the guide catheter as high as possible to provide support to the navigating catheter.
    - Point the guide catheter posteriorly and laterally, which is more likely to enable the Microcatheter and wire to head in the right direction.
    - Shape the tip of the microwire so that it has a larger advancing loop ('J' or 'shepherd's crook' shape). This will prevent it from going into smaller branches (with possible inadvertent perforation) and also allow clot maceration when treating venous sinus thrombosis.

Spinal Angiography

- For details on spinal angiography, see Chaps. 7 and 8.
- In brief, a Cobra or Mickelson catheter is used.

- Radiopaque markers attached to a plastic ruler are kept on one side to help demarcate the vertebral bodies.
- The parallax is removed by placing the desired markers and catheter tip in the center of the fluoroscopic field. The catheter tip will appear below the overlapping marker when in the superior edge of the field and above the overlapping marker when in the inferior edge as it is farther from the x-ray source.
- Usually, the catheter tip needs to be pointed slightly posteriorly and laterally to enter the ostium of the spinal artery.
- For efficiency, once an ostium is found, catheterized and angiography completed, it is pulled down maintaining the tip's position. It will jump into the ostium of the next vessel. One side is completed, and then the opposite side is addressed. This avoids the need to 'rediscover' the ostium position at each level.
- Due to the small size of spinal arteries, we perform hand injections.

Suggested Reading

Morris P. Practical neuroangiography. Philadelphia: Lippincott Williams & Wilkins; 2007. p. 36–85.

Venography and Intervention

7

Equipment

- The sheaths, catheters, wires etc. used for venography are the same as for standard angiography. Similar to the arterial side, the size and selection of equipment are dependent upon the purpose of procedure, e.g., a 5-Fr sheath and catheter are used when performing a diagnostic procedure, while at least a 6-Fr sheath will be required in an intervention.
- When anticipating a potential intervention, start with at least a 6-Fr sheath, even if performing a diagnostic procedure.

Access

- The technique of gaining access is similar to arterial access using modified Seldinger technique. However, the skin stab incision and vessel puncture are made medial to the arterial pulsations, as the femoral vein lies medial to the femoral artery.
- When successfully punctured, dark blood will emanate from the needle at low pressure and without the pulsations characteristic of arterial puncture.
- Place sheath in the vein using modified Seldinger technique in the same fashion, as when you catheterize the artery.
- Connect the sheath to a continuously running flush of heparinized saline and secure the sheath to adjacent skin using 2-0 silk suture.

© Springer International Publishing AG 2017
S.H. Khan and A.J. Ringer, *Handbook of Neuroendovascular Techniques*,
DOI 10.1007/978-3-319-52936-3_7

Navigation

- Navigate the catheter connected to a continuous heparinized saline flush over a leading wire using fluoroscopy.
- The course of inferior vena cava is usually to the right of aorta and leads to right atrium.
- The catheter is then advanced over wire into the superior vena cava.

Vessel Selection

- When performing roadmapping to assist with navigation, remember to wait at least 3 sec after the arterial injection, before acquiring fluoroscopy to get the roadmap, to avoid arterial contamination of the image.
- The guidewire is then directed to the patient's left (for left internal jugular vein [IJV]) or superiorly (for right IJV), depending on which IJV needs to be catheterized.
- Unlike the arteries, veins have valves and therefore, resistance might be encountered as the closed valve is encountered. Do not push through forcefully. Time the advancement and manipulation of wire with inspiration. Follow with the catheter.
- Once the IJV has been entered, the navigation is similar to arteries as the cranial venous sinuses do not have valves.

Intervention

- Venous intervention is usually required for conditions such as cerebral sinus thrombosis, and dural AVMs including carotid cavernous fistulae (CCF).
- Consider placing a 6- or 7-Fr sheath in the femoral vein.
- In case of intervention in cerebral sinuses, we usually position the guide catheter in the jugular bulb. This may be advanced higher if more support is required. However, usually the limit is the sigmoid sinus turn, beyond which it is very difficult to advance.
- The microcatheter is advanced over a 0.014″ or 0.016″ wire. For more wire support, consider the Headliner® (Microvention, Aliso Viejo, CA) as it is stiffer than Transend® and may be able to negotiate the sigmoid turn better.

Cranial Sinus Thrombosis

- First-line therapy involves anticoagulation except in high-risk cases. When 24 h of IV heparin fails, or the patient's clinical condition worsens, then endovascular intervention is a consideration.

Chemical Thrombolysis

- The objective of chemical thrombolysis is re-establishment of blood flow in the involved sinus, not complete reconstitution of the sinus. After placement of microcatheter in the involved sinus, administer 2–5 mg of TPA over a period of 15 min as the microcatheter is slowly retracted from distal to proximal aspect of the clot.
- Subsequently, commence a continuous infusion at a rate of 0.5–1 mg/h for 12–24 h.
- The TPA for continuous infusion is prepared by mixing 1 mg of TPA in 10 ml on normal saline, resulting in a concentration of 0.1 mg TPA per 1 ml saline. This solution is then administered at a rate of 10 ml/h.
- Another option is to place two microcatheters in the involved sinus: one at the distal aspect of the clot and another proximally. TPA at a rate of 0.5 mg/h can be infused through each catheter.
- While the patient is in the suite, angiography is performed every 15 min to assess the results of thrombolysis.
- Repeat angiography the following day.

Contraindications

- Hemorrhagic stroke (relative).
- Recent major surgery (relative).
- Radiologically demonstrable large ischemic infarct.

Mechanical Thrombectomy

- When it appears no headway is being made with chemical thrombolysis, or there is a need to reduce significant clot burden to hasten chemical thrombolysis, then mechanical thrombolysis may be used in conjunction with TPA (see Figs. 15.8 and 15.9, Chap. 15, Stroke). The following devices are currently available:

  - *Penumbra*® aspiration device (see Chap. 15, Stroke for technique details): Perhaps currently the best available interventional option for cranial sinus thrombosis (CST). Taking into consideration the size of the venous sinuses, use the largest available (currently 5Max, 0.064″) catheter and separator.

- *Pronto*® aspiration device (see Chap. 15 Stroke for technique details): Designed for peripheral vascular clot aspiration, this device works by manual aspiration thru multiple side holes using a large syringe
- *AngioJet*™: This device is designed specifically for venous clot aspiration, but due to its bulky catheters that are almost impossible to negotiate around the sigmoid. We do not use it.
- *Merci* catheter is also an option (see Chap. 15 Stroke for technique details).
- However, similar to arterial occlusions, in our experience it is not very effective.

Dural Arteriovenous Malformations/Fistulae

- The dural AVM may be better dealt with by occlusion from the venous aspect. This approach has been demonstrated to attenuate the arterial feeders. The initial obliteration of veins in dural AVM contrasts the approach for cerebral arteriovenous malformations, where such an approach would be detrimental.
- When opting for the venous route, ensure that the venous fistula is well developed enough not to tear or rupture by manipulation (e.g., an acute fistula/malformation). Usually, fistulae/malformations that have been present for a while can be dealt with via the venous route, with reasonable safety (also see Chap. 14 Vascular Malformations for further details).

Closure

- Once the procedure is complete and venous access is no longer required.
- Remove the sheath and apply manual pressure until bleeding stops.
- When possible perform femoral arterial access and venous access on separate limbs. It will diminish the likelihood of a femoral arteriovenous fistula formation.
- The postoperative care remains the same as for standard arterial angiography and intervention.

Techniques in Case of Difficult Navigation

Sigmoid Sinus

- The sigmoid sinus can be very difficult to navigate across, particularly with a larger catheter, e.g., AngioJet™ (Boston Scientific) or Penumbra (Penumbra, Inc.). Consider the following strategies in case of difficulties:

- Create a coaxial system.
- Advance the guide catheter as high as possible to provide support to the navigating catheter.
- Point the guide catheter posteriorly and laterally, which is more likely to enable the microcatheter and wire to head in the right direction.
- Try firm microwires e.g., Headliner.
- Place a buddy wire to help straighten out the sinus.
- If difficulty is being encountered with firm wires, switch to softer microwire, as sometimes this strategy may be successful.

Suggested Reading

Pearce M. Practical neuroangiography. Philadelphia: Lippincott Williams & Wilkins; 2007. p. 443–55.

Spinal Angiography and Intervention

8

Spinal Angiography

Indications and Case Selection

- Evaluation prior to biopsy or surgical intervention, e.g., evaluation of tumors suggestive of hypervascularity on MRI.
- Localization of origin of spinal cord arteries prior to transthoracic operative approaches or other extensive spinal instrumentation.
- Diagnosis of suspected vascular malformations or tumors.

Contraindications

- Uncorrected bleeding disorders.
- Thoracic aortic aneurysm (relative).

Preoperative Management

- Verify laboratory values including platelet count, BUN, CR, APTT, PT/INR, and ß-HCG for females of reproductive age group.
- In case of renal insufficiency, diabetes, CHF, etc., ensure usage of diluted non-ionic contrast agent and carefully pre-plan to maintain contrast load to minimum.
- Liquids only on morning of procedure.
- NPO (for ≈6 h) when procedure performed under general anesthesia (GA).
- Obtain informed consent for angiography.
- Ensure two IV lines inserted.
- Insert Foley. Patient will be more comfortable and cooperative with an empty bladder in case the procedure becomes prolonged.

© Springer International Publishing AG 2017
S.H. Khan and A.J. Ringer, *Handbook of Neuroendovascular Techniques*,
DOI 10.1007/978-3-319-52936-3_8

- Position patient on neuroangiography table.
- Attach patient to pulse oximetry and ECG leads for monitoring O_2 saturation, HR, cardiac rhythm respiratory rate, and BP.

Technique

Planning

- A complete spinal angiography would include external carotids, vertebral arteries (VA), thyrocervical trunks, costocervical, and intercostal arteries. Due to previous investigations, e.g., MRI indicating the location of lesion, usually a complete spinal angiography is unnecessary. It may occasionally be needed, e.g., in some cases of dural arteriovenous fistulae (DAVF).
- In case of tumors, plan investigation of 2 spinal levels above and below the expected pathology.
- In case of spinal arteriovenous malformation (AVM) or arteriovenous fistula (AVF), plan investigation of 4 levels above and below expected fistula site.
- Plan your procedure beforehand to minimize the amount of contrast used.
- The arteries that will need to be catheterized is based on the region of the spine being studied, as shown in Table 8.1.
- Remember the artery is being labeled with respect to the vertebral body (VB) at that level. Therefore, an artery labeled T5 may not necessarily be a true T5 since the intercostal arteries are not concordant with the VBs in the thoracic region.

Table 8.1 Arteries to be catheterized

Spinal region	Arteries to be catheterized
Upper cervical region C1–C4	Vertebral arteries Occipital arteries Ascending pharyngeal arteries Thyrocervical (anterior) trunks Costocervical (dorsal) trunks
Midcervical region C5–C7	Vertebral arteries Thyrocervical trunks Costocervical trunks Supreme intercostal arteries Ascending pharyngeal arteries
Upper thoracic region T1–T4	Supreme intercostal arteries Thyrocervical trunks
Thoracic and upper lumbar regions T5–L3	Intercostal/segmental artery of the involved level Intercostal/segmental arteries of two levels above and below the tumor site
Lower lumbar arteries L3–L4	Segmental arteries of two levels above and below the tumor site
Sacrum	Internal iliac arteries lateral sacral arteries (from internal iliac arteries) Median sacral artery (from aortic bifurcation)

- As the spine is a midline structure, the arteries on both right and left sides will need to be catheterized and studied.
- Infrequently, intracranial vessels also have to be studied when suspecting spinal dural arteriovenous malformation (DAVM). As an example, a DAVM of middle meningeal artery draining into a restricted venous compartment may cause distention of anterior and posterior spinal veins. This may cause venous hypertension of the spinal cord and myelopathy.

Procedure

- Fluoroscopy is performed, and the parallax is removed by placing the desired markers and catheter tip in the center of the fluoroscopic field.
- Ensure the VB spinal processes are aligned halfway between the spinal pedicles (on A-plane).
- Radiopaque markers attached to a plastic ruler are taped to the back of the patient after positioning the patient supine on operating table to help demarcate the vertebral bodies.
- It should be positioned to the right of the spine so as not to overlap the spine or the aorta.
- The lettering on the ruler is correlated with the VB, e.g., the letter 'Q' may be at T12 level. The angiography run performed will depict the radiopaque letter, and the artery at this level will therefore be identified as T12 (i.e., by the level) and documented. The reason for doing this is to eliminate any difficulties in identification during interpretation later.
- We use a preprinted table, as shown in Table 8.2, for documentation of reference letter and angiography scene number at each level.
- Prep and drape both femoral regions.
- Gain access to the femoral artery using modified Seldinger technique (see Chap. 2 for details on access).
- Immobilize a segment of the artery between the index and middle fingers.
- Infiltrate the skin overlying the immobilized segment and underlying tissue with local anesthesia using 1% lidocaine with epinephrine.
- Make a small stab incision in the anesthetized skin.
- Immobilize the artery, and with the bevel of single-wall needle leading, puncture the artery at 45° through the previously created stab.
- When blood emanates from the needle hub, stop and advance the provided wire into the needle hub and into the arterial lumen.
- Retract the needle over the wire. Make sure to maintain control of the wire at all times.
- Introduce the pre-assembled 4 Fr sheath with dilator over the wire into the artery.
- Withdraw the wire and dilator leaving the sheath in the artery.
- Cover the hub of the sheath with your thumb to prevent unnecessary blood loss.

Table 8.2 Reference letter and angiography scene number at each level

Letter	Level	Right	Left
	T1	a	a
	T2		
	T3		
	T4		
	T5		
	T6		
	T7		
	T8		
	T9		
	T10		
	T12		
	L1		
	L2		
	L3		
	L4		
	L5		
	L5 S1		

aDocument the number assigned to the angiography run here

- Introduce a J wire (60–70 cm) into the sheath until it is in the artery well beyond the sheath.
- Maintaining control of wire at all times, retract and completely withdraw the small sheath over the wire.
- Compress the artery with the same hand which is holding onto the wire to prevent bleeding from the enlarged entrance wound.
- Introduce the 5 Fr or larger sheath over the wire into the arterial lumen.
- Retract and remove the wire when the sheath has been positioned in the artery.
- Connect the hub of the sheath to a RHV which is attached to tubing with three-way stopcock and neonatal transducer to ensure the continuously running heparinized saline solution is at a rate of 30 ml/h. Make a wet connection so that no air bubbles enter the vascular system.
- Secure the sheath by suturing it to the skin using 2–0 silk.
- Prepare a Cobra catheter (AngioDynamics, Queensbury, NY). Other options when having difficulties are indicated shown in Table 8.3.
- We do not connect the diagnostic catheter to a flush system, and perform hand injections for angiography due to the frequency of injections performed. A one-way stopcock may be interposed between the catheter and syringe to prevent excessive blood loss. Meticulous catheter hygiene is maintained to prevent blood clot formation in the catheter, or embolism.
- Introduce the catheter into the sheath and advance over a glidewire.
- Once the diagnostic catheter is in the desired location, e.g., in the descending aorta for studying the thoracolumbar region, remove the guidewire.

Table 8.3 Scenario options

Scenario	Catheter
Standard	Cobra catheter, Mikaelsson
Difficulty catheterizing intercostal arteries in thoracic region	H-1-H
Difficulty catheterizing segmental arteries in lumbar region	HS-1
Difficulty catheterizing because of an ample or capacious aorta	HS-2 Mikaelsson

- Usually, the catheter tip needs to be pointed slightly posteriorly and laterally to enter the ostium of the spinal artery. Advance and retract it rostrally and caudally to find the ostium.
- When the ostium is engaged, inject a small amount of contrast to confirm. Additionally, you will note that the catheter tip ceases its bobbing movement with arterial pulsations, when it is in a vessel origin.
- Perform angiography. We hand-inject the contrast. Do so at a gentle gradually increasing rate.
- The scale with radiopaque markers placed at the side of the patient is used to label each artery.
- Remember, for practical convenience, the intercostal artery is labeled by the vertebral body at the same level.
- For efficiency, once an ostium is found, catheterized, and angiography completed, it is pulled down maintaining the tip's position. It will jump into the ostium of the next (caudal) vessel. The catheter tip may need to be rotated slightly posteriorly for more inferior branches and laterally for more cranial branches. Systematically complete one side in this fashion then address the opposite side. However, if the ostium on the opposite side is unintentionally catheterized, do not relinquish it before performing angiography. The idea is to perform the procedure efficiently in terms of time and contrast used.
- When an intercostal artery at the level of lesion is injected, it will demonstrate the osseous, epidural, and paraspinal extensions of the lesion.

Postoperative Management and Follow-up

- If the procedure was diagnostic only, the patient is monitored for approx 2 h and then discharged if he/she remains asymptomatic.
- Any inexplicable change in neurological examination should lead to thorough investigation including CT head and if indicated repeat angiography.
- Also monitor the access site for pseudo-aneurysm, vessel occlusion, etc.
- The patient should be ambulatory, able to void, and back to pre-procedure status at time of discharge.
- Site of vascular access should be documented, so that in a future study, the contralateral side is used.

- Any unusual aspect encountered during navigation including difficult vasculature and how it was addressed should be documented for future reference.

Spinal Interventional Procedures

Indications and Case Selection

- Embolization of spinal vascular malformations for cure or for preoperative embolization.
- As an adjunct to surgery, e.g., pre-surgical embolization for devascularization of vascular tumors. Such intervention may prove beneficial in benign or malignant (e.g., metastatic renal or thyroid tumors) spinal tumors.
- Benign lesions which may require intervention include hemangiomas, aneurysmal bone cysts, and very rarely osteoblastomas.
- Embolization following an unsuccessful attempted resection because of excessive bleeding.
- Palliation, for example, of inoperable tumors including or relief of symptoms such as pain.
- Incidental asymptomatic lesions should not be treated.

Contraindications

- If anticoagulant and/or antiplatelet therapy is contraindicated (relative).
- Severe vascular tortuosity or anatomy that would preclude the safe introduction or maintenance of a guide catheter, sheath, or interventional devices. This would include the anterior spinal artery (ASA), posterior spinal arteries, or spinal medullary arteries being visualized on pedicle injection, along with vascular supply to the lesion.
- Uncorrected bleeding disorders.

Preoperative Management

- Complete workup including metastatic workup in case of tumor. This includes CT and/or MRI to diagnose primary tumor, as well as, assess the extent of metastases.
- Verify laboratory values including platelet count, BUN, CR, APTT, PT/INR, and ß-HCG for females of reproductive age group.
- In case of renal insufficiency, diabetes, CHF, etc., ensure usage of diluted non-ionic contrast agent and carefully pre-plan to maintain contrast load to minimum.
- Liquids only on morning of procedure.
- NPO (for ≈6 h) when procedure performed under GA.

- Obtain informed consent for angiography, and the indicated interventional procedure.
- Ensure two IV lines inserted.
- Insert Foley. Patient will be more comfortable and cooperative with an empty bladder in case the procedure becomes prolonged.
- Position patient on neuroangiography table with lettered markers taped to back.
- Attach patient to pulse oximetry and ECG leads for monitoring O_2 saturation, HR, cardiac rhythm respiratory rate, and BP.

Technique

- We usually perform spinal angiography and intervention under local anesthesia with mild to moderate conscious sedation. The advantage of this is the availability of a neurological examination.
- If GA is elected, then SSEPs should be performed through the procedure.
- Unlike diagnostic spinal angiography, for interventional procedures the catheters are connected to a continuous flush of heparinized saline.
- Perform angiography to ensure the pedicle to be embolized does not concurrently supply the radiculomedullary, or radiculopial arteries. Perform highly selective angiography to determine this, since the tumor blush may obscure the spinal supply on less selective injections. If the pedicle concurrently supplies the cord, then it is not suitable for embolization.
- After selecting the segmental branch supplying the target for embolization, superselective catheterization is achieved with a microcatheter distal to the ostium to avoid reflux into the aorta. The microcatheter selected must be compatible with the embolic agent chosen (see below).

Postoperative Management and Follow-up

- Admit to NSICU for overnight observation.
- 0.9% NS + 20 meq KCl @ 150 cc/h X 2 h.
- Keep right/left leg (whichever side was used for procedure) straight X 2 h, with HOB elevated 15°.
- Check groins, DPs, vitals and neuro checks q 15 min X 4, q 30 min X 4, then q h.
- Advance diet as tolerated.
- Review/resume pre-procedure medications (except oral hypoglycemics, which are resumed 48 h after the procedure and when oral intake has been established).
- D/C next morning after mobilizing (if no complications/other ongoing medical concerns requiring hospitalization).
- F/u on outpatient basis in 4 weeks.
- F/u angiography at 3 months, e.g., if AVF was treated.

Spinal Fistulae

Indications and Case Selection

- Simple DAVF with single draining vein is usually treated surgically. This is because of the low rates of permanent cures and eventual recurrence with proximal feeding artery occlusion with agents such as PVA. With the advent of Onyx, the permanent cure rate may be >60%.
- Another consideration is inadvertent embolization of normal spinal vasculature through connections. During diagnostic procedure, if it is felt that the single fistula can be treated especially with onyx, without imperiling the normal spinal cord supply, then it may be a worthwhile attempt (Fig. 8.1).

Contraindications

- When embolization would also result in interruption of normal spinal arteries.

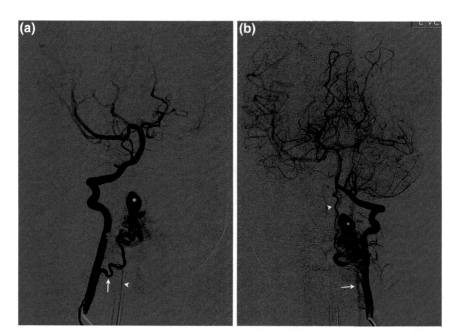

Fig. 8.1 **a** Right vertebral angiography demonstrates a high cervical cord DAVF. One of the main supplying branches (*arrow*) is demonstrated. The anterior spinal artery (*arrowhead*) is also seen with a pedicle supplying it arising from the VA. If the VA is followed rostrally to the basilar artery, it is noted that the posterior circulation is significantly supplying the anterior circulation. Left VA angiography **b** demonstrates additional arterial supply to the AVF from ASA (*arrowhead*). The asterisk (*asterisk*) demarcates a venous pouch or an aneurysmal dilatation. The *arrow* points to venous drainage further caudally

Preoperative Management

- As described above.
- Document patient's preoperative myelopathy and any other neurological deficit.

Technique

- Gain arterial access as indicated above (also see Chap. 2 for details on access).
- Advance Guide catheter over glidewire into the spinal artery pedicle.
- An Envoy catheter, Cobra catheter or any of the catheters indicated above may be used as the guide catheter provided it is of sufficient caliber (ideally, at least 5 Fr).
- Unlike the diagnostic spinal angiogram, in this case the guide catheter is connected to a continuously running flush of heparinized saline.
- Once the guide catheter is securely positioned in the pedicle, prepare a microcatheter (e.g., Marathon®, Micro Therapeutics, Inc., Irvine, CA) and connect it to a continuously running flush of heparinized saline.
- Ensure the system is free of air bubbles or foreign bodies.
- Advance the microcatheter over a microguidewire through the RHV of guide catheter. The microguidewire options include Mirage™ (0.008; ev3, Irvine, CA), Agility® steerable wires (0.010 Codman & Shurtleff, Inc., Raynham, MA), Transend, (0.010, Stryker Neurovascular, Fremont, CA) and Synchro2 (0.010 or 0.014, Stryker Neurovascular, Fremont, CA).
- If the guide catheter is of sufficient caliber (at least 5 Fr, preferably 6 Fr), perform a roadmap before the microcatheter is advanced beyond the distal tip of the guide catheter.
- If the guide catheter is of small caliber or there is considerable difficulty in injecting, then the roadmap should be performed prior to introducing the microcatheter.
- Using roadmap guidance, advance the microcatheter over the microwire to intended location.
- Remove the microwire.
- Perform angiography through the microcatheter to ascertain the normal spinal vasculature is not involved.
- If satisfied with the position of the catheter, embolization can commence.

Embolic Agents

PVA

- Not recommended for treatment of spinal fistula since the occlusion is only temporary and the fistula in all likelihood will recur.

Onyx

- Onyx embolization for endovascular cure of spinal fistula has been reported as far back as 2003.
- It may be more advantageous for this purpose than NBCA because of its higher viscosity. The greater viscosity enables better control in delivering the agent.
- A DMSO compatible microcatheter is required. Use one of the following:

    - Marathon™ (ev3 Neurovascular, Irvine CA)
    - Echelon™ (ev3 Neurovascular, Irvine CA)
    - Rebar™ (ev3 Neurovascular, Irvine CA)
    - Ultraflow™ (ev3 Neurovascular, Irvine CA)

- The following will also be required:

    - Onyx® 18, or Onyx® 34 (consider the latter for cases with brisk blood flow across fistula)
    - Onyx mixer

- Place the selected onyx bottles on the mixer, and set it at 8. The mixing has to be performed for at least 20 min, so it is efficient to initiate it beforehand.
- Once the microcatheter has been positioned as indicated above, then commence as follows.

Procedure

- When ready to perform embolization, perform a blank roadmap, i.e., step upon the pedal as if performing a roadmap, but not actually injecting contrast.
- Ensure the entire microcatheter system is free of blood.
- Draw up the DMSO into the provided yellow colored syringe.
- Disconnect the RHV from the microcatheter and attach a syringe with DMSO to the microcatheter. Make a meniscus-to-meniscus connection. Again, ensure there are no air bubbles or blood in the microcatheter. If needed, fill the hub of microcatheter with saline, to ensure a proper connection.
- Forewarn the patient that he/she may sense a 'garlic-like taste' in the back of the throat with DMSO injection. Additionally, during injection and for a day or two thereafter, the patient's breath and skin may carry the peculiar odor of DMSO.
- Very slowly, inject 0.3–0.8 ml of DMSO (depending on the dead space of the microcatheter), such that the entire catheter is primed with it. Rapid injection of DMSO may also cause pain and discomfort.
- While undertaking the placement of the microcatheter and its priming, Onyx 18 or 34 is prepared concurrently, bearing in mind the following:

– The numbers 18 or 34 following 'Onyx' are indicative of its viscosity at 40 °C.
– Onyx solidifies in 5 min after exposure to blood or saline. To prevent this solidification within the microcatheter itself, ensure that the catheter is free of contrast, saline, and blood during Onyx injection.
– The temperature of Onyx should be between 19–24 °C, when used. If it is frozen because it was stored at a cooler temperature, allow it to thaw at room temperature.

- Place the bottle of onyx on the Onyx mixer and set the mixer at 8. Keep the Onyx bottle on the mixer for at least 20 min. The mixing should continue until you are just ready to inject Onyx. This will cause a thorough mixing of Onyx and tantalum powder, which assists in satisfactory visualization of the deposited onyx.
- Immediately prior to injection, draw up Onyx into the provided white 1-ml syringes. To do so, hold the bottle upright (in contrast to when drawing up other fluids into a syringe, e.g., 1% Lidocaine), using an 18G or 20G needle. If any air is noted in the syringe, invert the bottle such that the bottle is superior and the syringe is below it. Inject the air from the syringe into the bottle. Turn the bottle upright again, so that the syringe is again on top and continue to draw up onyx. Draw a total of 1 ml of air-free onyx into the syringe.
- Detach the yellow DMSO syringe from the hub of the microcatheter.
- Hold the catheter hub vertically and overfill the hub with DMSO.
- Holding the Onyx syringe upright, make a meniscus-to-meniscus connection, ensuring that no air is introduced into the system.
- Maintain the syringe containing onyx in a vertical position. Maintain this position until the onyx passes beyond the hub of the microcatheter. After that, the syringe can be held in a more comfortable position.
- Inject Onyx slowly at a rate of 0.16 ml/min and not to exceed 0.3 ml/min. The injection should be slow and deliberate, using thumb pressure.
- When injecting, track the onyx under live fluoroscopy.
- The goal for embolization in case of spinal fistula is to deposit onyx in the proximal radicular vein.
- If there is reflux of onyx, wait for a couple of minutes to allow the Onyx to solidify. The solid Onyx plug may prevent further reflux. However, the reflux over the microcatheter should be no greater than 1 cm. Otherwise, it may become difficult to extract the catheter and lead to complications.
- When the fistulous connection is occluded, perform angiography to confirm the same.

NBCA

- Indicated for the embolization of brain and spinal cord vascular malformations, this is now used less commonly due to the tendency for rapid solidification resulting in proximal occlusion, but may prove useful in single-pedicle dural AV fistulae. In our opinion, due to better control on delivery, onyx is the agent of choice if the fistula is to be treated endovascularly.

- The indications for NBCA use in spinal fistulae are the same as for Onyx.

Additional Equipment/Devices

- Trufill kit comprising of NBCA/ethiodol/tantalum (Trufill, Cordis Endovascular).
- For NBCA administration, we recommend a small (1.5–1.8 Fr) flow-directed, non-reinforced catheter, e.g.,

  - Regatta (Cordis, Miami, FL).
  - Spinnaker Elite (Boston Scientific, Fremont, CA).
  - Ultraflow (ev3).
  - (See Chaps. 1 and 2 for additional equipment/devices for vascular access and navigation).

Procedure

- Advance and position the microcatheter, attached to a continuously running flush of heparinized saline, as instructed above.
- Prepare the NBCA mixture on a separate table using clean gloves. This is to prevent any contamination with ionic catalysts.
- Add the vial of tantalum powder to above mixture to enhance its radiopacity.
- For spinal fistula, we recommend a relatively concentrated NBCA preparation, i.e., a 1:1 or 1:2 Ethiodol: NBCA concentration.
- To do so mix 1 cc of NBCA with 1 cc of ethiodol or 2 cc of NBCA with 1 cc of ethiodol in a shot glass.
- Increasing the ratio of ethiodol to NBCA slows the rate of solidification permitting deeper penetration.
- Perform test injections using subtracted fluoroscopic observation (blank roadmap) to assess catheter position and optimal rate of injection.
- Choose the desired ratio of ethiodol/NBCA (typically between 50:50 and 80:20) based on the test injections, drawing the desired volume of each into a 3-ml syringe, mixing continuously until ready for injection.
- Ensure microcatheter lumen is devoid of ionic catalysts by irrigating with 5% dextrose.
- Obtain a blank roadmap; then, commence injecting NBCA slowly, under continuous visualization, over few seconds.
- Adjust the injection rate in order to obtain a solid caste without reflux.
- Stop injecting once the proximal aspect of draining vein of fistula is occluded

  - Injection may need to stop if reflux occurs, coating the microcatheter, which may make removal impossible.

- At higher concentrations (NBCA $\geq 50\%$), up to 0.5 g of tantalum should be added to the mixture and the injection rate is faster and injection time is shorter (1–3 s).
- If there is a large direct fistula, or rapid flow, induce hypotension and use a very high concentration of NBCA. Alternatively, coils may be used first to slow down the rate of blood flow, followed by NBCA.
- After completion of procedure, aspirate the microcatheter briskly and remove it quickly.
- Aspirate the guide catheter and examine it fluoroscopically.

Postoperative Management and Follow-up

- As indicated in section above.
- In addition, the patient is monitored for any persistence, return or worsening of symptoms, which would be an indication of recurrence of DAVF. In such a situation, the spinal angiogram is repeated.

Spinal Tumors

Indications and Case Selection

- Preoperative embolization of tumors for devascularization.
- Palliation of symptoms in untreatable tumors/metastases.
- Retarding tumor growth.

Contraindications

- Significant risk of neurological deficit as pedicle supplying tumor also supplying normal cord and superselective catheterization not possible.

Preoperative Management

- As indicated above.

Technique

- In case of spinal tumors, the vascular supply 2 levels above and 2 levels below should be studied. If the lesion is extensive, the number of pedicles catheterized and studied rostrally and caudally should be increased.

- For more effective embolization, first close the collaterals and less direct feeders, such that the tumor is left supplied by a single dominant pedicle. Do not occlude this pedicle proximally, to enable retreatment later, if needed.
- The guide catheter and microcatheter are positioned as indicated above.
- Microcatheter selection should depend upon the size of the PVA particles to be used, in order to prevent catheter occlusion by the particles. Preferably use a larger caliber catheter (e.g., 2.3 Fr). If possible, avoid using tapered tip Microcatheter, as it is more likely to occlude. We commonly use Marathon (ev3) while treating fistulae in the ECA branches.
- Other microcatheter considerations include Prowler Plus (Codman & Shurtleff, Inc., Raynham, MA) and Rapidtransit (Codman).

Embolic Agents

PVA

- Suitable for preoperative embolization.
- Do not embolize particles with the tip of the catheter in a wedged position, as this may result in intra-tumoral hemorrhage.
- Polyvinyl alcohol (PVA) is available in sizes ranging from 50 to 1000 μm.

Procedure

- Advance the microcatheter to its planned location.
- Inspect angiograms carefully for potentially dangerous collaterals, i.e., those that supply the spinal cord.
- Measure the feeding vessels and lesion to select the appropriate size particles.
- Bear in mind, the smaller the particles, the greater the likelihood of deep penetration into smaller vessels, e.g., pre-capillaries, resulting in cranial nerve deficits, etc.
- Proceed to prepare the PVA mixture on a separate table/space, taking care that other equipment used during procedure does not get contaminated with the particles. Once the mixture is prepared, change gloves. Take extreme precautions that the PVA particles do not inadvertently contaminate drapes, catheters, etc., leading to possibility of embolic complications.
- Inspect the PVA particles for uniformity of size.
- Inject 15 ml of non-ionic contrast and 5 ml saline into the bottle containing PVA. Conversely, it may be safer to remove the top of the bottle and empty the contents into a shot glass and then add the non-ionic contrast to it.
- Shake to suspend the particles in the contrast.
- Attach a 3-way stopcock to a 20-ml syringe.
- Draw up the suspension into the syringe.

- Attach a 3-ml syringe to the 3-way stopcock. The 3-ml syringe should be attached to the port in line with that which will be attached to the catheter. The larger 20-ml syringe is attached to the port perpendicular to these two.
- Ensure the syringes and stopcock system are free of air bubbles.
- Use the plungers of the small and large syringes to push the suspension back and forth between the syringes, while the stopcock is turned to close off the third (free) port, intended for the microcatheter. The movement will assist in keeping the PVA particles in suspension.
- Draw suspension into the 3-ml syringe from the larger syringe and turn the stopcock, so that the port with the 20-ml syringe is blocked.
- Change gloves and discard any towels, etc., contaminated by PVA particles.
- Detach the RHV from the microcatheter and make a meniscus-to-meniscus connection between the microcatheter and the free portal of the 3-way stopcock. Ensure the system is free of air bubbles.
- Place a towel on the drape under the microcatheter to ensure it catches any errant PVA particles and the operating field is not inadvertently contaminated by potential emboli.
- Confirm that the microcatheter tip has maintained its position. Perform angiography, if necessary.
- Make a blank roadmap.
- Gradually commence injecting the PVA from the 3-ml syringe under direct visualization.
- Monitor carefully to ensure there is no reflux. Also monitor closely to ensure the PVA particles are not flowing into the draining vein/sinus. If this is detected, stop immediately.
- As the feeding vessel is occluded, resistance may be felt during injection.
- Do not attempt to overcome this resistance by using greater force. Such attempts may lead to reflux, or untoward embolization of an unintended vessel.
- As needed, refill the 3-ml syringe from the 20-ml syringe by turning the stop-cock to the microcatheter and closing the system to the catheter. Then, aspirate the PVA suspension into the 3-ml syringe from the large syringe. To ensure uniform distribution of the PVA particles, agitate the suspension by initially drawing it back and forth between the two syringes. Once a smooth suspension is achieved, fill the 3-ml syringe for administration of PVA via the micro-catheter. During the agitation process, ensure that the stopcock is closed to the microcatheter, to avoid inadvertent and potentially catastrophic embolization.
- After the 3-ml syringe is filled, turn the stopcock to open the microcatheter to the 3-ml syringe and close it to the 20-ml syringe.
- Resume injecting PVA under direct vision.
- Once the vessel/nidus is occluded, perform angiography to confirm.
- If the catheter appears obstructed, do not attempt to open it in vivo by a forceful injection or passing microwire through it. Remove the microcatheter completely from the guide catheter, and inspect it. If occluded and unable to re-establish flow by irrigating it, replace it with a new microcatheter.

- When the embolization procedure has been completed, withdraw and remove the microcatheter while maintaining gentle suction upon it, so that the PVA particles still contained within it do not inadvertently embolize.
- Discard the microcatheter along with the protective towel placed under it.
- Complete post-procedure angiography.

Onyx

- Please refer to usage technique as described above for spinal fistulas.

Alcohol

- Alcohol is used infrequently for the vessel sclerosis in tumors or in treatment of AVM.
- It acts by immediate cytotoxic effect upon the vessel endothelium near the microcatheter tip and the resultant vessel thrombosis is manifest within 5–10 min.
- The risks associated with ETOH include significant toxicity of brain parenchyma (when injected in high concentrations) and pulmonary edema.
- A possible advantage is the dilution of alcohol downstream from the site of treatment, thereby avoiding injury to normal venous drainage.

Procedure

- All current microcatheters are compatible with alcohol.
- Alcohol is supplied in 5-ml vials.
- The volume of ETOH injected during one session should not exceed 1 ml/kg body weight.
- Use injection of contrast through the microcatheter to gauge the force needed for the alcohol injection in order to impact the entire vessel wall. Remember, unlike other agents, alcohol is not visible fluoroscopically during the injection so reflux must be estimated before injection.

Postoperative Management and Follow-up

- As indicated above.

Location Specific Considerations Including Difficult Access

Cervical

- When performing angiography for arteries such as thyrocervical trunk, a usual diagnostic catheter, e.g., 5 Fr front angled catheter (Terumo), will suffice. Cobra catheter is more suitable for studying intercostal arteries in the thoracic/lumbar regions.

- Study the spinal arterial supply on both sides.
- The competence of the circle of Willis as well as the dominant VA will need to be determined, in case one of the VAs needs to be sacrificed.
- Angiography will also allow the operator to determine the potential technical difficulties that may be encountered during embolization.
- When embolizing a cervical tumor, consider temporary balloon occlusion distally during embolization, for cerebral protection.

Thoracic

- The posterior portion of the vertebral body is usually best visualized by injecting the left intercostal artery.
- The anterior portion of the vertebral body is usually best visualized by injecting the right intercostal artery.
- The intercostal arteries arise from the aorta with a sharp superior angulation especially in T2 to T4 region. The pattern gradually changes with the caudal arteries such that the lumbar segmental arteries are directed horizontally or caudally.
- Table 8.4 lists some possible problems and solutions.

Table 8.4 Difficult access problems/solutions thoracic location

Problem	Solution
Difficulty catheterizing the intercostal artery	• Switch from Cobra catheter to an H-1-H catheter

Catheter jumps out of pedicle during angiography	• Inject gently with gradual rise of pressure
	• Switch from Cobra catheter to an H-1-H
	• Position catheter a little further in the pedicle. To do so, may need to rotate the tip further in the direction of the pedicle, concurrently with a gentle push
	  – In case using a Mikaelsson catheter, maintain a downward tension
	• Ensure the external segment of the catheter outside the sheath is stable and has not built countertorque that will undo the position of the tip
	• If still having difficulties
	  – Perform roadmap and introduce a soft wire into the pedicle and advance the catheter into the pedicle over it. If this fails then using roadmap, advance a coaxial system
	• Advance a microwire into the pedicle, and then, advance a microcatheter over the wire
	• Perform angiography through the microcatheter

Table 8.5 Difficult access problems/solutions lumbar location

Problem	Solution
Difficulty catheterizing the segmental artery	• Switch from Cobra catheter to an HS-1 catheter

Catheter jumps out of pedicle during angiography	• Inject gently with gradual rise of pressure
	• Switch from Cobra catheter to an HS-1
	• Position it a little further in the pedicle. To do so, may need to rotate the tip further in the direction of the pedicle, concurrently with a gentle push
	  – In case using a Mikaelsson catheter, maintain a downward tension
	• Ensure the external segment of the catheter outside the sheath is stable and has not built countertorque that will undo the position of the proximal tip
	• If still having difficulties
	  – Perform roadmap and introduce a soft wire into the pedicle and advance the catheter into the pedicle over it. If this fails, then, using roadmap, advance a coaxial system
	• Advance a microwire into the pedicle and then advance a microcatheter over the wire
	• Perform angiography through the microcatheter

Lumbar

• Lumbar segmental arteries are more likely than thoracic intercostal arteries to have a conjoined pedicle. Therefore, on injection both the right- and left-side branches will be visualized.
• The origin of lumbar segmental arteries is directed horizontally or caudally. This pattern gradually changes to a superiorly directed origin of the intercostal arteries in the thoracic region.
• Table 8.5 lists some possible problems and solutions.

Suggested Readings

1. Berenstein A, Lasjaunias P, Ter Brugge KG. Surgical neuroangiography, vol. 2.2. Heidelberg: Springer-Verlag; 2004. p. 874–911.
2. Morris PP. Practical neuroangiography. Philadelphia: Lippincott Williams & Wilkins. 2007. pp. 36–85; 396–403; 456–65.
3. Song JK, Gobin YP, Duckwiler GR, Murayama Y, Frazee JG, Martin NA, Viñuela F. N-butyl 2-cyanoacrylate embolization of spinal dural arteriovenous fistulae. AJNR Am J Neuroradiol. 2001;22:40–7.
4. Warakaulle DR, Aviv RI, Niemann A, Byrne JV, Teddy P. Embolisation of spinal dural arteriovenous fistulae with Onyx. Neuroradiology. 2003;45:110–2.

Embolization for Epistaxis and Cranial Tumors

9

Epistaxis

Indications and Case Selection

- Refractory epistaxis that has not responded to treatment including manual compression, nasal packing, local vasoconstrictors, endoscopic cauterization, or surgical ligation of sphenopalatine arteries.

Preoperative Management

- Verify laboratory values including platelet count, BUN, CR, APTT, PT/INR, and ß-HCG for females of reproductive age group.
- In case of renal insufficiency, diabetes, CHF, etc., ensure usage of diluted nonionic contrast agent and carefully pre-plan to maintain contrast load to minimum.
- Liquids only on morning of procedure.
- NPO (for ≈6 h) when procedure performed under General anesthesia.
- Obtain informed consent for angiography and embolization ECA branches.
- Ensure two IV lines inserted.
- Insert Foley. Patient will be more comfortable and cooperative with an empty bladder in case the procedure becomes prolonged.
- Position patient on neuroangiography table.
- Attach patient to pulse oximetry and ECG leads for monitoring O_2 saturation, HR, cardiac rhythm respiratory rate, and BP.

© Springer International Publishing AG 2017
S.H. Khan and A.J. Ringer, *Handbook of Neuroendovascular Techniques*,
DOI 10.1007/978-3-319-52936-3_9

Equipment

- 4 Fr micropuncture kit.
- 6 Fr short sheath (may use a 22-cm sheath, or a shuttle sheath if the patient's vasculature is particularly tortuous).
- 5 or 6 Fr MPC Envoy Guide catheter.
- Rotating hemostatic valves (2). Ensure the RHV attached to the guide catheter is ≥ 0.096″ or 2.44 mm.
- Pediatric transducers (30 ml/h; 2).
- Diagnostic catheter: Terumo® angled glide catheter 5 Fr (for diagnostics).
- Angled glidewire (0.035; Terumo).
- Syringes 10 cc (at least 3), 20 cc (at least 4), 3 cc (for ACT).
- Three-way stopcock: 3.
- Torque device.
- Marathon or a 0.021″ or larger microcatheter (e.g., Prowler Plus, rapidtransit, echelon).
- 0.008″ Mirage (with marathon microcatheter) or 0.014″ microwire (e.g., Transend, synchro, agility).
- When using PVA particles, select the larger catheters, e.g., rapidtransit, Prowler Plus,
- PVA particles (250–300 μm), or
- Trisacryl gelatin microspheres (Embospheres; BioSphere Medical, Inc., Rockland, ME, USA), or
- Onyx 18 (must use with DMSO compatible microcatheter, i.e., marathon, echelon, rapid transit, ultra-flow, headway Duo).
- Continuous heparinized saline flush systems (6000 IU Heparin per 1000 ml saline).
- Telfa strip.
- Mandrel for shaping microwire tip.
- Angioseal™ closure device (6 Fr). Use larger size if a larger sheath is inserted.

Vascular Access

- Gain arterial access with micropuncture needle, using modified Seldinger technique.
- Make an exchange over wires to place a 6 Fr short sheath.
- Connect the sheath to a continuously running flush of heparinized saline after confirming that the entire flush system is free of air bubbles.
- Secure the sheath to the patient's skin using 2-0 silk suture.
- Prepare a 5 Fr diagnostic catheter by wiping it with moist Telfa to activate the hydrophilic coating.

- Connect the catheter to a continuously running flush of heparinized saline and ensure that the system is free of air.
- Our preference particularly in someone with relatively straightforward vasculature is to forgo the diagnostic catheter and start right away with a 5 or 6 Fr MPC Envoy guide catheter. This will save a few steps and time that would otherwise be spent in switching catheters. Prepare the guide catheter as described above for diagnostic catheter.
- Using fluoroscopy, advance the guide catheter into the aortic arch, ensuring that the tip of the glidewire is always leading.
- Catheterize the common carotid artery (CCA). If known, start with the side of the bleeding nostril.
- Remove the guidewire and perform baseline angiography to include the cerebral vasculature, in addition to external carotid artery (ECA) and its branches.
- When feasible, use the same angiogram as roadmap (smart mask) to advance the guide catheter (over the wire) into the ECA, then retract, and remove the wire.
- Ensure the system is bubble-free.
- Perform external carotid angiography by hand injection (to prevent pain) with gentle and progressive increase in pressure through the course of injection. If the contrast is injected vigorously, it will cause pain and may also result in the catheter kicking out of the ECA.
- Study the baseline and ECA angiography performed to understand any anatomical variations, e.g.,

  - Confirm whether the ophthalmic artery arises off the internal carotid artery (ICA) or middle meningeal artery (MMA).
  - Confirm whether the anterior cerebral artery (ACA) arises off the ICA or MMA.
  - Assess any anastomosis to cerebral or retinal circulation, e.g., retrograde filling of the ophthalmic artery to the carotid via the facial artery.

- Look for any unusual causes of epistaxis, e.g., AVM, tumor, pseudoaneurysm of sinonasal arteries or ICA aneurysm that has ruptured through dehiscence of sphenoid sinus.
- When the cause of epistaxis remains unknown, then prepare to embolize ECA branches on both sides.
- When possible, use the previously performed angiogram as a roadmap. Otherwise, perform a new roadmap and use the same to position the guide catheter securely in the proximal ECA.
- Prepare a microcatheter by attaching it to a continuously running flush of heparinized saline. Ensure there are no bubbles in the system.
- Advance a microwire through the RHV of the microcatheter, until its tip emerges from the distal end of the catheter.
- Give the tip of the microwire an appropriate shape to aid in navigation.
- The caliber of the microcatheter should be large enough to not get occluded by 250–300 μm PVA particles. When in doubt, it is preferable to use a larger

caliber catheter, e.g., 2.3 Fr. If possible, avoid using tapered tip microcatheter, as it is more likely to occlude. We commonly use rapidtransit, echelon, or Prowler Plus, while embolizing the ECA branches. It is not necessary and may be confusing when navigating near the skull base, to use dual-marker tip micro-catheters. We prefer single (tip)-marker catheters, unless planning to deploy coils.

- If the intention is to use Onyx, then ensure the microcatheter selected is DMSO compatible.
- Using fluoroscopy and roadmapping, advance the microcatheter over the microwire and position it at the site of intended occlusion, or as close as possible.
- Generally, the pterygopalatine portion of the IMA is embolized distal to the deep middle temporal artery.
- When the facial artery is embolized, it is done distal to glandular and labial branches.

Procedure

Particle Embolization

(a) *PVA Particles*

- Advance the microcatheter to its planned location, positioning it at or, as close as possible to the site of intended occlusion.
- Remember, the smaller the particles, the greater the likelihood of deep pene-tration into smaller vessels, e.g., pre-capillaries, which could result in compli-cations such as cranial nerve deficits.
- Very large particles (>300 μm) will result in premature catheter occlusion.
- Prepare the PVA mixture on a separate table/space, taking care that other equipment used during procedure does not get contaminated with the particles. Once the mixture is prepared, change gloves. Take extreme precautions that the PVA particles do not inadvertently contaminate drapes, catheters, etc., leading to the possibility of embolic complications.
- Inspect the PVA particles for uniformity of size.
- Inject 10 ml of nonionic contrast and 5 ml saline into the bottle containing PVA. Conversely, it may be safer to remove the top of the bottle and empty the contents into a shot glass and then add the nonionic contrast to it.
- Shake to suspend the particles in the contrast.
- Attach a three-way stopcock to a 20-ml syringe.
- Draw up the suspension into the syringe.

(b) *Embospheres*

- Alternatively, embospheres come packaged in a 30-ml syringe with 10 ml saline. Simply add contrast to this syringe to create the desired dilute contrast solution.
- Then, for either PVA particles or embospheres, the procedure continues as follows:
- Attach a 3-ml syringe to the three-way stopcock. The 3-ml syringe should be attached to the port inline with that which will be attached to the catheter. The larger 20- or 30-ml syringe containing the particle and dilute contrast mixture is attached to the port perpendicular to these two.
- Ensure the syringes and stopcock system are free of air bubbles.
- Use the plungers of the small and large syringes to push the suspension back and forth between the syringes, while the stopcock is turned to close off the third (free) port, intended for the microcatheter. The movement will assist in keeping the embolic particles in suspension.
- Draw suspension into the 3-ml syringe from the larger syringe and then turn the stopcock, so that the port with the large syringe is blocked.
- Change gloves and discard any towels contaminated by particles.
- Detach the RHV from the microcatheter and make a meniscus-to-meniscus connection between the microcatheter and the free portal of the three-way stopcock. Ensure the system is free of air bubbles.
- Place a towel on the drape under the microcatheter to ensure it catches any particles and the operating field is not inadvertently contaminated by potential emboli.
- Confirm that the microcatheter tip has maintained its position. Perform angiography if necessary.
- Make a blank roadmap, to mask bone at the skull base and permit visualization of injected contrast mixture.
- Gradually commence injecting the PVA or embospheres from the 3-ml syringe under direct visualization.
- Monitor carefully to ensure there is no reflux. Also monitor closely to ensure the particles are not flowing into the draining vein/sinus. If this is detected, stop immediately.
- As needed, refill the 3-ml syringe from the large syringe by turning the stopcock to the microcatheter and closing the system to the microcatheter. Then aspirate the suspension into the 3-ml syringe. To ensure uniform distribution, agitate the suspension by initially drawing it back and forth between the two syringes. Once a smooth suspension is achieved, fill the 3-ml syringe for administration via the microcatheter. During the agitation process, ensure that the stopcock is closed to the microcatheter, or the results could be catastrophic.
- After the 3-ml syringe is filled, turn the stopcock to open the microcatheter to the 3-ml syringe and close it to the large ml syringe.
- Resume injecting embolic suspension under direct vision using the blank roadmap.

- As the embolized vessel is occluded, there is flow arrest and resistance is felt during injection or one may see stasis or reflux on the blank roadmap.
- The microcatheter may become occluded during embolization, resulting in a dramatic increase in resistance for injection and loss of visible contrast on the road map. Do not attempt to overcome this resistance by using greater force. Such attempts would lead to reflux, or untoward embolization of an unintended vessel, e.g., internal carotid vasculature. Remove the microcatheter completely from the guide catheter and inspect it. If occluded and unable to re-establish flow by irrigating it, replace it with a new microcatheter. Once the vessel/nidus is occluded, perform angiography to confirm.
- When the embolization procedure has been completed, withdraw and remove the microcatheter while maintaining gentle suction upon it, so that the embolic material still contained within it does not inadvertently embolize.
- Discard the microcatheter along with the protective towel placed under it.
- Complete post-procedure angiography.

Location-Specific Considerations

- Particle embolization of ECA branches is relatively safe. However, vigilance should still be exercised, to prevent inadvertent embolization to ICA and its branches.
- Do not try to overcome resistance by forceful injection. This may result in reflux of embolus into ICA.
- Look out for collaterals whereby the particles may inadvertently embolize to ICA circulation.

Postoperative Management and Follow-up

- Admit to NSICU or a similar monitored unit for at least overnight observation. Further ICU stay, dependent upon clinical condition.
- Typically, nasal packing is left intact overnight and removed for inspection for bleeding the next day.
- 0.9% NS + 20 meq KCl @ 150 cc/h × 2 h, then decrease to 100 cc/h if patient is NPO.
- Keep the accessed extremity straight for 2 hours (in case of angioseal closure) or 6–8 hours (in case manual compression was applied), with the head elevated no more than 15°. This is achieved by placing a pillow under the patient's head. Remember, there should be no flexion in the femoral region. If greater head elevation is required, place bed in reverse-Trendelenberg position.
- Check groins, DP's, vitals and neuro checks q 15 min × 4, q 30 min × 2, then q hr.

- Advance diet as tolerated.
- Review/resume pre-procedure medications (except oral hypoglycemics) when good PO intake is established).

Onyx

- This may be used as an alternative to embospheres and PVA particles for the treatment of epistaxis.
- Position a 6 Fr MPC Envoy guide catheter in the ECA as described above.
- Select a DMSO compatible microcatheter, e.g., Marathon™ (ev3 Neurovascular, Irvine CA), Echelon™ (ev3 Neurovascular, Irvine CA), Rebar™ (ev3 Neurovascular, Irvine CA), and Ultraflow™ (ev3 Neurovascular, Irvine CA), and connect it to a continuously running flush of heparinized saline.
- Advance the microcatheter over a microwire to the intended location using fluoroscopy and roadmapping.
- Ensure the Onyx (usually Onyx 18) is shaken on a mixer (set at 8) for at least 20 min, so that the tantalum powder is well mixed with Onyx and easy to visualize during deposition.
- Draw up DMSO into the yellow syringe provided in the Onyx kit.
- Slowly irrigate the catheter with at least 0.3 ml of DMSO or a volume greater than the labeled dead space for the catheter.
- While DMSO is being injected, Onyx is drawn up into the provided white syringe (3 white syringes are provided in each kit). Draw Onyx with the bottle inferior to the syringe and the syringe held upright over it. Discard any air aspirated into the syringe by inverting the bottle above the syringe and injecting the air back into bottle.
- Ensure the Onyx syringe is free of air.
- After irrigation of the microcatheter, overfill the hub of the microcatheter with DMSO.
- Make a wet meniscus-to-meniscus connection of the DMSO with Onyx, ensuring no air is introduced into the microcatheter.
- Obtain a blank roadmap.
- Begin injecting Onyx.
- Initially hold the syringe upright with hub pointing down until Onyx is in the catheter, to avoid streaming. At this point, the syringe can be held in a more comfortable position.
- Inject Onyx very gradually at a rate of around 0.16 ml/min and no greater than 0.3 ml/min. Slow injection results in better deposition of Onyx while a faster injection will result in Onyx reflux.

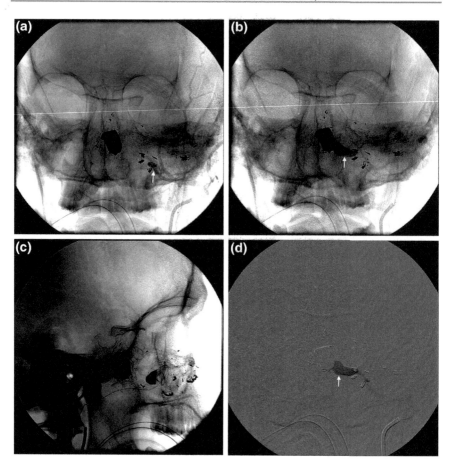

(images continued on next page)

Fig. 9.1 A 45 years old with recurrent epistaxis after gunshot wound. The bullet fragment and shrapnel can be appreciated. Attempts at removal of bullet were also unsuccessful because of the epistaxis. An unsubtracted angiogram performed through guide catheter demonstrates the disruption of the internal maxillary artery (**a**, *arrow*). Microangiography in anteroposterior and lateral views demonstrates a traumatic pseudoaneurysm (**b, c**). Onyx deposition into the pseudoaneurysm (*arrow*) can be appreciated because of admixture of tantalum powder in it. The microcatheter is also appreciated on the blank roadmaps (**d, e**). Post-intervention angiography (subtracted) demonstrates obliteration of the pseudoaneurysm (*arrow*, **f, g**). This resulted in complete resolution of epistaxis. Subsequently, the large bullet fragment was successfully extracted

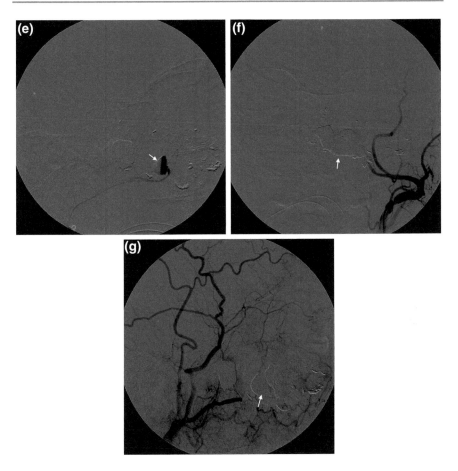

Fig. 9.1

- If Onyx reflux occurs, wait for a couple of minutes to allow the Onyx to solidify. The solid Onyx plug may prevent further reflux as the Onyx infiltrates a route with less resistance. The reflux over the microcatheter should be no greater than 1 cm, or not beyond a significant vascular bend traversed by the catheter. Otherwise, it may become difficult to extract the catheter and lead to complications.
- Once the contents of the syringe are completely injected, disconnect the syringe and replace with the next Onyx syringe making a 'meniscus-to-meniscus' connection. Again, ensure that no air or other substances such as blood and contrast gain entrance into the microcatheter. If needed, use Onyx or DMSO (not saline) to overfill the hub of microcatheter.
- Once the treatment is complete, wait a few seconds, slightly aspirate the syringe, and gently pull the microcatheter to separate from the cast.

- In case resistance is encountered because the tip of microcatheter is adherent in the Onyx plug, maintain a constant, gentle but firm tension upon it, until a sensation of 'giveway' happens when the tip of microcatheter breaks free from Onyx. Do not rapidly tug as this may fracture the catheter.
- Confirm the targeted vessel is occluded by performing an angiogram.
- Perform post-procedure angiography, after retracting the guide catheter into the common carotid. If there is any possibility that there may be Onyx in the guide catheter, e.g., the Onyx reflux close to or all the way back to the guide catheter, exchange catheters before doing post-embolization angiography. This will prevent inadvertent embolization into the ICA vasculature (Fig. 9.1).

Tumors

Indications and Case Selection

- Preoperative devascularization of vascular tumors including meningiomas. Hemangiopericytomas, juvenile nasopharyngeal angiofibromas, glomus jugulare tumors, hemangioblastomas, vascular metastases.
- Devascularization is commonly performed for meningiomas usually 24 h–1 week preoperatively. Not only does the devascularization result in attenuation of operative blood loss, frequently the tumor is rendered softer and easier to remove by creating necrosis after several days.

Contraindications

These are relative.

- Observable collaterals between ECA and ICA. The inadvertent deposition of embolic material into cerebral circulation may prove catastrophic.
- If a decision is made to embolize the ICA supply to a tumor, the benefits of devascularization must be weighed against the risks including, stroke.
- Iodine allergy. Pre-medicate if embolization is necessary.

Preoperative Management and Procedure

- These are the same as described above for epistaxis.
- Specifically for tumors, embolization is continued until most or all, of the tumor blush is resolved (Fig. 9.2).

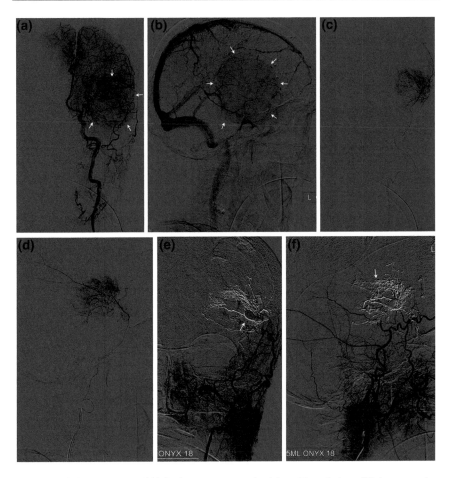

Fig. 9.2 A left common carotid injection, anteroposterior (**a**), and lateral views (**b**) demonstrating a tumor blush (*arrows*) in a meningioma. Super selective angiography after catheterization of middle meningeal branch of the ECA demonstrates tumor supply but no obvious intracranial collaterals (**c**, **d**). Embolization was performed using Onyx 18. Post-embolization ECA angiography shows no blood supply to tumor (**e**, **f**). The Onyx cast is easily appreciated (*arrow*)

Postoperative Management and Follow-up

- This is the same as described above for epistaxis.
- Specifically for tumors, steroid administration may be necessary to address associated edema, e.g., in case of meningiomas. In case of a large tumor where embolization may cause life-threatening progression of edema, in addition to steroids, early surgery (within 24–48 h) may be needed.

Extracranial Angioplasty and Stenting

10

Subclavian Artery Angioplasty and Stenting

Indications and Case Selection

- Symptomatic subclavian artery stenosis, e.g., stenosis resulting in subclavian steal syndrome.

Contraindications

- If anticoagulant and/or antiplatelet therapy is contraindicated.
- Severe vascular tortuosity or anatomy that would preclude the safe introduction or maintenance of a guide catheter, sheath, or interventional devices.
- Hypersensitivity to the metal used in the stent, e.g., steel, nickel, or nickel-titanium.
- Uncorrected bleeding disorders.

Preoperative Management

- Verify lab values including platelet count, BUN, CR, APTT, PT/INR, and ß-HCG for females of reproductive age.
- In case of renal insufficiency, diabetes, CHF, etc., ensure usage of diluted non-ionic contrast agent and carefully pre-plan to maintain contrast load to minimum.
- Plavix 75 mg PO daily starting 3 days before procedure or
- Plavix 300 mg (4 tabs) PO LD on morning of procedure or
- If unable to administer Plavix in a timely fashion, another option is:
- Abciximab (Rheopro®) in a L.D. of 0.25 mg/kg followed by continuous IV infusion of 0.125 µg/kg/min (to a maximum of 10 µg/kg/min) for 12 h, then

© Springer International Publishing AG 2017
S.H. Khan and A.J. Ringer, *Handbook of Neuroendovascular Techniques*,
DOI 10.1007/978-3-319-52936-3_10

d/c. Start this after arterial access has been secured. Administer Plavix 75 mg PO the same evening and then 75 mg PO daily.

- ASA 81–325 mg PO daily.
- Liquids only on morning of procedure.
- NPO (for ≈6 h) when procedure performed under GA.
- Obtain informed consent for angiography, angioplasty, and stenting.
- Ensure two IV lines inserted.
- Insert Foley. Patient will be more comfortable and cooperative with an empty bladder in case the procedure becomes prolonged.
- Position patient on neuroangiography table.
- Attach patient to pulse oximetry and ECG leads for monitoring O2 saturation, HR, cardiac rhythm respiratory rate, and BP.

Drugs

- 0.9% NS + 20 meq KCl @ 75 cc/h (adjust to higher rate as needed).
- Fentanyl 25–100 µg IV prn.
- Versed 0.5–1 mg IV prn.
- Heparin IV per physician instructions. (See "Technique" below.)

Devices

- Micropuncture kit 4 Fr.
- 6-Fr shuttle sheath (80 cm; may use longer catheter if patient is tall), which may be advanced initially over dilator into the descending aorta and then into subclavian artery proximal to the stenosis over 6-Fr H1 slip catheter. A shuttle sheath is preferable because it will provide greater support and considerably decrease the likelihood of the apparatus collapsing into the aortic arch at critical time points, e.g., during stent deployment.
- 6-Fr H1 slip catheter.
- Rotating hemostatic valves (2). Ensure the RHV attached to the guide catheter is $\geq 0.096''$ or 2.44 mm.
- Pediatric transducers (30 ml/h; 2).
- Diagnostic catheter: Terumo® front-angled glide catheter 5 Fr (for diagnostics).
- Front-angled glidewire (0.035; Terumo).
- Balloon dilatation catheter (non-compliant) with pre-mounted stent, e.g., Express® LD Stent Delivery System (Boston Scientific, Natick, MA) or
- Balloon dilatation catheter: non-compliant balloon for pre-stent dilatation, if needed, e.g., Ultra-thin™Diamond™ (Boston Scientific, Natick, MA). This can be used with the 0.035 glidewire and therefore may prove convenient. Another option is Aviator™ Plus (RX) (Cordis), which will use 0.014 microwire and is an exchange (RX) catheter.
- The size of the balloon dilatation catheter is based on the vessel size, as explained in "Procedure" section.

- Syringes 10 cc (at least 3), 20 cc (at least 4), 3 cc (for ACT).
- Three-way stopcock: 3.
- Torque device.
- Telfa strip.
- Mandrel for shaping microwire tip.
- Angioseal™ closure device (6 Fr). Use larger size if a larger sheath is inserted.

Vascular Access

- Gain arterial access with a micropuncture needle, using modified Seldinger technique.
- Insert a glidewire into the descending aorta.
- Attach a 6-Fr shuttle sheath to a continuously running flush of heparinized saline and confirm that the system is free of air bubbles.
- Insert the provided dilator into the shuttle sheath and then introduce this assembly onto the glidewire.
- Using fluoroscopy, advance the shuttle sheath into the aortic arch, ensuring that the tip of the glidewire is always leading.
- Retract and remove the dilator.

Intervention

- Administer 5000 IU heparin IV. Perform ACT approximately 20–30 min later; use a 15-cc syringe, draw 10–15 cc of blood from the sheath, and then immediately attach a 3-cc syringe to draw 1–2 cc of blood, which is sent for ACT.
- May return the blood drawn prior to ACT sample back to the patient via the sheath, as long as the distal tip of the sheath is proximal to the subclavian-carotid vasculature.
- Check ACT hourly throughout the procedure and administer heparin IV to maintain an ACT of 300–350.
- Attach a 6-Fr H1 slip catheter to a continuously running flush of heparinized saline and confirm that the system is free of air bubbles.
- Advance the slip catheter over the guidewire into the sheath.
- Ensure that the distal tip of glidewire remains in its position, leading the catheter.
- Using fluoroscopy, continue to advance the slip catheter until it emerges from the distal tip of the shuttle sheath.
- Ensure that during navigation, the glidewire is leading.
- Navigate the glidewire into the subclavian artery and advance the slip catheter over it.
- Use roadmapping, as necessary.
- Ensure that the manipulation remains proximal to the stenosed segment.
- Cross the lesion using the glidewire. Advance the wire into the subclavian, not vertebral artery.

- Once the slip catheter is in the proximal subclavian, advance the shuttle sheath over the slip catheter and glidewire.
- After the shuttle sheath is positioned in the proximal subclavian, retract and remove the glidewire and slip catheter from the shuttle sheath.
- Perform angiography.
- Measure the length and breadth of stenosed segment to select the appropriate sized angioplasty balloon and stent.
- When ready to perform the procedure, do a roadmap.
- When possible, we prefer using a balloon-mounted stent (e.g., Express LD, Medtronic).
- If a balloon-mounted stent is intended for use, ensure that the stenosed segment is of adequate width, e.g., when using Express LD system the vessel width at the site of the stenosis should be at least 2 mm. If not, then first perform pre-dilatation angioplasty to gain adequate caliber. Once appropriate caliber is gained, proceed with angioplasty and stenting. As an example, if the vessel at the site of stenosis has a diameter of <2 mm, first use 4-mm Viatrac 14 Plus for pre-dilatation and then use Express LD balloon-mounted stent.
- Select the appropriate length stent system based on the distance of the stenosed vessel from the access site (usually femoral artery). Express LD comes in two lengths: 75 and 135 cm.
- Open package and remove contents using sterile precautions.
- Remove the hoop containing stent system.
- Remove the stent system from the hoop.
- Confirm that the stent is located between the proximal and distal balloon markers.
- Do not use if the system is damaged in any way.
- Flush the stent system's guidewire lumen with normal saline.
- Prepare the inflation device system with diluted contrast medium. The manufacturer recommends 50:50 contrast dilution with normal saline. However, we use a 2/3:1/3 dilution and find it more convenient due to better visualization.
- Additionally, the manufacturer recommends priming the balloon with contrast prior to insertion. We routinely perform this in vivo and will describe it as such.
- Cross the stricture site with a 0.035 guidewire.
- If needed, advance a pre-dilatation balloon catheter over the wire and perform angioplasty.
- Remove the pre-dilation balloon catheter and advance the Express® LD balloon-mounted stent system over the wire.
- Using fluoroscopy and roadmapping, position the stent system across the lesion.
- When satisfied with stent position, attach the inflation device and syringe with contrast medium to the balloon catheter via a stopcock.
- Close the stopcock to inflator and then vigorously aspirate the syringe to remove any air from the balloon catheter. Release the plunger slowly to replace the air with dilute contrast. Repeat this maneuver once or twice.
- Now close the stopcock to the syringe, such that it is open to the inflation device.

- Deploy the stent by slowly inflating the balloon to the nominal pressure (usually 8 atm). Always double check the measurement card provided for this purpose during inflation.
- In order to overcome the stricture, higher pressure may be required. However, do not exceed the rated burst pressure (12 atm).
- Use fluoroscopy to visualize the stent as it is being deployed.
- Once the stent is deployed completely, deflate the balloon. Apply negative pressure if need be for complete deflation. Confirm complete deflation fluoroscopically.
- Slowly withdraw the balloon catheter after it is deflated. It is our experience that some resistance is encountered at the onset of removal as the balloon disengages from the stent, but it is very transient and usually inconsequential. However, do not continue to pull the catheter if the resistance perseveres. Determine the cause of resistance fluoroscopically and if need be, perform angiography.

  - If correctly placed, the stent should cover the entire extent of stricture.
  - If significant stenosis persists that needs to be addressed, perform post-stenting angioplasty using the balloon catheter that came with the stent, or an alternative catheter, e.g., Viatrac.

- Do not expand the stent beyond its maximum diameter.
- Do not give up guidewire access across the lesion, until completely satisfied that the lesion has been addressed.
- Perform Post-procedure cerebral angiography.

Vessel Perforation or Arteriovenous Fistula

Indications and Case Selection

- A covered stent is required in case of treatment of cervical vessel or when treating an arteriovenous fistula, e.g., between internal jugular vein and ICA or VA.
- The diameter of the vessel should be ≥ 2.75 and ≤ 12 mm.
- For vessels up to 12 mm an 'over the wire' (OTW) Jostent (Abbott Vascular, Santa Clara, CA) is used. It is a stainless steel stent with a polytetrafluoroethylene graft, which is shorter than the stent length. If used intracranially, extreme caution should be exercised as covering the ostia of perforators may cause devastating infarcts. Additionally, these are 'stiffer' to deploy than devices meant for intracranial usage.

Preoperative Management

- Same as indicated above. However, in case of free perforation antiplatelet agents and Heparin to elevate ACT are deferred, until the stent is deployed. After successful stent deployment, the patient may be loaded with Reopro and an infusion started.

Drugs

- 0.9% NS + 20 meq KCl @ 75 cc/h (adjust to lower or higher rate as needed).
- Fentanyl 25–100 µg IV prn.
- Versed 0.5–1 mg IV prn.
- Heparin IV per physician instructions. (See "Technique" below.)

Devices

- Micropuncture kit 4 Fr.
- 7 Fr Guide catheter, e.g., Envoy (Cordis).
- Rotating hemostatic valves (2). Ensure the RHV attached to the Guide catheter is ≥ 0.096″ or 2.44 mm.
- Pediatric transducers (30 ml/h; 2).
- Front-angled glidewire (0.035; Terumo).
- Syringes 10 cc (at least 3), 20 cc (at least 4), 3 cc (for ACT).
- Three-way stopcock: 3.
- Torque device.
- Telfa strip.
- Mandrel for shaping microwire tip.
- Angioseal™ closure device (8 Fr).
- In addition to above for vascular access and guide catheter placement, specifically for Jo stent deployment, the following will be needed.

    - 20 ml syringe.
    - Microguidewire (max. diameter 0.014″).
    - Jostent of appropriate size and length based on angiographic measurements.
    - Inflation device.
    - Three-way stopcock.

- The selected stent should be at least 1 mm beyond lesion on either end (i.e., the stent is distal to the lesion distally and proximal to the lesion proximally) for complete coverage.
- Table 10.1 indicates the available diameters, lengths, and other important particulars of Jo Stent.

Table 10.1 Jostent

Diameters (mm)	2.75, 3.0, 3.5, 4.0, 4.5, 5.0
Lengths (mm)	12, 16, 19, 26
Maximum guidewire	0.014″
Shaft size	Proximal: 3.1 Fr Distal: 2.6 Fr
Minimum deployment pressure	14 atm
Rated burst pressure	16 atm

Vascular Access

- Vascular access is gained as described above using a 21G entry needle and 4-Fr micropuncture set.
- A 6-Fr or 7-Fr Guide catheter (e.g., Envoy) connected to a continuously running flush of heparinized saline, may be used instead of the shuttle sheath.
- Advance the Guide catheter over a 0.035 guidewire (e.g., 0.035 glidewire) through a short sheath using fluoroscopy and roadmapping.
- Position the distal tip of the guide catheter proximal to the lesion and remove any slack.
- Ensure that the tip of guide catheter is close enough to the lesion to enable stable stent deployment. However, there should be enough space between the lesion and guide tip to enable unobstructed deployment.
- Remove the system carefully from its packaging maintaining sterile precautions.
- Remove the delivery system out of the sterile hoop ensuring it is not kinked, or bent in the process.
- Hold the delivery system just proximal to the balloon (at the proximal balloon bond site) with one hand, and with the other hand, gently remove the stent protector and stylet located distally.

Intervention

Ex Vivo Preparation of Balloon

- Fill a 20- or 30-ml luer lock syringe with diluted contrast medium (2/3:1/3 concentration).
- Attach the syringe to inflation device using a three-way stopcock and aspirate the contrast medium into the inflation device leaving 2–3 ml in the syringe.
- Ensure that the entire inflation system is free of air bubbles.
- Attach the system to the balloon inflation port of the delivery system.
- Turn the stopcock so that the inflator is occluded and there is direct communication between syringe and balloon catheter.
- Aspirate to remove air from the system, holding the syringe upright. Gently allow the plunger to return toward its original position so that air is replaced by contrast in the stent system.
- Repeat the process, until air bubbles are no longer visible during aspiration.

- Allow the ambient pressure to return to the balloon before detaching the syringe.
- A meniscus will appear in the balloon inflation port when the syringe is detached.
- Purge the aspirated air from the inflation system by inverting the syringe and injecting out the air.
- If air bubbles continue to be aspirated despite multiple aspirations, discard the system and prepare another.
- We usually perform an in vivo preparation, which is described below in the sequence it is undertaken during procedure.
- Moisten the stent system by soaking it in a bowl containing heparinized saline (DO NOT wipe down with moist gauze sponge as the stent graft may be disrupted by gauze fibers).
- Visually confirm that the stent graft is located between the proximal and distal stent markers.

Stent Delivery

- Place a 0.014″ microguidewire into the lumen of the balloon catheter.
- Ensure the appropriately positioned guide catheter (distal tip of the guide catheter should be proximal to the lesion) is stable.
- Advance this system through the RHV of the guide catheter.
- Using fluoroscopy and roadmapping, advance the delivery system to the target lesion and position it optimally such that the distal radiopaque marker on the balloon catheter should be distal to the lesion and the proximal marker, proximal to the lesion.
- Ensure that the distal marker is at least 1 mm distal to the lesion.
- Once optimal positioning is confirmed sufficiently tighten the RHV around the system. Do not over tighten, which may impede the proper functioning of the delivery system.
- If ex vivo balloon preparation was performed, then securely attach the inflation system to the balloon inflation port by making a wet meniscus to meniscus connection. To do this, fill the port with diluted contrast to replace any air, and then make a meniscus to meniscus connection with the inflation device.
- Ensure that inadvertent, premature deployment of the balloon catheter does not occur during attachment.

In Vivo Balloon Preparation

- If ex vivo preparation was not performed, then do in vivo preparation as follows:

  - Fill a 20- or 30-ml luer lock syringe with diluted contrast medium (2/3 contrast:1/3 saline).
  - Attach the syringe to inflation device using a three-way stopcock and aspirate the contrast medium into the inflation device leaving 2–3 ml in the syringe.

- Ensure that the entire inflation system is free of air bubbles.
- Securely attach the system to the balloon inflation port of the delivery system.
- Turn the stopcock so that the inflator is occluded and there is direct communication between syringe and balloon catheter.
- Aspirate to remove air from the system, holding the syringe upright. Gently allow the plunger to return toward its original position so that air is replaced by contrast in the stent system.
- Repeat the process, until air bubbles are no longer visible during aspiration.

Stent Deployment

- Prior to stent deployment, confirm that the stent is appropriately positioned and the guide catheter and balloon catheter are free of slack.
- Turn the stopcock so that it is off to the syringe and open to inflation device and balloon catheter port.
- Place the compliance chart in front of you.
- Turn the inflator slowly (approximately 1 atm per 15 s) to gradually inflate the balloon. Inflate to a minimum of 14 atm to expand the stent by balloon inflation.
- Use the compliance chart to achieve the appropriate inflation pressure for a particular stent size.
- Do not exceed the rated burst pressure or expand the stent beyond its actual size.
- Maintain the inflation pressure for 15–30 s for full expansion and adequate approximation of the stent to vessel wall. Underexpansion may result in stent graft movement or lack of proper coverage of perforation.
- After completion of stent deployment, deflate the balloon completely by applying negative pressure, if needed. Wait at least 15 s to ensure complete deflation.
- Confirm fluoroscopically that the balloon is completely deflated.
- Fully open the RHV of the guide catheter.
- Maintaining negative pressure, withdraw the balloon catheter from the deployed stent. Ensure that the guidewire and guide catheter maintain their position.
- Close the RHV around the guidewire, once the balloon catheter is removed.
- Perform angiography to confirm complete apposition of stent against vessel wall.
- If complete apposition was not achieved, then use a non-compliant, high-pressure balloon of the same size (or slightly larger) and length as the balloon of the delivery system to perform a second stent expansion.
- Do not overdilate the vessel to the extent that dissection may occur.
- The final post-procedure angiogram should demonstrate the stent diameter to be the same as (or slightly larger) than the vessel proximal and distal to the stent.
- Observe the patient (especially if procedure done under moderate sedation) and perform periodic angiographic assessment within the initial 30 min after stent deployment.

Table 10.2 Some problems encountered and solutions

Problem	Solution
Resistance encountered during advancement of balloon catheter through guide catheter	Do not force your way forward. If possible and already achieved, maintain guidewire access across the lesion and remove the delivery system (balloon catheter and stent) as a single unit. Identify the cause of resistance. If required, replace the system with a new one
A single stent cannot be positioned to cover the lesion adequately	If needed, deploy two stents in a telescopic fashion to cover the lesion entirely. Preferably, deploy the distal stent first, followed by the proximal stent. This will eliminate the need to cross the just deployed proximal stent with a stent delivery system that could result in its dislodgment

- Perform post-procedure cerebral angiography to rule out any embolic complication.
- Do not perform MRI for approximately 8 weeks (until the stent has completely endothelialized), to avoid the risk of stent movement.

Problems Encountered and Solutions

- Table 10.2 shows some problems encountered and solutions.

Carotid Artery Angioplasty and Stenting

Indications and Case Selection

- *Carotid Stenosis*: If a patient has expected survival of less than 5 years; patients with malignancies and other life-threatening conditions should be considered for endovascular treatment instead of carotid endarterectomy.
- *Carotid Dissection/Pseudoaneurysm*: e.g., due to trauma. In such a case stenting (with or without coiling) may be performed to appose the walls of the injured artery. Angioplasty is not done. Intervention is needed when the dissection is symptomatic; the intimal flap faces the flow of blood, in which case the dissection/associated false lumen is likely to expand; and pseudoaneurysm, will be at a risk of rupture if not treated.

Contraindications

- If anticoagulant and/or antiplatelet therapy is contraindicated.
- Severe vascular tortuosity or anatomy that would preclude the safe introduction or maintenance of a guide catheter, sheath, or interventional devices.

- Hypersensitivity to nickel-titanium.
- Uncorrected bleeding disorders.
- Lesions in the ostium of CCA.

Preoperative Management

- Verify lab values including platelet count, BUN, CR, APTT, PT/INR, and ß-HCG for females of reproductive age group.
- In case of renal insufficiency, diabetes, CHF, etc., ensure usage of diluted non-ionic contrast agent and carefully pre-plan to maintain contrast load to minimum.
- Plavix 75 mg PO daily starting 3 days before procedure **or**
- Plavix 300 mg (4 tabs) PO LD on morning of procedure **or**
- If unable to administer Plavix in a timely fashion, another option is:
- Abciximab (Rheopro®) in a L.D. of 0.25 mg/kg followed by continuous IV infusion of 0.125 µg/kg/min (to a maximum of 10 µg/kg/min) for 12 h, then d/c. Start this after arterial access has been secured. Administer Plavix 75 mg PO the same evening and then 75 mg PO daily.
- ASA 81–325 mg PO daily.
- Liquids only on morning of procedure.
- NPO (for ≈6 h) when procedure performed under GA.
- Obtain informed consent for angiography, angioplasty, and stenting.
- Ensure two IV lines inserted.
- Insert Foley. Patient will be more comfortable and cooperative with an empty bladder in case the procedure becomes prolonged.
- Position patient on neuroangiography.
- Attach patient to pulse oximetry and ECG leads for monitoring O2 saturation, HR, cardiac rhythm respiratory rate, and BP.

Carotid Stenosis

Drugs

- 0.9% NS + 20 meq KCl @ 75 cc/h (adjust to higher rate as needed).
- Fentanyl 25–100 µg IV prn.
- Versed 0.5–1 mg IV prn.
- Heparin IV per physician instructions. (See "Technique" below.)

Devices

- Micropuncture kit 4 Fr.
- 6-Fr short sheath (10 cm); use long sheath if tortuous vasculature, e.g., a 6-Fr shuttle sheath which may be advanced initially over dilator into the descending

aorta and then into common carotid over 6-Fr H1 slip catheter. A shuttle sheath is also preferable because it will provide greater support and significantly decrease the likelihood of the apparatus collapsing into the aortic arch at critical time points, e.g., during stent deployment.

- 6-Fr H1 slip catheter.
- Rotating hemostatic valves (2). Ensure the RHV attached to the Guide catheter is ≥ 0.096″ or 2.44 mm.
- Pediatric transducers (30 ml/h; 2).
- Guide catheter: 6-Fr Envoy® MPC guide catheter (90 cm).
- Diagnostic catheter: Terumo® front-angled glidecath 5 Fr (for diagnostics. May use Envoy guide catheter for the same purpose).
- Front-angled glidewire (0.035; Terumo).
- Embolic protection system (Guidant, Accunet). The package containing this product has three pouches which contain the following: RX Accunet™ delivery system comprising of 0.014″ guidewire with filter basket, peel away delivery sheath, introducer tool, torque device with peel away adapter, and flushing tool.
- The other two pouches contain filter basket recovery catheters. One has a shapeable tip, while the other is low profile and more flexible.
- Selection of filter basket size will depend upon the diameter of carotid artery. (See chart in "Technique" section.)
- Balloon dilatation catheter: Aviator™ Plus (RX) (Cordis, Warren, NJ, USA).
- It is a rapid exchange (RX) catheter.
- It is available in 4–7 mm balloon diameter range. Select the appropriate size for the vessel being treated, based on the table provided with the product.
- Carotid stent: Acculink™ (Guidant). See tables in "Procedure" section for selecting the appropriate size to the vessel being treated, in untapered or tapered stents.
- Syringes 10 cc (at least 3), 20 cc (at least 4), 3 cc (for ACT and angioplasty balloon preparation).
- Three-way stopcock: 3.
- Torque device.
- Telfa strip.
- Mandrel for shaping microwire tip.
- Angioseal™ closure device (6 Fr). Use larger size if a larger sheath inserted.

Vascular Access

- Attach a 6-Fr shuttle sheath to a continuously running flush of heparinized saline and confirm that the system is free of air bubbles.
- Insert the provided dilator into the shuttle sheath.
- Gain access with micropuncture needle using modified Seldinger technique.
- Insert a glidewire into the descending aorta.
- Remove the 4-Fr sheath over the wire, maintaining wire access to the vasculature.
- Introduce the shuttle sheath-dilator assembly onto the glidewire.

- Using fluoroscopy, advance the shuttle sheath into the aortic arch, ensuring that the tip of the glidewire is always leading.
- Retract and remove the dilator.
- Administer 5000 IU heparin IV. Remember to perform ACT approximately 20–30 min later. Using a 15-cc syringe, draw 10–15 cc of blood from the sheath and then immediately attach a 3-cc syringe to draw 1–2 cc of blood, which is sent for ACT.
- May return the blood drawn prior to ACT sample back to the patient via the sheath, as long as the distal tip of the sheath is proximal to the carotid vasculature.
- Check ACT hourly throughout the procedure and administer heparin IV to maintain an ACT of 300–350.
- Attach a 6-Fr H1 slip catheter to a continuously running flush of heparinized saline and confirm that the system is free of air bubbles.
- Advance the slip catheter over the guidewire into the sheath if an exchange length wire has been used. Ensure that the distal tip of glidewire remains in its position.
- If the guidewire is not exchange length, remove the wire from the shuttle sheath, introduce it into the H1 catheter, and then advance this system into the sheath.
- Using fluoroscopy, continue to advance the slip catheter until it emerges from the distal tip of the shuttle sheath.
- Ensure that during navigation the glidewire is in the lead.
- Navigate the glidewire into the common carotid artery (CCA) and advance the slip catheter over it.
- Use roadmapping, as necessary.
- Ensure that the manipulation remains proximal to the stenosed segment.
- If greater wire purchase is needed, advance the glidewire into the external carotid artery not internal carotid artery (ICA).
- Once the slip catheter is in the proximal CCA, advance the shuttle sheath over the slip catheter and glidewire.
- After the shuttle sheath is positioned in the CCA, retract and remove the glidewire and slip catheter from the shuttle sheath.

Intervention

Placement of Embolic Protection Device

- Perform pre-intervention cervical and cerebral angiography in AP and lateral views.
- Select the working views.
- Measure the diameter of stenosis and the length of the affected segment.
- Measure the vessel diameter proximal and distal to the stenosis.
- Use these measurements to select the appropriate size embolic protection device. See Table 10.3.

Table 10.3 Accunet

Filter size fully expanded (mm)	Reference vessel diameter minimum to maximum range (mm)
4.5	3.25–4.0
5.5	4.0–5.0
6.5	5.0–6.0
7.5	6.0–7.0

- As an example, if the stenosis is measured as 3.28 mm, use the 4.5-mm embolic protection device.

Preparation of Embolic Protection Device

- Transfer the embolic protection system, e.g., RX ACCUNET™ (Guidant) system from its package in an aseptic fashion.
- Hold the dispenser hoop containing the embolic protection device and the flush tool in one hand.
- Loosen the RHV on the flush tool.
- Hold the flush tool upright and attach it to a 10-cc syringe containing heparinized saline (see Fig. 10.1).
- Flush gently to remove air from the filter and confirm that the fluid exits from the RHV.
- After confirming that no part of the light blue distal section of the sheath is within the RHV, tighten the RHV on the delivery sheath (see Fig. 10.1).

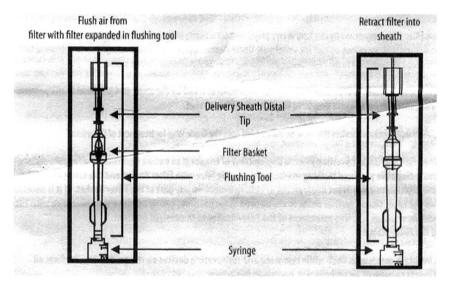

Fig. 10.1 Courtesy Abbott™ (Abbott Vascular, Santa Clara, CA)

Fig. 10.2 Courtesy
Abbott™ (Abbott Vascular,
Santa Clara, CA)

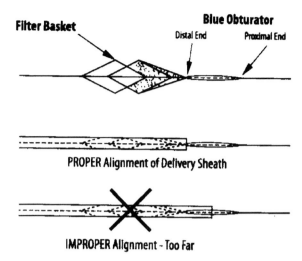

- Release the flushing tool and delivery sheath from the dispenser hooks.
- Also release the proximal end of the wire from the dispenser hook.
- Ensure the system is undamaged, prior to its use.
- Flush the sheath with heparinized saline to remove air from it. Confirm that the fluid exits from the proximal end of the sheath.
- Place a torque device on the proximal end of the guidewire of the embolic protection system and tighten it.
- Carefully pull back on the torque device while observing the flushing tool, to pull the filter basket into the delivery sheath, until the distal tip of the delivery sheath aligns with the proximal end of the blue filter obturator (Fig. 10.2). DO NOT pull in the filter basket any further.
- Loosen the RHV of the flushing tool and slide the flushing tool off the delivery system.
- Loosen the torque device and position it so that the proximal end of the light blue delivery sheath is within the central collet tube of the peel away adapter of the torque device. After this positioning, tighten the torque device.

Delivery of Embolic Protection Device

- Ensure the guide catheter (shuttle sheath) is well positioned and stable in the CCA.
- The tip of the guide catheter must always be kept in view during the procedure to ensure that it does not prolapse into the aortic arch.
- If needed, shape the tip of the RX Accunet™ embolic protection system (EPS) guidewire.
- Insert the tip of the guidewire into the introducer tool and then advance these as a unit into the RHV of guide catheter, until the delivery sheath has entered the guide catheter.

- Remove the introducer tool.
- Advance the delivery sheath slowly after the delivery tool is removed from the RHV.
- The presence of delivery tool there may result in air entrapment.
- Using fluoroscopy advance the tip of the sheath and cross the lesion, with the guidewire leading.
- The guidewire, filter basket, and delivery sheath are slowly advanced as a unit.
- Independent advancement of the guidewire may result in premature deployment.
- Use the torque device to torque the guidewire. Do not torque the delivery sheath.
- Position the filter basket at least 4 cm distal to the lesion in a relatively straight segment of the blood vessel. The radiopaque markers on the system aid in this positioning.
- In case difficulty is encountered during advancement of the EPS, stop and determine the cause. The following maneuvers may help:

  - Make the patient rotate his head from side to side. This may re-orient the carotid artery.
  - If the EPS cannot cross the lesion, then withdraw it and first pre-dilate with a 2-mm balloon.
  - A stiff 0.014″ buddy wire may be inserted to straighten the carotid. Once the EPS has been advanced to its appropriate position, remove the buddy wire, prior to deployment of the filter basket.

Deployment of Filter Basket

- Ensure the radiopaque markers of the filter basket are distal to the lesion and proximal to the petrous segment of ICA.
- Confirm that position is appropriate.
- Loosen the torque device on the guidewire.
- Feed the proximal light blue end of the delivery sheath into the port of the peel away adapter located on the torque device (see Fig. 10.3).
- Advance the torque device until it abuts against the darker blue part of the sheath, where the slit in the sheath begins.

Fig. 10.3 Courtesy Abbott™ (Abbott Vascular, Santa Clara, CA)

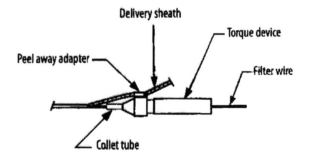

- Tighten the torque device to the wire.
- Remove all slack from the system.
- Loosen the RHV of the Guide catheter if one other than shuttle sheath is used.
- In case of a shuttle sheath (which has a hemostasis valve), reposition the previously retracted introducer tool in the valve. This will enable free movement of the delivery sheath. Even in case of shuttle sheaths, we prefer using an RHV instead of the valve that comes with the shuttle sheath.
- Stabilize the torque device with the left hand, keeping the hand resting over the delivery sheath, distal to the torque device.
- Grab the proximal, light blue end of the delivery sheath that has been fed through the peel away adapter with the right hand.
- Observing with fluoroscopy, use your right hand to pull the end of the sheath approximately 3 cm in a horizontal direction away from the patient. The sheath will peel away. Fluoroscopy will demonstrate the expansion of the filter basket by separation of the radiopaque markers.
- Avoid excessive movement of the filter basket during unsheathing. To ensure this, remove all slack from the system, prior to commencing unsheathing.
- The slight advancement of guidewire during unsheathing may also be required to avoid excessive movement of filter basket during unsheathing.
- Maintain the guidewire in a stable position, while continuing to peel back and retract the delivery sheath from the wire. When the light blue part of the delivery sheath exits the RHV of guide catheter, close the RHV. In case of shuttle sheath, remove the introducer tool after the light blue part of the delivery sheath exits the hemostasis valve.
- Confirm the expansion of the filter basket in two projections, e.g., AP and lateral.
- Perform angiography to confirm the position of the filter basket and adequate flow distal to the basket.
- Ensure that the radiopaque proximal bushing markers on the guidewire will be at a sufficient distance from the distal markers on the stent.
- If needed, gently advance the guidewire, to move the filter basket further away from the lesion.
- If during the interventional procedure, the distal flow of contrast is diminished due to filter basket filling with embolic debris, remove and replace the EPS. (See section on Recovery of Filter Basket.)

Pre-stent Angioplasty

Preparation

- Remove the contents of the Aviator Plus dilatation catheter from its package and transfer them onto the table maintaining sterile precautions. The contents are as follows:

- (i) Aviator ™ RX dilatation catheter in its protective tube, (ii) flushing needle in its protective sheath, (iii) compliance card.
- Hold package tube/tray in one hand and gently grasp the hub of the catheter, to remove it from the tube.
- Ensure the catheter is not kinked, bent, or otherwise damaged.
- Slide the forming tube off the balloon at the distal aspect of the catheter, without any twisting.
- Note that the balloon has radiopaque markers to aid in its positioning in the stenosed segment. The proximal shaft of the balloon catheter also has radiopaque markers that aid in gauging balloon catheter position relative to guide catheter tip. These are at 90 and 100 cm from the distal tip.
- Take a syringe containing heparinized saline and attach it to the flushing needle. Remove the protective sheath from the flushing needle. Insert the flushing needle into the distal tip of the catheter and flush the catheter, until the heparinized saline is seen exiting the guidewire exit notch located about 25 cm proximal to the distal tip.
- Submerge the balloon catheter in heparinized saline to activate its coating.
- In order to maintain the smooth contour, we do not prime the balloon until it is across the stenosed segment. This is contrary to manufacturers' instructions, but we have not experienced any difficulties.
- Fill a 20-cc syringe with 15-cc contrast and 5-cc heparinized NS (2/3:1/3 concentration).
- Attach a three-way stopcock to the inflation device and connect the syringe containing contrast medium to the sideport of the stopcock.
- Aspirate the contrast into the inflation device, leaving only 1–2 cc within the syringe.
- Purge any air out of the barrel and tubing of the inflation device, all the way to the distal portal of the stopcock.
- Leave inflation device on the table, until needed.

Deployment

- Backload the dilatation catheter onto the guidewire of the previously placed Acculink EPS.
- Ensure that the guidewire exits the notch 25 cm proximal to the catheter tip.
- Advance the balloon catheter over the wire into the shuttle sheath. In case guide catheter is used, open the RHV and advance the balloon catheter into it. Then tighten the RHV just enough to prevent excessive blood loss and not cause a hindrance in advancing the balloon catheter.
- Take care that the position of the guidewire is maintained during this maneuvering. Occasionally, confirm the same by fluoroscopy.
- Continue to advance the dilatation catheter over the guidewire until the proximal marker on the balloon catheter aligns with the hemostatic valve. This indicates that the balloon catheter tip has reached the tip of shuttle sheath/guide catheter.

- Perform roadmapping for further navigation and appropriate deployment of the balloon catheter system.
- Using fluoroscopy and roadmap, continue to advance the balloon catheter over the guidewire until it is appropriately positioned across the stenosed segment.

Angioplasty

- Recover the inflation device from the table.
- Use the distal-free port of the stopcock attached to the inflation device (which is in line with the inflation device) connection with the inflation hub of balloon catheter.
- Ensure that this connection is secure so that it will not disconnect during angioplasty.
- Close the stopcock to the inflation device.
- Aspirate the syringe (with nozzle pointing down) attached to the sideport of the stopcock to purge air out of the balloon catheter system.
- Slowly release the plunger of the syringe, so that the air is replaced with the contrast left in syringe for purpose. Repeat this step once or twice.
- Close the stopcock to syringe and open it to the inflation device.
- Place the compliance card in front of you in the operating field where you can easily look at it, while performing angioplasty.
- Initially, inflate the balloon to a very low pressure (1 atm) and again confirm that it is appropriately positioned across the stenosed segment. Also look at the radiopaque markers for confirmation of balloon position. These markers are more easily visualized on the native image. Using the compliance card slowly begin inflating the angioplasty balloon using the balloon inflation device.
- Inflate slowly by turning the screw provided on the inflation device at a rate ≤ 1 atm/15 s (to 'stretch' not 'crack' the vessel).
- Keep track of and document the inflation time (during which the blood flow will be interrupted by the balloon).
- Step on fluoroscopy pedal frequently to visualize progression of angioplasty.
- During inflation, the balloon may acquire a 'waist' due to vessel stenosis. This resolves with the progression of angioplasty.
- Once the goal pressure is reached, deflate the device.
- Confirm complete balloon deflation fluoroscopically.
- In order to achieve complete deflation, you may need to open the stopcock to the syringe and vigorously aspirate. Close the stopcock to syringe while aspiration is fully applied.
- Confirm complete balloon deflation fluoroscopically.
- Perform f/u angiography to evaluate results of angioplasty.
- If needed, repeat the angioplasty followed by angiography.
- Note that the minimum recommended lumen for Acculink™ stent is 2.5 mm, so pre-stent angioplasty must achieve dilatation at least to this extent.

- Do not exceed the recommended balloon pressures on the compliance card.
- Once angioplasty is completed and balloon completely deflated, withdraw the balloon catheter over guidewire. Use fluoroscopy to ensure the guidewire and the EPS do not move down as well.
- Once the balloon catheter exits from the hemostatic valve of the guide catheter, wipe it clean with moist Telfa and store it in a basin, keeping it submerged in heparinized saline.
- If the guide catheter has a RHV, ensure it is tightened adequately following balloon catheter withdrawal.
- If needed, maintain the balloon catheter in coiled position by inserting the proximal shaft into the hub clip (Fig. 10.4).

Selection of Stent

- Select the correct stent size, taking into account vessel measurements proximal and distal to the lesion.
- For Acculink™ untapered stent, the stent sizes available and reference vessel diameters are indicated in Table 10.4.
- For tapered stents, that are used when there is a difference between the calibers of proximal (CCA) and distal (ICA) vessel measurements, the stent sizes available and reference vessel diameters are indicated in Table 10.5.
- When selecting the length of stent, choose one that will extend at least 5 mm beyond the stenotic lesion at either end.

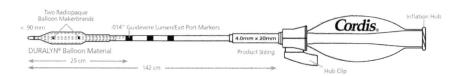

Fig. 10.4 Courtesy Cordis (Cordis, Bridgewater, NJ)

Table 10.4 Acculink stent—untapered

Unconstrained stent diameter (mm)	Stent length (mm)	Reference vessel diameter (mm)
5	20, 30, 40	3.6–4.5
6	20, 30, 40	4.3–5.4
7	20, 30, 40	5.0–6.4
8	20, 30, 40	5.7–7.3
9	20, 30, 40	6.4–8.2
10	20, 30, 40	7.1–9.1

Table 10.5 Acculink stent—tapered

Unconstrained stent diameter (mm)	Stent length (mm)	ICA reference vessel diameter (mm)	CCA reference vessel diameter (mm)
6–8 taper	30, 40	4.3–5.4	5.7–7.3
7–10 taper	30, 40	5.0–6.4	7.1–9.1

Preparation of Stent

- Remove the stent from its pouch using sterile precautions, as follows:

  - Remove the handle from the package before removing the shaft from the hoop.
  - Lay the device on a flat surface and inspect to confirm it has no kinks or other damage.
  - Inspect the stent through its delivery system and ensure it is fully covered by the sheath.
  - Also ensure the stent does not overlap the proximal marker.
  - Do not remove the distal mandrel from the inner lumen.

- The stent (see Fig. 10.5) delivery catheter has a radiopaque tip. The distal and proximal radiopaque markers on the catheter demarcate the position of the stent during fluoroscopy.
- Ensure the dial on the housing assembly is in locked (closed) position (Fig. 10.6a).
- Attach a 10-cc syringe with heparinized saline to the flush port at the proximal end of the assembly. Inject saline into the system (Fig. 10.6b). Confirm that the flush exits through the wire exit notch distally.
- Now tightly pinch the exit notch to enable the flush to exit at the distal end, as well as at the mandrel.
- Remove the mandrel by gently twisting and pulling (see Fig. 10.7).
- Ascertain that you are not holding the sheath while removing the mandrel.
- Continue to flush after the removal of the mandrel.
- If the mandrel does not come out easily or flush solution is not seen at the stent sheath junction, do not use the device.
- Keep the system on a flat surface until ready for use.

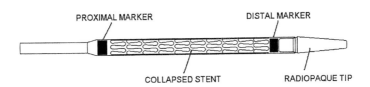

Fig. 10.5 Courtesy Abbott™ (Abbott Vascular, Santa Clara, CA)

(a)

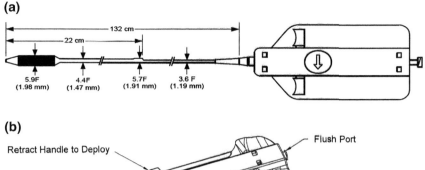

(b)

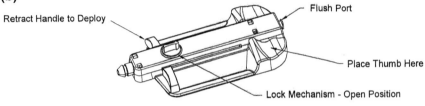

Fig. 10.6 Courtesy Abbott™ (Abbott Vascular, Santa Clara, CA)

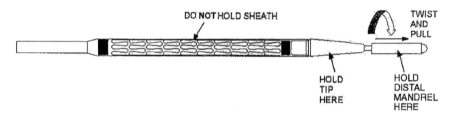

Fig. 10.7 Courtesy Abbott™ (Abbott Vascular, Santa Clara, CA)

Stent Delivery

- Backload the stent delivery system onto the EPS guidewire. The guidewire will emerge through the exit notch approximately 22 cm from the distal tip.
- If using a shuttle sheath, ensure the funnel introducer is placed onto the system prior to backloading the guidewire.
- If using guide catheter, ensure the RHV is open and back bleeding is observed.
- Secure the guidewire and sheath position with one hand (usu. left) and use the other hand to advance the delivery system to the lesion site, with the aid of fluoroscopy.
- Observe the radiopaque markers, which indicate the location of the stent.
- Using roadmapping, advance the stent system over the guidewire until the stent is positioned across the lesion, with the distal markers distal to the lesion and proximal markers proximal to it.
- At this point ascertain the positions of the following:

    - The EPS, which should be well distal to the lesion.
    - Radiopaque tip of the delivery catheter, which is distal to the lesion.

- Distal marker that indicates distal end of the stent. This should be distal to the lesion.
- Proximal marker that indicates proximal end of the stent. This should be proximal to the lesion. (However, if the lesion is unusually long, then the proximal markers may be at the lesion. In such a situation, the plan will be to deploy multiple stents to cover the entire lesion, with the stents partially overlapping each other.)

- Perform angiography and adjust position of stent if needed, until satisfied with position.
- Ensure that the RHV is closed just enough to prevent loss of blood, but still enables unhindered adjustment and maneuvering of the stent delivery catheter. Ensure the shuttle sheath and RHV hub are free of any static blood, which may clot. Flush the Guide catheter, if need be.
- Repeat angiography after each stent catheter adjustment.
- Ensure that all slack has been removed and the system is completely straight.
- Perform angiography to ascertain satisfactory final position.
- Ensure that the vessel distal to the lesion is visualized.
- Place the housing/handle of the delivery system on the patient's leg or adjacent stable surface.
- Ensure the funnel introducer is inserted in the shuttle sheath valve or the RHV of shuttle sheath is adequately open.
- Now deploy stent under continuous fluoroscopy as follows:
- Position your thumb in the proximal groove provided in the handle. Place two fingers (usu. index and middle) on the pullback handle (Fig. 10.8)
- Turn the safety lock counterclockwise to the deployment position, symbolized by an open padlock icon. The arrow on the lock will point in the direction the handle will move.
- Ensure that the guidewire, sheath/guide catheter do not move during stent deployment.
- Immobilize the guidewire, sheath/RHV, by holding them in place with the other hand (usu. left).
- While pressing down with the thumb to prevent motion, retract the handle.
- Watch the stent deployment fluoroscopically.

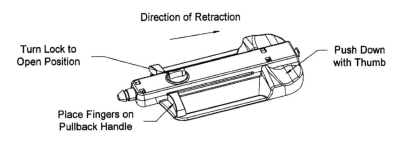

Fig. 10.8 Courtesy Abbott™ (Abbott Vascular, Santa Clara, CA)

- Once stent deployment is complete, re-advance the sheath, and re-lock the delivery system before removal into the sheath/guide catheter. If inserted, remove the funnel introducer from the hemostatic valve, and then remove the delivery system from the patient.
- Ensure that the guidewire and associated EPS remain in position and are not inadvertently retracted.
- If significant difficulty is encountered during handle pullback before the stent is deployed, re-lock the handle and remove the device.
- Perform angiography to confirm satisfactory results of angioplasty and stenting.
- If needed, the stent can be post-dilated. This may achieve good stent position to vessel wall. Take care not to expand the stent past the unconstrained maximum diameter. Post-stent angioplasty can be performed using the previously used Aviator™ plus catheter. If the use of another catheter is desired, consider Viatrac® (Abbott Vascular, Abbott Park, USA); see section "alternatives" for additional details.
- After completion of angioplasty and stenting, recover the EPS as follows.

Selection of Recovery Catheter

- Two types of recovery catheters are provided in the package.

  - The RX ACCUNET™ 2 is low profile and more flexible. This is usually our first choice.
  - The RX ACCUNET™ has a shapeable tip design and may provide torquability and steerability at its tip, in case of more difficult vasculature.

- Never discard the second catheter off the sterile field. Just in case the selected catheter is damaged during use, the second will be available.
- Remove the selected recovery catheter from its dispenser hoop.
- Using a 10-cc syringe with heparinized saline, flush the recovery catheter to remove air. This can be done by aligning the tip of the syringe with the tip of the recovery catheter. Alternatively, attach a leur lock syringe to the distal end of the flush tool. Insert the distal 3 cm of the recovery catheter into the proximal end of the flush tool. Tighten the RHV of the flush tool very lightly and flush gently, until all air is removed.
- Confirm the fluid emanating from the exit notch.
- Ensure that the RHV of the flush tool is not closed on the clear tip area of the recovery catheter.
- When using the shapeable recovery catheter, the distal 3 cm of the catheter may be shaped. Keep the shapeable ribbon on the outside curve. Place the bend at the proximal part of the shaping ribbon (which is the area where the orange catheter body transitions into the clear tip area).

Recovery of the Filter Basket

- Once the angioplasty and stenting has been completed, remove all interventional devices from the guidewire.
- Backload the selected and prepared recovery catheter onto the proximal end of wire and advance the system through the open RHV into the guiding catheter or shuttle sheath.
- While advancing the recovery catheter, do not rotate the recovery catheter more than 90° in either direction, or it may entangle the guidewire.
- Using fluoroscopy, carefully advance the recovery catheter through the deployed stent
- After navigating the recovery catheter through the stent, gently advance the recovery catheter over the filter basket until the radiopaque tip of the catheter just covers the four radiopaque markers on the filter basket. The collapse of the basket will cause these markers to come closer to each other (see Fig. 10.9).
- Do not pull the basket completely into the recovery catheter.
- Hold tension on the guidewire and grasp the recovery catheter. Retract the two devices as a single unit with no movement relative to the catheter or guidewire. Keep observing fluoroscopically to ensure the filter basket does not redeploy.
- If there is an RHV on the guide catheter, ensure it is fully open to facilitate the devices being removed as a single unit.
- Confirm and document angiographically the adequacy of cervical angioplasty and stenting (Figs. 10.10 and 10.11).
- Perform standard AP and lateral views to confirm and document that cerebral vasculature has remained the same as pre-intervention angiography and that there is no complication, e.g., vessel cutoff, indicative of embolism.

Fig. 10.9 Courtesy Abbott™ (Abbott Vascular, Santa Clara, CA)

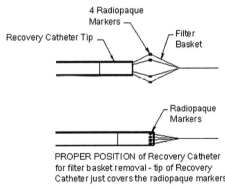

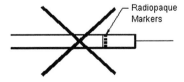

PROPER POSITION of Recovery Catheter for filter basket removal - tip of Recovery Catheter just covers the radiopaque markers

IMPROPER POSITION - Recovery Catheter tip advanced beyond radiopaque markers

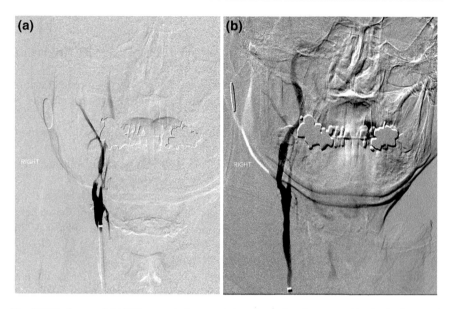

Fig. 10.10 Severe right ICA stenosis in an octagenerian before treatment (**a**). Angioplasty and stenting resulted in satisfactory resolution (**b**). The patient noticed an immediate improvement and indicated he could 'think more clearly'

- If angiography indicates satisfactory results, retract the guide catheter to the femoral artery and perform angiography in ipsilateral oblique (45°) view.
- If the femoral angiography indicates arteriotomy is proximal to the femoral bifurcation and the caliber is ≥ 4 mm, perform angioseal closure.
- If difficulty is encountered in negotiating the stent with the recovery catheter, consider the following:

    - Have the patient move her/his neck from side to side. The movement may re-orient the carotid artery.
    - Adjust the position of the shuttle sheath/guide catheter. The change in position may provide better support or re-orient the catheter tip in a different direction.
    - Insert another guidewire (buddy wire) to straighten the stented area.
    - If using RX Accunet™ shapeable tip recovery catheter, the tip may be shaped to allow it to deflect off stent struts and be maneuvered across bends. To deflect the tip of the catheter, rotate the proximal luer of the recovery catheter up to 90° in either direction. If there is difficulty with negotiating the stent, shape the tip of the catheter in another direction or modify the degree of angulation.
    - Consider using the alternate recovery catheter, if difficulties are encountered in navigation with the initially selected catheter.
    - If stent struts are obstructing the advance of recovery catheter, post-dilate the stent.

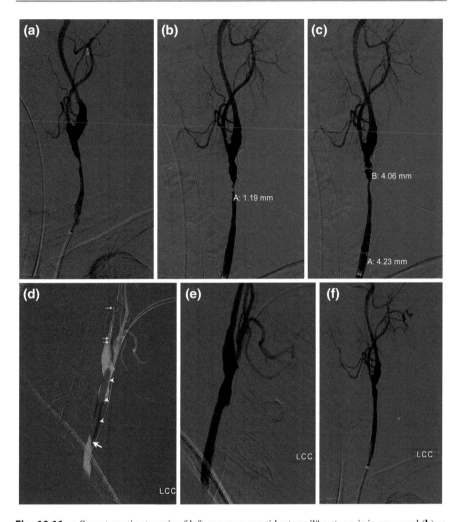

Fig. 10.11 **a** Symptomatic stenosis of left common carotid artery. The stenosis is measured (**b**) as well as, the artery proximal and distal to the stenosis (**c**). Angioplasty and stenting was performed. **d** A saved roadmap image during post-stenting angioplasty. The markers on embolic protection device are visible (*single arrow*), as is its guidewire (*double arrows*). A marker on the guidewire is manifested just superior to the *double arrows*. The shadow (*arrow heads*) is the expanded balloon. The extent of resolution of stenosis can be appreciated by comparing the caliber of the artery before angioplasty and the width of the balloon. The *thick arrow points* to an area of stenosis not covered by the balloon. It was addressed during repeat angioplasty by slightly retracting and repositioning the balloon. **e** Lateral view post-angioplasty and stenting demonstrates significant reconstitution of vessel lumen. Compare it to the lumen (*white*) in the roadmap in (**d**). **f** Post-intervention oblique view demonstrating the resolution of stenosis (compare to Fig. 'a')

- In case difficulty is encountered in retrieving the filter basket, consider the following:

  - A resistance is felt during collapsing the filter basket into the RX Accunet™ two recovery catheters, this may be expected. It is because of a built-in stop in the catheter that causes resistance to be felt when the catheter has been advanced far enough over the filter basket. The stop mechanism is not present in the RX Accunet™ recovery catheter. Therefore, one has to rely solely on angiography to ensure the filter basket is not pulled too far into the recovery catheter.
  - If needed, use a simultaneous push–pull maneuver (push catheter, pull basket).
  - Ensure the tip of recovery catheter is distal to stent before performing this maneuver.
  - If both recovery catheters fail in retrieval, consider using a suitable guide catheter or balloon catheter to recover the device.
  - Do not attempt to retract an uncollapsed filter basket through the stent.
  - If unable to retract the filter basket through the guide catheter, stabilize the filter basket and recovery sheath at the guide catheter tip by tightening down the RHV. Remove the filter basket, guidewire, recovery catheter, and guide catheter as a unit.
  - If filter basket gets entangled or detached in stent, then surgical conversion or collapsing the basket with a second stent may be required.

Postoperative Management and Follow-up

- Admit to NSICU for overnight observation.
- 0.9% NS + 20 meq KCl @ 150 cc/h X 2 h.
- Keep right/left leg (whichever side was used for procedure) straight X 2 h, with head elevated no more than 15°.
- Check groins, DPs, vitals and neurochecks q 15 min X 4, q 30 min X 4, then q hour.
- Plavix 75 mg PO daily X 4 weeks.
- ASA 81–325 mg PO daily.
- Advance diet as tolerated.
- Perform baseline TCDs on POD 1 or within first few days of procedure prior to patients' discharge and repeat at 6 months (at which time any recurrent stenosis is most likely to show up) and then annually.
- Review/resume pre-procedure medications (except oral hypoglycemics). These are best resumed 48 hours after procedure and when good PO intake is established.
- Discharge next morning after mobilizing (if no complications/other ongoing medical concerns requiring hospitalization).
- Follow-up on outpatient basis in 4 weeks.
- Follow-up angiography at 3 months.

Alternative Balloon Dilation Catheters

- In addition to Aviator Plus RX (Cordis Endovascular), other balloon dilatation catheters include RX Viatrac 14 Plus (Abbott Vascular, Abbott Park, USA). Their usage technique and performance are comparable.
- Details for Viatrac 14 Plus are tabulated in Table 10.6. The common measurements are indicated in first row.
- Compliance chart (see Table 10.7) for Viatrac 14 Plus.

Carotid Dissection/Pseudoaneurysm

In traumatic ICA dissections, the procedure is same as that described for carotid stenosis above. However, angioplasty is usually not performed, and therefore, an embolic protection device need not be used. Coils may or may not be used, depending on nature of dissection (Fig. 10.12). Whereas, frequently the apposition

Table 10.6 Viatrac 14 Plus balloon catheter

RX Viatrac 14 Plus catheter lengths (cm): 80 and 135; balloon lengths (mm) 15, 20, 30, 40 mm; nominal pressure (atm) 8; burst pressure (atm) 14; min Guide catheter 6 Fr (0.067″); max guidewire (in.) 0.014

Balloon diameter (mm)	Crossing profile (in)	Prox/distal shaft diameter (Fr)	Min sheath size (Fr)
4.0	0.036	3.3/3.3–2.9	4
4.5	0.037	3.3/3.3–2.9	4
5.0	0.038	3.3/3.3–2.9	5
5.5	0.041	3.3/3.3	5
6	0.043	3.6/3.3	5
6.5	0.048	3.6/3.5	5
7.0	0.049	3.6/3.5	5

Table 10.7 Compliance chart for Viatrac 14 Plus balloon catheter

Balloon size (mm)	Inflation pressure (atm)																	
	2	3	4	5	6	7	8	9	10	11	12	13	14	15	16	17	18
4	3.58	3.68	3.76	3.84	3.9	3.96	4	4.04	4.08	4.11	4.14	4.16	4.19	4.21	4.23	4.26	4.28
4.5	3.88	4	4.11	4.2	4.36	4.43	4.5	4.56	4.61	4.66	4.7	4.75	4.79	4.83	4.87	4.92	4.97
5	4.34	4.47	4.59	4.69	4.83	4.92	5	5.07	5.14	5.21	5.27	5.34	5.4	5.46	5.53	5.6	5.68
5.5	4.94	5.06	5.17	5.26	5.35	5.43	5.5	5.57	5.63	5.68	5.74	5.79	5.84	5.9	5.95	6.01	6.08
6	5.35	5.49	5.62	5.73	5.83	5.92	6	6.07	6.13	6.19	6.24	6.29	6.34	6.39	6.45	6.5	6.56
6.5	5.76	5.93	6.08	6.21	6.32	6.42	6.5	6.57	6.63	6.68	6.73	6.77	6.81	6.85	6.88	6.92	6.97
7	6.23	6.39	6.54	6.67	6.79	6.9	7	7.09	7.18	7.26	7.34	7.41	7.49	7.58	7.66	7.76	7.86

(a)

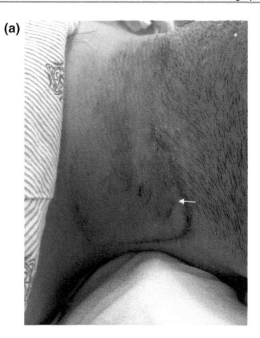

(images continued on pages 147 and 148)

Fig. 10.12 A 35-year-old involved in an MVA where his vehicle crashed into a tree. A bruise across the *left side* of his neck persisted a few days after the accident (**a**, *arrow*). The extent of it was outlined by *ink marking*. The *asterisk* in the *upper right-hand corner* of the picture indicates the patients chin. Subtracted angiography, left ICA, lateral view, demonstrates the outpouching of an aneurysm (**b**, *arrow*). A catheter is appreciated further proximally in the vessel. An enterprise stent was placed across the aneurysm in the ICA. The markers on the rostral and caudal ends of the stent are identified by *arrows* (**c**). The wire upon which the stent was mounted can also be appreciated, its tip rostral to the distal stent markers. The aneurysm was coiled a few days later (**d**). The *short arrow* points to coils filling the aneurysm. The markers on the rostral and caudal ends of the stent are identified by *curved arrows*. The *long thin arrow* points to the proximal marker on the miccrocatheter. The distal marker on the tip of the miccrocatheter is in the aneurysm, amidst the coils loops. The *short thin line* just distal to the indicated proximal marker is on the pusher used to advance coils into the aneurysm. This position of the pusher marker with respect to the proximal marker on catheter indicates that the coil is fully deployed and ready for detachment. Almost a month later, the patient represented with symptoms suggestive of carotidynia, after he forcefully turned his neck during lawn mowing. Imaging demonstrated recurrence of aneurysm. Angiography demonstrates the aneurysm is much larger than at original presentation (**e**). The previously placed coils are obviously compacted (*arrow*). The aneurysm was coiled again (**f**). This resulted in almost immediate resolution of his symptoms. Additionally, an Acculink stent, which had not been available during previous intervention, was placed across the neck of the aneurysm, extending rostrally and caudally, beyond the previously placed stent. The AP and lateral views of interval angiography performed a month later demonstrates the aneurysm continues to remain occluded (**g** and **h**, *arrow*). The same is demonstrated in magnified view (**i**)

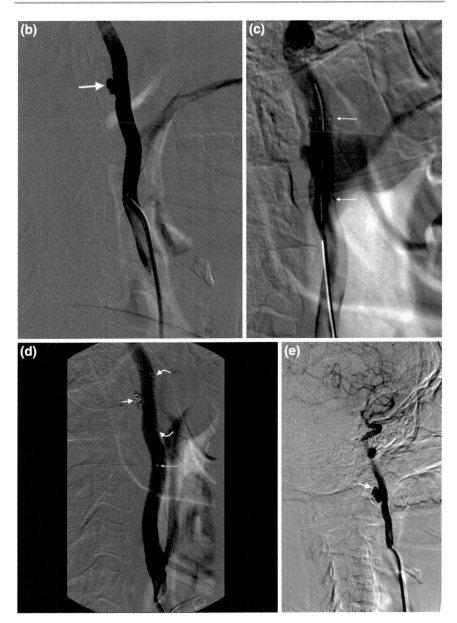

Fig. 10.12 (images continued on next page)

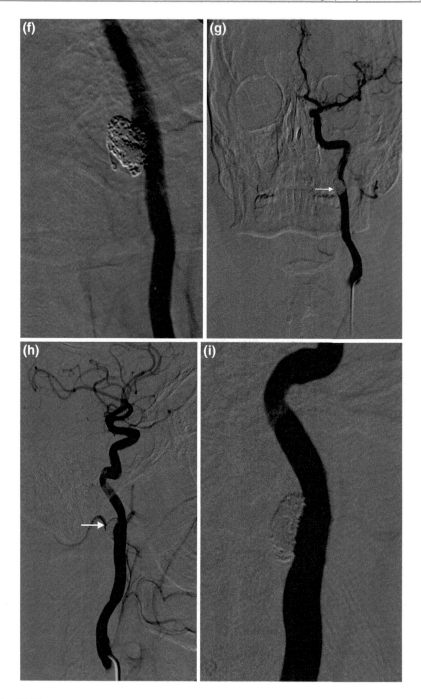

Fig. 10.12

of the layers of vessel wall of injured segment by the radial force of the stent suffices, in case of pseudoaneurysm this may not be enough. In case multiple stents are deployed for appropriate coverage and the dissection is still not cured, in such a situation placement of coils later may prove difficult or no longer possible. Should that occur, consider using Headway 17 microcatheter (MicroVention Inc, Tustin, CA).

- The sequence of procedure after placing shuttle sheath in the carotid is as follows:

  - Advance the appropriate size Acculink over a 0.014 microwire and position the stent across the lesion.
  - Perform angiography to confirm appropriate positioning and repeat angiography every time after stent is adjusted.
  - Remove any slack.
  - Deploy stent as explained above under 'stenting.' Then remove the apparatus
  - If coiling is indicated, advance an Excelsior SL10 Microcatheter (or similar microcatheter) over a 0.014 or 0.010 microwire, e.g., Transend or Synchro2, standard or soft into the aneurysm and perform coiling using previously described technique (see Chap. 12).
  - If needed, additional stents can be deployed across the lesion.

- Postoperative management is same as described for angioplasty and stenting.
- Depending on the size of the vessel, in addition to Acculink, other stent options include Enterprise (Codman), Neuroform (Stryker), and Pipeline (Medtronic). A covered stents, e.g., JoStent Graftmaster (Abbott) is also a consideration.

Suggested Readings

1. Chaloupka JC, et al. Recurrent carotid blowout syndrome: diagnostic and therapeutic challenges in a newly recognized subgroup of patients. AJNR Am J Neuroradiol. 1999;20:1069–77.
2. Kadkhodayan Y, Jeck DT, Moran CJ, Derdeyn CP, Cross DT 3rd. Angioplasty and stenting in carotid dissection with or without associated pseudoaneurysm. AJNR Am J Neuroradiol. 2005;26:2328–35.
3. Package Insert, Guidant RX Accunet™ Embolic protection System.
4. Package Insert, Cordis Aviator™ PLUS percutaneous transluminal angioplast (PTA) balloon dilatation catheter.
5. Package Insert, Jostent GRAFTMASTER with HYDREX Coating System, Abbott Vascular, Santa Clara, CA.

Intracranial Angioplasty and Stenting

11

Indications and Case Selection

- Patient with intracranial stenosis that is symptomatic despite best medical management.
- Focal (as opposed to diffuse) stenosis.
- Accessible lesion, i.e., proximal to A2, M2, P2.

Contraindications

- Congenitally hypoplastic vessel.
- Stenosis $\leq 50\%$ where best medical management has not been attempted.
- Tandem lesions (relative) where angioplasty and stenting of proximal lesion will prove clinically futile, due to the impact of more distal and inaccessible lesions.
- Patients in whom antiplatelet and/or anticoagulant therapy cannot be used.

Preoperative Management

- Verify laboratory values including platelet count, BUN, CR, APTT, PT/INR, and
- ß-HCG for females of reproductive age group.
- In case of renal insufficiency, diabetes, CHF, etc., ensure usage of diluted non-ionic contrast agent and carefully pre-plan to maintain contrast load to minimum.
- Plavix 75 mg PO daily starting 3 days before procedure or
- Plavix 300 mg (4 tablets) PO loading dose (LD) on morning of procedure or
- If unable to administer Plavix in a timely fashion, another option is:
- Abciximab (Rheopro®) in a LD of 0.25 mg/kg followed by continuous IV infusion of 10 µg/kg/min for 12 h and then d/c. Administer Plavix 75 mg PO the same evening and then 75 mg PO daily.

© Springer International Publishing AG 2017
S.H. Khan and A.J. Ringer, *Handbook of Neuroendovascular Techniques*,
DOI 10.1007/978-3-319-52936-3_11

- ASA 81–325 mg PO daily.
- Liquids only on morning of procedure.
- NPO (for ≈6 h) when procedure performed under general anesthesia (GA).
- Obtain informed consent for angiography, angioplasty, and stenting.
- Ensure two IV lines are inserted.
- Position patient on neuroangiography table.
- Attach patient to pulse oximetry and ECG leads for monitoring O_2 saturation, HR, cardiac rhythm, respiratory rate, and BP.

Angioplasty and Stenting

Equipment

Drugs

- 0.9% NS + 20 meq KCl @ 75 cc/h (adjust to higher rate as needed).
- Fentanyl 25–100 µg IV prn.
- Versed 0.5–1 mg IV prn.
- Heparin IV per physician instructions (see 'Technique' below).

Devices

- Micropuncture kit 5 Fr.
- 6 Fr Short sheath (10 cm); use long sheath if tortuous vasculature.
- Guide catheter: 6 Fr Envoy® MPC guide catheter (90 cm).
- Diagnostic catheter: Terumo® front-angled glidecath 5 Fr (for diagnostics, may use Envoy guide catheter for same purpose if intervention anticipated).
- Microwire (exchange length): Transcend EX 0.014 300 Floppy (preferable) or
- Transcend EX 0.014 300 ES.
- Angioplasty: Gateway™ PTA balloon catheter (size: $\leq$ artery proximal and distal to the stenosis).
- Inflation device with manometer.
- Stent: Wingspan™ stent system (size: ={or slightly oversized} than the artery proximal and distal to the stenosis. Length should extend at least 2 mm beyond the proximal and distal aspect of stenosis).
- Rotating hemostasis valve (RHV) and adaptor: 4.
- Syringes 10 cc (at least 3), 20 cc (at least 4), and 3 cc (for ACT and angioplasty balloon preparation).
- Three-way stopcock: 3.
- Torque device.
- Telfa strip.
- Mandrel for shaping microwire tip.
- Angioseal™ closure device.

Technique

- Gain access with micropuncture needle using modified Seldinger technique.
- Using J-wire, exchange for a 6 Fr short sheath.
- Insert 6 Fr short sheath over J-wire (see Chap. 2, Specifics for Micropuncture Technique section) or
- Insert a 6 Fr long sheath if the patient's vascular anatomy is known to be tortuous.
- Secure sheath in position using 2-0 silk suture.
- Administer 5000 IU Heparin IV once the sheath is secured.
- Approximately 20–30 min. later, using a 15-cc syringe, draw 10–15 cc of blood from the sheath and then immediately attach a 3-cc syringe to draw 1–2 cc of blood, which is sent for ACT.
- Blood drawn prior to ACT sample may be returned back to the patient via the sheath, if the distal tip of the sheath is proximal to the cervical vasculature.
- Check ACT hourly throughout the procedure and administer heparin IV, to maintain an ACT of 300–350.

Preparation of Guide catheter

- Attach an RHV to the hub of a 6 Fr Envoy® guide catheter.
- Attach a three-way stopcock to the sidearm of RHV.
- Connect the heparinized saline flush line (6000 IU/1000 ml) to the three-way stopcock (in line with RHV sidearm).
- Ensure the entire saline flush system is free of any air bubbles.
- Ascertain all connections are secure and will not fall apart during procedure.
- Leave the third port of the stopcock (which is perpendicular to RHV sidearm) for contrast administration, etc.
- Introduce a glidewire (with its coating already activated by lubrication in saline) through the hub of the RHV into the guide catheter.
- Allow the flush system to run fast until it is ascertained that there are no air bubbles in the system, including the guide catheter.

Insertion of Guide catheter

- Ensure the tip of the glidewire™ is not extending beyond the tip of the guide catheter.
- Introduce the guide catheter through the hub of the sheath.
- Push in the glidewire™ so that it extends ahead of the tip of the guide catheter in the lumen of blood vessel.
- Advance the catheter under fluoroscopic guidance, with the guidewire leading.
- Complete diagnostic imaging if not already done (refer to cerebral angiography for details).
- [For diagnostic angiography, a Terumo® 5 Fr front-angled glidecath may be used. However, this will require removal and exchange for a guide catheter following completion of diagnostic study. In the interest of saving time, using an Envoy® guide catheter for diagnostic purposes is very reasonable in unchallenging anatomy].

- Ensure the cervical vasculature is included in the diagnostic study in order to be cognizant of any asymptomatic pathology, e.g., stenosis or atherosclerotic plaque.
- Study the vessel with pathology last, so that the Envoy® guide catheter will not require re-navigation.
- In case diagnostic imaging is already available, position the guide catheter straightaway to provide support in the vessel of interest, e.g., in internal carotid artery (ICA) for ICA, middle cerebral artery (MCA), or anterior cerebral artery (ACA) stenosis, remaining proximal to the lesion.
- Measure the length and width of stenosis on angiogram.
- Select an angioplasty balloon that is ≤ the size (breadth) of the artery proximal and distal to the stenosis.
- Select a stent that is equal to or slightly greater in caliber than the size of the artery proximal and distal to the stenosis. The length of the stent should extend at least 2 mm beyond the proximal and distal aspect of Stenosis.
- Prior to starting intervention, again ensure the guide catheter is appropriately positioned to support the angioplasty microcatheter and stent systems.

Preparation of PTA Balloon Catheter for Angioplasty

- Two sterilely draped tables positioned end to end and free of clutter are used to support the length of the interventional devices.
- Place the balloon catheter on the preparation table using sterile precautions.
- Lubricate the balloon catheter system in its protective hoop using heparinized 0.9% NS.
- Remove the balloon catheter from its protective hoop and place it on the table, placing sterile towels on the catheter if necessary, to keep it secure and extended along its length.
- Remove the stylet from the distal tip of the catheter.
- Attach a syringe with heparinized normal saline (NS) to the hub of the catheter and flush the catheter, until NS drops are noted at the distal tip of the catheter.
- Place a 0.014" Transend™ wire on the preparation table using sterile precautions.
- Irrigate the wire in its protective hoop, using the portal provided.
- Backload the stiff end of the wire into the distal tip of the angioplasty catheter, until it emerges from the hub of the catheter.
- Now, gently grasp the stiff end of the wire at the hub and pull it out until only a few cm of wire extends beyond the distal tip of catheter.
- Using a mandrel, shape the distal tip of the microwire to enable easy navigation to the stenosis.
- Withdraw the tip of the wire into the distal tip of the catheter, such that there is no wire extending beyond the catheter tip.
- Ensure the wire does not get kinked during manipulation.
- Remove the balloon protector from the distal tip of the angioplasty catheter by sliding it off.
- Take a 3-cc syringe containing contrast and heparinized NS in 2/3 and 1/3 concentration and attach it to a three-way stopcock.
- Attach the stopcock to the balloon port (the sidearm of the angioplasty catheter).

- Hold the syringe with the nozzle pointing down and aspirate for 5 seconds to remove air from the balloon and then release the plunger.
- Close the stopcock to the balloon and disconnect the syringe and evacuate air from the syringe.
- Reconnect the syringe to stopcock, open the stopcock to the balloon. Re-aspirate and release plunger, until bubbles no longer appear.
- If bubbles persist, do not use the system.
- Detach the syringe after air purgation is complete.
- Lubricate the balloon catheter shaft to activate the hydrophilic coating.

Preparation of Inflation Device with Manometer

- Fill a 20-cc syringe with 15 cc contrast and 5 cc heparinized NS (2/3:1/3 concentration).
- Attach a three-way stopcock to the inflation device and connect the syringe containing contrast medium to the sideport of the stopcock.
- Aspirate the contrast into the inflation device, leaving only 1–2 cc within the syringe.
- Purge any air out of the barrel and tubing of the inflation device, all the way to the distal portal of the stopcock.
- Leave the inflation device on table, until needed.

Deployment of PTA Balloon Catheter for Angioplasty

- Attach the hub of the balloon catheter to an RHV such that the proximal tip of the microwire in the catheter extends out from the hub of the RHV.
- Ensure the balloon catheter is continuously flushed with heparinized NS via the sideport of the RHV attached to a three-way stopcock which connects to the tubing of the flush system.
- Ensure there are no air bubbles in the balloon catheter and that NS is dripping continuously from its distal tip.
- Ensure the distal tip of the microwire is not extending beyond the tip of balloon catheter.
- Loosen the knob of the RHV attached to the guide catheter and carefully insert the balloon catheter through it.
- Tighten the knob of RHV again, so that a seal is created around the balloon catheter, but it can still be advanced through the guide catheter without any difficulties.
- Once the distal aspect of balloon catheter is within the lumen of guide catheter, advance the microwire so that it leads the balloon catheter.
- Continue to advance the balloon catheter and wire assembly until the proximal markings on the balloon catheter align with the hub of the guide catheter RHV. This alignment indicates that the balloon catheter tip has reached the distal tip of the Guide catheter.
- Perform fluoroscopy to confirm location of the microcatheter, wire, and guide catheter.

- Perform angiography to visualize the stenosis using the free port of the stopcock connected in the guide catheter system and select the appropriate working views for treating the lesion
- Attach a torque device to the guidewire.
- Using road map guidance, advance the wire with constant half rotatory motion to cross the lesion.
- Ensure there is adequate length of wire distal to the lesion.
- Advance the balloon catheter over the wire using road map guidance.
- The two marker bands on the distal aspect of the balloon catheter tip which indicate the proximal and distal ends of the angioplasty balloon are positioned across the lesion.
- Confirm appropriate positioning by visualizing the marker for the tip of the balloon catheter, followed by the two marker bands indicating either end of the angioplasty balloon. For better visualization of markers, also use native imaging and magnification as necessary.
- Perform angiography to ascertain appropriate positioning of the balloon relative to the stenosis.
- Repeat angiography every time the position of the balloons is adjusted, until completely satisfied with the position of the balloon.
- Recover the inflation device from the table.
- Use the distal free port of the stopcock attached to the inflation device (which is in line with the inflation device) to make a wet (meniscus to meniscus) connection to the balloon port of the balloon catheter.
- Ensure that this connection is secure so that it will not disconnect during angioplasty.
- Close the stopcock to the inflation device.
- Aspirate the syringe (with nozzle pointing down) attached to the sideport of the stopcock to purge air out of the balloon angioplasty system.
- Slowly release the plunger of the syringe, so that the air is replaced with the contrast left in syringe for purpose. Repeat this step once, or twice.
- Close the stopcock to syringe.
- Reconfirm balloon position fluoroscopically.
- Using the chart provided with the balloon catheter, slowly begin inflating the angioplasty balloon, utilizing the balloon inflation device. For example, to perform an angioplasty to 1.57 mm using a 1.5 mm balloon, slowly inflate to 9.0 atm.
- Inflate the balloon slowly, by turning the screw provided on the inflation device at a rate ≤ 1 atm/15 s (to 'stretch' not 'crack' the vessel).
- Step on fluoroscopy pedal frequently to visualize progression of angioplasty.
- During inflation, the balloon may acquire a 'waist' due to vessel segment stenosis. This resolves with the progression of angioplasty.
- Once the goal pressure is reached, deflate the device.
- Confirm complete balloon deflation fluoroscopically.
- In order to achieve complete deflation, you may need to open the stopcock to the syringe and vigorously aspirate. Close the stopcock to syringe while aspiration is fully applied.
- Confirm complete balloon deflation fluoroscopically.
- Perform f/u angiography to evaluate results of angioplasty.
- If needed, repeat the angioplasty.

Removal of PTA Balloon Catheter

- Confirm that the balloon is completely deflated by visualizing fluoroscopically.
- Make sure not to lose wire access across lesion during catheter removal.
- Loosen the knob of the RHV attached to the Guide catheter.
- Under continuous fluoroscopy, begin catheter withdrawal, while the microwire remains in position across the lesion.
- This is a two-person maneuver: One operator controls the balloon catheter at the hub of the guide catheter RHV and the second operator withdraws the balloon catheter over the wire, while constantly observing the tip of the wire on the monitor to ensure it is not withdrawn inadvertently.
- The first operator is responsible for stepping on the fluoroscopy pedal until the catheter successfully exits the RHV of the guide catheter.
- The entire assembly is kept straight to ensure adequate control and maneuverability.
- The second operator progressively steps away from the first, to keep the system straight while withdrawing the catheter over the wire.
- Be vigilant to ensure the wire or catheter is not contaminated during the process by coming into contact with unsterile surfaces.
- As soon as the distal tip of the balloon catheter exits the hub of RHV, the first operator grabs the wire and secures it by forming a loop and holding it just next to the hub. The RHV knob is tightened around the wire. Then, the first operator uses a moist Telfa™ strip to wipe off the extraneous wire from RHV and toward the outer end, as the second operator completes the removal of the catheter of the wire. The second operator may receive the Telfa from the first operator, to wipe off the wire more within her/his reach.
- Wipe off the balloon catheter with heparinized NS and store in a bowl with the same solution, in case it may be required for reuse.
- Maintain wire access across lesion for the next step of advancing the stent.

Selection of Appropriate Gateway™ Stent

- Study the angiogram to select the appropriate size of stent.
- Measure the normal vessel diameter proximal and distal to the lesion. Select a stent that measures the normal size of the vessel. If needed, a slightly oversized stent may be selected. However, ***do not*** undersize the stent since that will risk dislodgement from intended location of deployment.
- The length of the stent should be such that at least 2 mm of the stent extends proximal and distal to the lesion, e.g., for a vessel with a diameter of 4.4 mm and a lesion length of 4 mm, use a 4.5 mm stent (which expands to 4.9 mm) with a 9 mm length (see table for sizing guidelines).

Preparation of Gateway™ Stent

- Open the pouch and transfer the packaging tray to the preparation table under sterile precautions.
- Examine the system to rule out any damage.

- Using a 15-cc syringe, flush the dispenser hoop with saline.
- Carefully pull out the proximal hub aspect of the system from the tray.
- Locate the rotating hemostatic valve of the outer body and tighten it onto the inner body of the stent system.
- Now, transfer entire system out onto the table from the tray and dispenser hoop.
- Inspect the stent delivery system for any damage or flaws.
- Inspect to ensure that the stent is preloaded into the distal tip of the system.
- Locate the hub of the inner body, which is the most proximal aspect of the system, and attach an RHV to it.
- Flush the lumen of the inner body with heparinized saline.
- Loosen the previously tightened RHV of the outer body and flush the lumen of the outer body with heparinized saline to purge air from the system.
- Gently advance the pusher of the inner body of the system until the proximal radiopaque marker band bumper is just proximal to the stent.
- Re-tighten the RHV of outer body to lock onto the inner body, so that the entire system will move as a single unit.
- There is an option of connecting heparinized saline flush to the sideports of the RHVs of the outer and inner bodies.

Deployment of Gateway™ Stent

- Fluoroscopically, ascertain that the guidewire is still across the lesion.
- Perform angiography in working view.
- Backload the stent system onto the guidewire.
- Loosen the hub of the RHV of the guide catheter and advance the stent system into it.
- When the stent system is just within the tip of the guide catheter, perform a roadmap to assist in navigation.
- Advance the stent system over the guidewire until the stent crosses the lesion and the distal marker bands on the stent are just distal to the lesion.
- At this point, ascertain the positions of the following: distal tip of the guidewire, distal marker bands on the distal tip of the stent, proximal marker band on the stent pusher/bumper
- The distal tip of the guidewire should be crossing the lesion and well distal to the distal marker bands on the stent.
- The distal marker bands on the stent should be just distal to the distal aspect of the lesion.
- The proximal marker band should be proximal to the lesion.
- Perform angiography and adjust position of stent if needed, until satisfied with its position.
- Repeat angiography after each adjustment.
- Loosen the RHV valve of the outer body and slightly withdraw the hub of the outer body until the stent is directly aligned with the lesion. Tighten the RHV and if needed pull back on the system to ensure that all slack has been removed and the system is completely straight.

- Perform angiography to ascertain satisfactory final position. Ensure that the vessel distal to the lesion is visualized.
- Loosen the RHV of the outer body.
- Now, deploy stent under continuous fluoroscopy as follows:
- Keep the inner body hub stationary with one hand.
- Continue to withdraw the hub of the outer body with the other hand.
- Visualize the marker band at the distal end spread out into multiple smaller markers, indicating the opening of the stent.
- Continue deployment in a smooth motion until the stent is completely deployed.
- Do not attempt to move the stent or advance the outer body once the deployment is underway.
- After completion of deployment, re-tighten the RHV of the outer body and gently withdraw the entire system maintaining wire access across the lesion.
- Once the system is out of the guide catheter RHV, secure the wire, stop fluoroscopy, and remove the system off the wire. This is a two-person procedure.
- Perform angiography to ascertain satisfactory result before giving up wire access.
- Withdraw the guidewire.
- Perform standard AP and lateral cerebral angiography. Rule out any vessel cut off or change in comparison with pre-procedure angiogram, which may be indicative of embolism.
- Retract the guide catheter to the femoral artery and perform femoral angiogram in $\approx 45°$ ipsilateral oblique view.
- If the arteriotomy is proximal to femoral bifurcation and the vessel size is ≥ 4 mm, perform closure with angioseal.
- Clean and dress site.
- Break sterile operating field.

Problems Encountered During Angioplasty and Solutions

Table 11.1 shows some problems and solutions during angioplasty.

Table 11.1 Problems/solutions during angioplasty

Problem	Solution
Balloon catheter will not move forward despite advancing it This may be consequent to the guide catheter losing its position and dropping back into the ECA, CCA, or further proximally	• Locate the tip of the Guide catheter. In case it has dropped down, loosen the hub of the RHV attached to the Guide catheter • Remove the redundancy in the system by pulling back the balloon catheter and wire concurrently, until the loops are gone and the system is straightened out • Advance the guide catheter over the microcatheter and microwire back into its intended position

(continued)

Table 11.1 (continued)

Problem	Solution
Unable to cross the lesion with the balloon catheter	• Use a smaller size balloon catheter to cross the lesion • Perform angioplasty to 'pre-dilate' the lesion • Then, re-attempt deployment of the balloon catheter of intended size
Disconnection of inflation device during angioplasty	• Attach large barrel syringe to balloon (side) port of catheter and aspirate to completely deflate balloon prior to withdrawal
Lack of flow distal to angioplasty on f/u angiography. This is probably due to acute vasospasm caused by the angioplasty	• Maintain wire access across the lesion • Rapidly deploy the stent across the lesion • Consider repeating the angioplasty
Proximal portion/tip of guidewire contaminated by touching unsterile surface, e.g., the injector or IV poles during angioplasty The maintenance of wire access across the lesion is imperative. Therefore, the wire must not be withdrawn and discarded	• Use an alcohol swab to wipe off the exposed wire. As extra precaution, repeat wipe with a second swab

Problems Encountered During Stenting and Solutions

Table 11.2 shows some problems and solutions during angioplasty.

Table 11.2 Problems/solutions during stenting

Problem	Solution
Difference in size of vessel proximal and distal to stent	• Choose a stent using the larger size measured, e.g., basilar artery measures 4 mm and PCA is 2 mm. The size of the stent should be ≥ 4 mm
Resistance in advancing the stent system	• Ensure the system is straight to remove any excessive tension build up in the system. Slightly retract the stent system and guidewire to remove any tension or redundancy • Check that the guide catheter is positioned adequately to support the system. If not, advance it forward • If there are any loops in the stent system, straighten them out • Use a soft (floppy) guidewire which enables easy maneuverability of the stent system rather than the more firm support guidewires • Ensure that the flush system is functioning • Once the stent system is advancing, continue to advance it even if it goes distal to the lesion because it is easier to move the system from distal to proximal location than vice versa • If inordinate resistance continues despite corrective maneuvers, consider possibility of damage to the guidewire from use and discard it for a new wire. At the same time, examine and consider replacing the stent system with a new one as well

(continued)

Table 11.2 (continued)

Problem	Solution
Feeling of resistance during deploying stent	• Some resistance is usually encountered and expected. However, if the resistance is excessive, check to ensure the entire system is straight and there is no tension buildup. Slightly retract the system and guidewire to remove excessive tension • Check the position of the guide catheter to ensure that it is providing adequate support. If not, advance it further up. • If excessive tension persists, consider discarding the stent system and replacing it with a new system. If deployment is already underway, do not attempt to re-sheath the stent. Complete the deployment
Loss of position during deployment	• If the stent has migrated distally, it may be possible to carefully pull back the entire system as deployment is taking place until it is back in the desirable location. Then, continue with the deployment. If any difficulty is encountered in the retraction, just deploy the stent in its current location. Then, deploy a second stent to cover the desired location • In case the stent has migrated proximal to the lesion while deployment is underway, **_do not_** attempt to push it forward to its intended location. Just deploy it maintaining wire access and then use an additional stent to cover the more distal site
Only partial coverage of lesion by the stent	• Maintain guidewire access across the lesion. Discard the used stent system. Bring a new system into the field, which should be ≥ length from the first system. Deploy the second stent within the first (telescoping) so that the entire lesion is covered including at least 2 mm of normal vessel on either side
Resistance during retraction of system following stent deployment	• Ensure the entire system (inside and outside the patient) is straight and there is no tension buildup. Slightly retract the system and guidewire to remove excessive tension • Maintain guidewire access at all times across the lesion • If tension persists, loosen the RHV of the outer body of the stent system and pull back the hub of the inner body, until its tip is in contact with the tip of the outer body. Re-tighten the RHV of the outer body and remove the entire stent system
Breakage/mechanical failure of stent during deployment	• If the stent is only partially deployed and still partially sheathed, consider retracting the entire system along with the stent outside the patient or, if complete retraction is not possible, retracting to deploy the stent in a more neutral location, e.g., ECA or its branches • In case the stent is completely outside the sheath, retract and discard the stent system. Introduce a microcatheter (e.g., Excelsior SL 10 or Prowler Plus) over the wire. Use the microcatheter to introduce an alligator snare or a similar retrieval device. Engage the stent with the snare and advance the microcatheter forward to secure the grip on the stent, positioned at the tip of the microcatheter. If possible, withdraw the stent, snare, and microcatheter simultaneously into the guide catheter. Once within the guide catheter, remove the stent, snare, and microcatheter all together. If the stent cannot be retracted into the guide catheter, maintain it at the tip of the catheter and pull out the entire system.

Indication and Choice of Balloons and Stents

- For atherosclerosis use Gateway™.
- For aneurysms use Enterprise™ or Neuroform™.

For intracranial ICA stenosis:

- Balloon system: Gateway™ PTA balloon catheter.
- Stent system: Wingspan™ stent system, Neuroform™ stent system.
- See Table 11.3 for sizing guidelines for Wingspan stent system.

Table 11.3 Sizing guidelines for Wingspan stent system

Sizing guidelines for Wingspan stent system

Labeled stent diameter (mm)	Labeled stent length (mm)	Maximum diameter of expansion (mm)	Vessel diameter (mm)	Useable length of delivery system (cm)	Maximum guidewire diameter	Minimum Guide catheter internal diameter
2.5	9	2.8	>2.0 and ≤ 2.5	135	0.36 mm (0.014 in)	1.63 mm (0.064 in)
	15					
	20					
3.0	9	3.4	>2.5 and ≤ 3.0			
	15					
	20					
3.5	9	3.9	>3.0 and ≤ 3.5			
	15					
	20					
4.0	9	4.4	>3.5 and ≤ 4.0			
	15					
	20					
4.5	9	4.9	>4.0 and ≤ 4.5			
	15					
	20					

Postoperative Management and Follow-up

- Admit to NSICU for overnight observation.
- 0.9% NS + 20 meq KCl @ 150 cc/h × 2 h.
- Keep right/left leg (whichever side was used for procedure) straight × 2 h, with head of bed elevated ≤ 15°.
- Check groins, DP's, vitals, and neuro checks q 15 min × 4, q 30 min × 4, then q h
- Plavix 75 mg PO daily × 4 weeks.
- ASA 81–325 mg PO daily.
- Advance diet as tolerated.
- Review/resume pre-procedure medications.
- D/c next morning after mobilizing (if no complications/other ongoing medical concerns requiring hospitalization).
- F/u on outpatient basis in 4 weeks.
- Perform F/u angiography at 3 months, 6 months, 1 year, and 2 years post-procedure.
- Case examples are shown in Figs. 11.1 and 11.2.

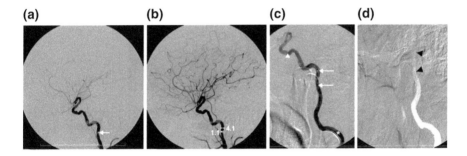

(a) **(b)** **(c)** **(d)**

Fig. 11.1 Intracranial angioplasty and stenting. **a** Severe intracranial stenosis of right ICA (*arrow*). **b** The stenosis is measured as 1.1 mm, while the normal arterial diameter distally is 4.1 mm. A 4.5 X 9 mm stent was selected. **c** Angioplasty balloon is in position. There is good wire access across the lesion with the tip of wire in the carotid siphon (*arrow head*). The distal marker on the angioplasty balloon is distal to the stenosis, and the proximal marker lies proximal to the lesion (*arrows*). The tip of the supporting Guide catheter is appreciated much proximally in the ICA (*asterisk*). **d** Stent following successful deployment. The radiological markers on the tines have separated out (*arrowheads*)

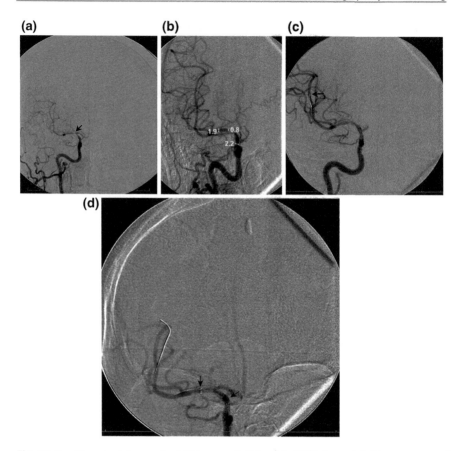

Fig. 11.2 a Stenosis at the proximal M1 segment of the right MCA (*arrow*). **b** Measurements of the breadth of normal blood vessel proximal and distal to the stenosis. The stenosis (0.8 mm) is also measured out. The appropriate length of stent would be one that extends 2 mm beyond the stenotic lesion both proximally and distally, and the diameter should be >2.2 mm (Fig. 11.2a, b reprinted with permission from [1]). **c** Good wire purchase with the tip (*arrow*) well distal to the lesion. A good purchase is highly desirable for undertaking angioplasty and stenting. **d** Stent deployment following angioplasty. The *arrows* point to the proximal and distal markers of the expanded stent

Suggested Reading

Khan SH, Ringer AJ. Technique of angioplasty and stent placement in acute ischemic stroke. J Neurol Res. 2011;1(3):81–9.

Treatment of Aneurysms

12

Location-Specific Considerations

Anterior Communicating Aneurysm

- Shape the tip of the microwire into a lazy 'S' or 'Shephard's crook' shape as shown, to assist in navigation.

Posterior Communicating Aneurysm

- Shape the tip of the microwire to a 'C' shape by giving a bend to the wire at the tip and then another bend further proximally.

Some Current Choices of Coils and Indications

1. Bare Platinum Coils, e.g., GDC®

   - The most commonly used coil type.

   - Available as standard, soft, and ultra-soft. The firmness or rigidity in these types is dependent upon the amount of platinum used in the coil, i.e., the lesser the platinum, softer the coil.

© Springer International Publishing AG 2017
S.H. Khan and A.J. Ringer, *Handbook of Neuroendovascular Techniques*,
DOI 10.1007/978-3-319-52936-3_12

- Effective and perhaps most straight forward to deploy.

- The size and length of coil chosen for deployment depends upon the size of aneurysm.

- A thicker (0.018″, 0.038 cm) and firmer coil such as standard GDC 18 is best deployed in a large, unruptured aneurysm.

- GDC 10 (0.010″, 0.025″ cm thick) is more commonly used.

- Table 12.1 indicates various coil diameters and examples of microcatheters to be used based on these.

- The framing coil should preferably be 'standard' and the size large enough to cover the circumference of the aneurysm.

- Soft and ultra-soft coils are usually deployed later on during the coiling or as 'finishing' coils, when standard coils become more difficult to deploy in aneurysm or do not stay within confines of the aneurysm.

- The size and length of the coil selected progressively decreases as coil embolization progresses. Usually, the framing coil is the largest and longest coil.

- Recently, Target® (Stryker Neurovascular, Fremont, CA) coils have been introduced as an alternative/replacement for GDC. Target coils are considered to cause less 'microcatheter' kickback toward the end of coiling.

2. Hydrocoil® Embolic System

- Hydrocoils® are coated with hydophilic gel that expands upon contact with blood. The principle is that the gel takes up and obliterates the inevitable space between coils.
- The hydrocoil should initially be advanced into a bowl of warm Ringer's lactate to soften it. Once the coil is noted to curl up more readily, it is retracted back into its sheath, then advanced through the microcatheter, and deployed within the aneurysm.
- Deployment should not take long (e.g., more than 5 min), as the coil may expand within the microcatheter requiring removal of the occluded catheter.

Table 12.1 Various coil sizes and examples of microcatheters to be used with each

Coil/guidewire diameter/thickness (inches)	microcatheter
0.010–0.012	Excelsior SL-10®; Prowler 10®
0.014	Prowler 14®
0.018	Excelsior 1018®; Prowler Plus®

- Extra care is taken to keep the microcatheter free of blood, to prevent premature expansion of coils within the microcatheter. To this end, a two-way stopcock is placed between the RHV and microcatheter hub. The two-way stopcock is 'closed' to microcatheter when the RHV is opened to introduce the coil and it is then 'opened' to advance the coil into the microcatheter, after tightening the microcatheter RHV to the extent that the coil can be advanced with ease, but blood will not reflux back into the catheter.
- The microcatheter is kept free of blood at all times.
- Perhaps the best aneurysm obliteration results are achieved with hydrocoils.
- Hydrocoils are associated with headaches in some patients. Theses headaches may respond to a short course of steroids.

3. Matrix® Coils

- These coils are coated with a copolymer, which upon hydrolysis induces inflammatory response.
- Of the three coil types, these are most associated with aneurysm residuals and recurrence. We no longer use them.

Coil Embolization

Indications and Case Selection

- Posterior circulation aneurysms, which include those of posterior communicating artery (per ISUIA data).
- For coiling, the aneurysm should usually be larger than 5 mm.
- Anterior circulation aneurysms in a WFNS grade III or IV patient, if technically amenable to endovascular intervention.
- Anterior circulation aneurysms that are anatomically challenging from an open surgical approach.
- Patient preference in anterior circulation aneurysms.
- Recurrent aneurysm when previously coiled.
- Incompletely clipped aneurysm (not always feasible for coiling).
- A wide-necked aneurysm may be made amenable to coiling by stent placement across the neck, or using a balloon catheter.

Preoperative Management

- ASA 325 mg on morning of procedure (in elective unruptured aneurysms).

- Verify laboratory values including platelet count, BUN, CR, APTT, PT/INR, and ß-HCG (in pre-menopausal females).
- Liquids only on morning of procedure.
- NPO (for ≈6 h) when the procedure is to be performed under general anesthesia.
- Continue prescribed medications (including ASA and anti-hypertensives).
- Insert 2 IV lines.

Equipment

- Rotating hemostatic valves (two).
- Fluid delivery system (for sheath, catheter, and microcatheter).
- Pressure tubing 12″ (for connection between injector and diagnostic/guide catheter).
- Low pressure tubing (3, i.e., for sheath, guide catheter, and microcatheter).
- Injector syringe 150 ml.
- Syringes (20 ml; 3; 10 ml; 3).
- Fluoroscope band bag.
- Transducer 30 ml/min (for each heparinized saline flush system; usually 3, i.e., for sheath, diagnostic/guide catheter and microcatheter).
- 1% lidocaine + syringe with 18G and 22G needles (for local anesthesia).
- Single-wall needle 18G or micropuncture kit.
- Sheath, e.g., Terumo 6 Fr 10 cm.
- 2-0 Silk suture.
- Diagnostic catheter, e.g., Terumo® 5-Fr angled catheter.
- Guidewire, e.g., Terumo® angled glidewire 0.035 150 cm.
- Codman 6 Fr Envoy® MPC 90 cm (or alternatively, 6-Fr Neuron Select™ catheter (Penumbra) with 5-Fr H1 Neuron catheter (Penumbra).
- Microguidewire Transcend Ex 182 cm or Synchro2 200 cm.
- microcatheter Excelsior® (1010, 1016 or 1018, depending on size of aneurysm and the coils intended to be used).
- Coil Detacher.
- Coils, e.g., GDC® (Stryker Neurovascular, Fremont, CA), Microplex® (Microvention, Tustin, CA), Hydrocoil® (Microvention), Target® (Stryker Neurovascular), Barricade™ (Blockade Medical, Irvine, CA).
- Angioseal closure device (St Judes Medical, St Paul, MN).
- Neuropack.

Technique

- Gain access to femoral artery using modified Seldinger technique.
- Insert 6-Fr short sheath over J-wire.

- The sheath is connected to a continuously running flush of heparinized saline.
- Ensure all flush systems are free of air bubbles and other foreign bodies.
- Secure the sheath to the patient's skin using 2-0 silk suture.
- If the location of the aneurysm is already known or the patient's vasculature is anticipated not to be tortuous, consider proceeding with the guide catheter straight away. Otherwise, a 5-Fr angled catheter is attached to a continuously running flush of heparinized saline that is free of any air.
- Advance a 0.035 angled glidewire into the diagnostic catheter.
- Insert the catheter through the sheath.
- With the guidewire leading, catheterize the vessels and complete the diagnostic imaging, if not already done (see Chap. 11 Intracranial Angioplasty and Stenting for details).
- Retract and remove the diagnostic catheter.
- Attach a 6-Fr envoy guide catheter to the flush system that was previously used by the diagnostic catheter and make sure that there are no air bubbles or foreign bodies in the system.
- Insert the 0.035 angled glidewire into the guide catheter.
- Insert the envoy through the sheath and advance over wire to the vessel of interest, e.g., right ICA for right ophthalmic aneurysm or vertebral artery for basilar tip aneurysm.
- For guide catheter placement, in general select the vessel that will provide the most direct access to the aneurysm.
- Perform 3D angiography and select working views.
- As shown in Fig. 12.1, measure the aneurysm including the widest circumferential diameter (a) of the aneurysm sac, longitudinal measurement from apex to base of aneurysm (b), and the width of the neck of aneurysm (c).

Fig. 12.1 Measurements to be performed during aneurysm coiling include the widest circumferential diameter (**a**) of the aneurysm sac, longitudinal measurement from apex to base of aneurysm (**b**) and the width of the neck of aneurysm (**c**)

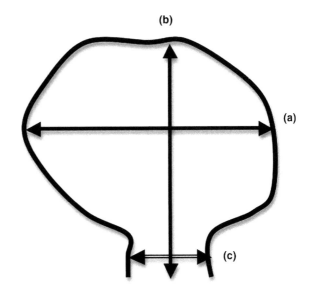

- If the aneurysm is multi-lobulated, then it should be measured as above, or each lobe treated and measured as a separate aneurysm.
- The working views should enable good visualization of the neck of the aneurysm, as well as adjacent vessels to enable safe coil deployment.
- Additionally, the view should also include the tip of the guide catheter, so that the surgeon remains cognizant of its location. If it is displaced downwards during the procedure, it may need to be re-advanced up to its original position to provide stability.
- The microcatheter used for coiling has 2 radiopaque markers at its distal aspect. The distal marker at the tip of the catheter helps guide the tip through the vessels into the aneurysm. The proximal marker indicates when the coil has been completely placed in the aneurysm. When the marker on the pusher just crosses this proximal marker on the microcatheter (to form a 'T'), the coil is ready for detachment. Any further pushing of the coil may cause the pusher itself to enter the aneurysm and rupture it.
- These proximal and distal catheter markers must be visible at all times during positioning of the microcatheter in the aneurysm. If the distal marker becomes difficult to visualize due to the coils placed within the aneurysm, remain cognizant of the position of proximal marker at all times. Ensure that it does not inadvertently move further forward.
- Attach the microcatheter to the flush system, e.g., Excelsior 1018 microcatheter if using 18 coils, with or without smaller coils. We most commonly use Excelsior SL 10 esp. for smaller aneurysms and ruptured larger aneurysms. If a concurrent lesion may require treatment, e.g., an AVM, with its feeding vessel bearing aneurysm/s, then a DMSO compatible microcatheter, e.g., Echelon-10 is used.
- Insert a microguidewire into the microcatheter. We commonly use 0.014 or 0.010 Synchro2 or Transend Microguidewire.
- Advance the microwire tip beyond the catheter tip.
- Shape the tip of wire using the provided mandrel, and then withdraw the tip back into microcatheter. The shape of the microwire tip will depend upon the location of the aneurysm. The most commonly used tip shape is 45°. For access to anterior communicating aneurysms, a 'shepherd's crook' shape is suitable. A 'C' shape is used for posterior communicating artery. Pre-shaped microwires are also available.
- After shaping, retract the wire into the microcatheter.
- Administer heparin 5000 IU IV, after the guide catheter has been positioned. In case of a ruptured aneurysm, we administer the heparin bolus only after the first coil has been successfully detached in the aneurysm.
- Send an ACT approximately 15 min after administration of heparin, and repeat ACT hourly. Aim to maintain the ACT between 250 and 300 s throughout the procedure by administering additional heparin as needed.
- Using fluoroscopy, advance the microcatheter and microguidewire through the guide catheter, until just short of the guide catheter tip.

- Perform roadmapping through the envoy, while the microcatheter is proximal to guide catheter tip in the appropriate working views.
- Navigate the microcatheter over the microwire preferably using two orthogonal views (Fig. 12.2).
- Advance the tip of microcatheter into aneurysm over the microwire.
- Advance and retract the microwire through the catheter tip once or twice, to ensure that the catheter is stable and will not harpoon during coil deployment, nor will it displace when the coil is being advanced.
- Then, remove the microwire completely.
- Obtain roadmapping in the working view selected for coiling. It will show the aneurysm, its neck, and related vessel/s well. This working view may be the same as or different from the projection/s used for navigation to the aneurysm.
- It is important to be able to definitively visualize that the coils are deposited within the aneurysm and are not compromising the adjacent vessels.
- It is also important that all catheters remain stable during the procedure, e.g., if the guide catheter is displaced downward, re-advance it.
- To do this, remove all slack from the system and tighten the RHV of the microcatheter. Loosen the RHV of the guide catheter, and visualizing under fluoroscopy, advance the guide catheter forward, while stabilizing the microcatheter and ensuring it does not move.

(a)   **(b)**

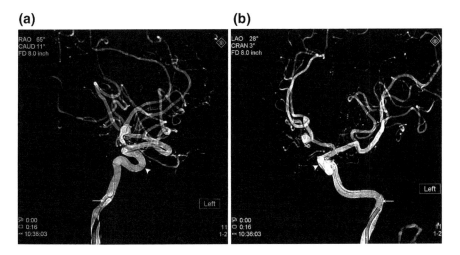

Fig. 12.2 Roadmaps in two orthogonal planes for navigating into the anterior communicating aneurysm. The guide catheter is in the distal cervical ICA, just short of skull base. The microwire is appreciated in the microcatheter (*arrow*). The *arrowhead* points to carotid siphon. The importance of visualization in two planes is demonstrated. The carotid siphon (*arrowhead*) can be navigated well using the (**a**) view, but not (**b**) view. Both working views are oblique (note the projection angles in the *upper left corner*). Conversely for accessing the anterior communicating artery, the oblique view (**b**) is better. Therefore, for accessing the aneurysm, both planes need to be utilized

Coiling

- Aneurysm coiling should preferably be performed with a biplane and usually working views in two planes are required to ensure safe coiling.
- During the procedure, alternately visualize coil deposition in both planes to ensure coils remain within the aneurysm.
- Select the first (framing) coil. We most frequently use GDC® coils.
- The size of the framing coil should be consistent with the diameter of the aneurysm, e.g., if the aneurysm is 6 mm in diameter, select a standard bare platinum coil that has a primary loop diameter of 6 mm, or slightly larger. The length of the coil will also depend on the size of the aneurysm, e.g., for a large aneurysm use the longest coil that you anticipate can be placed within the aneurysm. Therefore, a '6X9' GDC coil indicates that the loop formed by the coil is 6 mm in diameter, while the total length of the coil is 9 cm (i.e., first number [loop] is expressed in mm and the second [length] in cm).
- Prepare coils as follows:
- Remove the coil from containing plastic ring.
- 'Unlock' the sheath. This involves sliding off the black plastic piece on Hydrocoil® embolic system (Microvention, Inc., Tustin, CA) or twisting the proximal end of sheath in clockwise direction at the crimped site on GDC® or Matrix® coils (Stryker Neurovascular, Fremont, CA).
- Advance the coil out into a bowl of warm lactated Ringer's solution.
- Withdraw the coil back into its sheath after soaking for 15–30 secs to soften it.
- In case of Hydrocoils™, check that the detachment system is functional prior to coil insertion: the light will turn green on detachment mechanism, when proximal end of coil is inserted into detacher. DO NOT press detacher button during this test.
- Using road mapping, advance the first coil as a framing coil. As indicated above, the dimensions of the primary loop of this coil should be close to aneurysm size. We usually use a coil equal to the diameter of the aneurysm, or slightly larger.
- The coil is completely within the aneurysm once the marker on the coil pusher (that looks like a small line on the monitor) crosses the proximal marker (a dot) on microcatheter tip, forming a 'T.' The limbs of the 'T' should be perfectly abutted, such that there is no space between them (indicating the pusher in too far out). Nor should the vertical limb of the 'T' lie on either side of the dot on the catheter, indicating that the coil is not completely out of the microcatheter.
- After the coil is completely deployed, perform angiography to ensure the coil is positioned adequately and is within the aneurysm.
- If satisfied with coil deployment, detach the coil using the specific system provided for the purpose. It may be noted that detachment devices differ for different coil brands.
- For GDC system, it comprises of a detachment box and two cables (black and red).

- The detachment box is mounted on a pole preferably attached to the angio table. Or, it can be positioned on an independent pole, as long as care is taken, that this will not result in any problems, if the angio table is moved.
- Ensure the box has a fresh battery that is working.
- One end of each cable is plugged into the indicated slot on the detachment box. Maintain sterile precautions and ensure that the parts of the cables that will be on the operating field are not contaminated.
- Attach a sterile 18–22G needle to the other end of the black (ground) cable and partially insert the needle into the patient's thigh. Make sure that the femoral nerve and vessels are avoided.
- Turn 'on' the detachment box.
- The other end of the red coil is clipped onto the outer end of the coil pusher, once the coil has been deployed and is ready for detachment. Make sure that this attachment is performed right at the tip/end of the pusher.
- Press the button on the box to initiate detachment. A beeping sound will indicate that the coil has detached from the pusher.
- Turn 'off' the detachment box.
- Step on fluoroscopy as the pusher is withdrawn from the catheter. Once it is confirmed that the pusher did indeed detach from the coil (demonstrated by the coil maintaining its position, as the pusher alone is seen to retract). After confirmation of actual detachment, the rest of the pusher can be withdrawn without using fluoroscopy. Rarely, the coil does not detach, in which case after confirming suitable positioning detachment is attempted again.
- The first or 'framing' coil attempts to cover the entire circumference of the aneurysm (Fig. 12.3).
- The rest of the coils are deployed largely within the framing coil (Fig. 12.4).
- If the framing coil is well placed, further usage of road mapping for the following coils may not be required, as long as the coils are deposited within the confines of the framing coil (Fig. 12.3). Additionally, the frequency of angiography during deployment of additional coils may also be decreased. In short, live fluoroscopy alone may suffice, as long as the coil being deployed remains within the perimeter created by the framing coil.
- Otherwise, periodically perform angiography to verify unimpeded flow through adjacent arteries. If there is doubt about whether the coil is within vessel lumen vs aneurysm, perform angiography with the axis of projection same as that of the blood vessel as if 'looking down the barrel of a gun.'
- Complete coiling is indicated by an angiogram demonstrating a lack of filling of the aneurysm or complete obliteration of aneurysm by coils (Fig. 12.4).
- Do not attempt to place further coils into aneurysm beyond this point.
- We have noted that the tip of the microcatheter is progressively pushed out of the aneurysm by the deposited coils. At this point, if the aneurysm is no longer filling with contrast, do not attempt to re-advance the microcatheter back into the aneurysm.

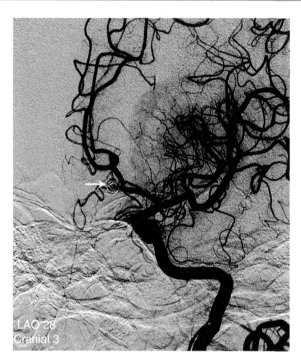

Fig. 12.3 A 5.6 × 7.5 mm anterior communicating aneurysm with a neck measuring 3.7 mm (same patient as shown in Fig. 12.2). A GDC 10 360° standard SR 5X9 mm framing coil has been placed that covers the entire aneurysm (*arrow*). Subsequent coils are deployed within the created 'basket.' Compare image to Fig. 12.2b

(a)   **(b)**

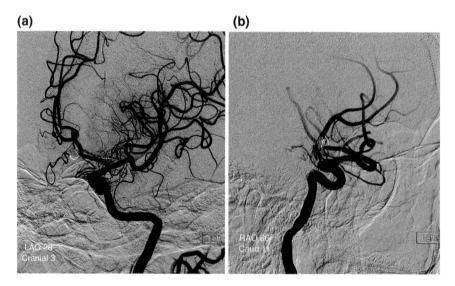

Fig. 12.4 Two orthogonal projections **a** and **b** utilized for coiling of the aneurysm (same patient as shown in Figs. 12.2 and 12.3). Complete coiling of AComm aneurysm is achieved with no entry of contrast into the aneurysm. The coils are confined within the aneurysm, and the adjacent vessels are unaffected

- If there is residual filling, then attempt to replace the microcatheter into the aneurysm, using the microwire.
- After completion of coiling, perform angiography in standard half Townes and lateral views (or same projections and magnification as baseline angiography), prior to the removing and discarding the microcatheter.
- Ensure that there is no unanticipated finding such as a vessel occlusion or 'cutoff' by emboli, when compared to pre-coiling angiogram.
- If embolic occlusion is present, use the microcatheter to administer Reopro or TPA.
- If the angiogram is unremarkable, remove the microcatheter.
- Retract the guide catheter into the femoral vessels.
- Position the fluoroscopy tube at 33–45° ipsilaterally over the femoral region.
- Perform angiography.
- If arteriotomy is proximal to the femoral bifurcation and the vessel is ≥ 4 mm in caliber, perform angioseal closure.

Retrieving and Storing a Deployed Bare Platinum Coil

- If a decision is made to remove a coil that has been partially or completely deployed (but not detached) in an aneurysm and it is anticipated that it may be required further on during the procedure, do the following:
- Insert the proximal (outer) end of the pusher into the coil sheath. Note that one vacant coil sheath should always be stored on the operating table, anticipating this possibility. The crimped end of the sheath, in case of GDC coils, is cut off to make the maneuver of coil re-sheathing unhindered.
- Continue to feed the coil pusher into the sheath while using fluoroscopy to ensure that the coil is exiting the aneurysm into the microcatheter as anticipated, at the other end. It also must be ensured that the exiting coil does not cause herniation of a previously detached coil, or any other untoward event.
- Continue feeding the pusher into the sheath until its proximal end emerges from the proximal other end of the sheath. During this process, the operator must have direct access to some part of the pusher at all times.
- Take hold of the emerged end of the pusher. Loosen the RHV to enable the insertion of the distal end of the sheath, which is closest to the RHV, halfway into it. Then, gently tighten the RHV around the sheath, ensuring that movement of pusher within the sheath is unimpeded.
- Continue retracting the pusher and monitor fluoroscopically until the coil completely exits the aneurysm.
- Watch the hub closely as the coil is pulled back.
- Stop retracting, once the entire coil enters the sheath.
- Loosen the RHV and recover the sheath. Re-tighten the RHV again.
- Gently loop the sheath with the coil within and put it aside on the operating table.

- After the next coil is deployed, store its sheath on the operating table to ensure a spare sheath is available at all times.
- Note that this retrieval and storage cannot be performed for expanding coils, e.g., hydrocoils. If a decision is made to remove such a coil, it must be retrieved and discarded approximately within 5 min of initiating deployment. During retrieval, it may be discovered that the coil has expanded to the extent that it gets stuck within the microcatheter. In such a situation, DO NOT attempt to forcefully pull the pusher. The microcatheter will need to be removed along with the coil and then replaced by another.

Problems Encountered During Coiling and Solutions

- Table 12.2 shows some possible problems/solutions.

Table 12.2 Problems/solutions during coiling

Problem	Solution
microcatheter kicks out of the aneurysm as the coil is being deployed	• Gradual retraction of the coil frequently causes the microcatheter tip to reenter the aneurysm. At this point, the following may be attempted
	• Advance the coil more gradually into the aneurysm. A slower or faster deployment, or the coil loops depositing differently within the aneurysm, either of these may result in complete deposition of coil within the aneurysm
	• Alternatively, advance the microcatheter slightly over the coil and then resume deploying the coil. Or
	• Remove the coil entirely and replace with a shorter and/or softer coil
	• If attempts to replace the microcatheter tip within the aneurysm do not succeed, then retract and remove the coil entirely. Advance the microwire through the microcatheter and then attempt to re-catheterize the aneurysm
	• Conversely, if a majority of the aneurysm is coiled and re-catheterization is proving difficult, consider postponing completion of coiling to another day. With a small residual remaining, the patient is more protected against SAH compared to an untreated aneurysm
Coil herniates out into blood vessel after detachment	• This usually occurs when the coil is of a smaller diameter than the aneurysm. Ascertain that the coil is stable (non-pulsatile) within the aneurysm before detaching it. If herniation of a detached coil appears imminent, rapid deployment of a second coil may prevent the initial coil from herniating.

(continued)

Table 12.2 (continued)

Problem	Solution
	If just the tip of the coil has herniated into the vessel, assess if it is stable and further herniation will not occur. When that is the case and the vessel does not appear compromised, then a small herniation may be accepted. If a significant amount of the coil has herniated, further herniation is unavoidable, or the blood flow in vessel appears compromised, consider placement of a stent to trap the coil against the vessel wall. If complete coil herniation has occurred, then consider attempting to remove it by using a snare device (e.g., alligator) or if that is unsuccessful, then placing a stent to trap the coil against vessel wall and restoring the vessel lumen
Coil penetrates through the aneurysm sac into the subarachnoid space	• DO NOT reflexively pull the coil back. Continue to deploy the coil. If the tip of the microcatheter also penetrated the aneurysm wall, then gradually pull it back as the coil is being deployed, in order to plug the aneurysm perforation with the coil. Continue coil deployment such that part of the coil is outside the aneurysm and the rest within. Perform angiography and then detach the coil. Deploy and detach additional coils, if needed

Stent-Assisted Coiling

Indications

- Broad-necked saccular aneurysms where coils cannot be kept within an aneurysm without a stent.
- Fusiform aneurysms.
- Residual or recurrent aneurysms where coils cannot be kept within an aneurysm without a stent (Fig. 12.5).
- Trapping a herniated coil against the vessel wall (Fig. 12.6).
- Flow diversion (complete overlapping of, e.g., three stents is required to achieve this)
- Stenting is usually performed for broad-based unruptured aneurysms because of the associated requirement of ASA + Plavix for the initial month. When necessary, we have performed stenting in ruptured aneurysms (that were coiled) with usage of ASA + Plavix, without any untoward consequences.
- In unruptured aneurysms, the procedure can be done in a staged fashion, as sometimes it may be difficult passing the catheter through the tines of recently placed stent. Persistence in this regard may lead to displacement of stent. When staged, stenting and coiling may be done a month apart to enable endothelialization of the stent.

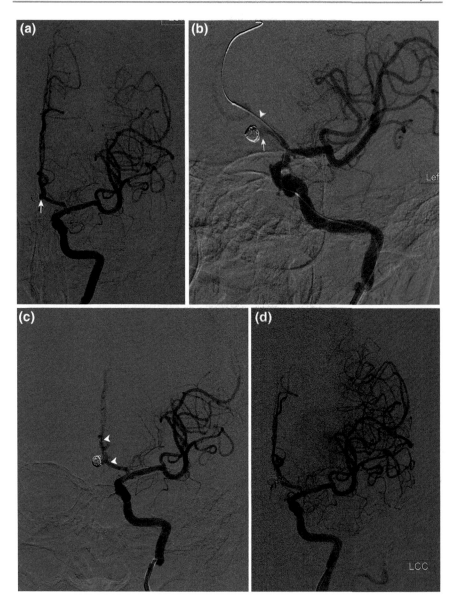

Fig. 12.5 A previously coiled anterior communicating aneurysm demonstrating recurrence (*arrow*) (**a**). For safe coiling of residual aneurysm (*arrow*), a prowler select plus catheter has been positioned (*arrowhead*), to enable the Enterprise stent to straddle the neck of the aneurysm (**b**). The microwire is advanced well ahead into the pericallosal artery for adequate support. *Arrowheads* indicate the tine markings on either end of the fully deployed stent (**c**). Even though the greater part of the stent is distal to the aneurysm, the neck of the aneurysm is completely covered by the stent. **d** The residual aneurysm was successfully coiled, and the contrast no longer enters the proximal aneurysm. Contrary to the impression on this projection, the coils were not in the vessel lumen. Hence, the satisfactory contrast flow to the vessel and branches distally. The presence of stent prevented the coil loops from herniating and compromising adjacent ACA lumen

Fig. 12.6 Complete herniation of detached coil out of the anterior communicating aneurysm into the pericallosal artery (**a**). A Prowler Select Plus microcatheter has been advanced in an attempt to trap the errant coil against the vessel wall, using a stent. The microwire is advanced well ahead of the catheter to provide support. The lumen of the effected vessel is not well visualized. A filling defect (*arrowhead*) is noted in the proximal aspect of the contralateral vessel.
b Angiography performed one year later demonstrates complete restoration of vessel lumen with good flow. The markings on either end of the stent are appreciated (*arrowheads*) that have successfully trapped the errant coil. A stent has also been deployed in the contralateral vessel (*arrowheads*), as the filling defect did not resolve with Reopro™ alone. There is complete restoration of vessel lumen

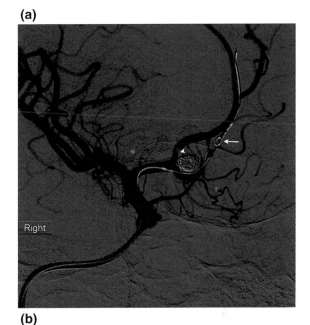

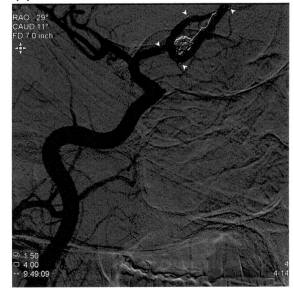

Contraindications

- Most contraindications are relative, and a risk benefit assessment is performed on a case-by-case basis:

  - ICH.
  - Provocative tests demonstrating intolerance to occlusion.

  - Recent major surgery.
  - Pregnancy.
  - Contraindication to anticoagulants and/or thrombolytics.
  - Nickel allergy.

Additional Equipment

In addition to the equipment described under 'Coil Embolization', consider

- Prowler Select Plus (0.021" inner diameter, 5 cm distal length) (Codman Neurovascular, Miami, FL).
- Transend or Synchro2 Microwire (0.014, or 0.010).
- Enterprise Vascular Reconstruction Device and Delivery System (Codman Neurovascular). This is our preferred device.
- The unconstrained diameter of Enterprise stent is 4.5 mm. The available lengths (in mm) are 14, 22, 28, and 37, respectively (see Table 12.3).

Technique

- Access to femoral artery and navigation is performed as described above.
- A guide catheter is prepared and positioned in ICA or VA proximal to the lesion. The guide catheter should be positioned as close to the lesion as safely possible to ensure stability of the system during deployment. However, it should be at least a cm (usually more) away from the site of stent placement to enable smooth deployment.
- Prepare a Prowler Select microcatheter by attaching it to an RHV and removing the shaping wire from its distal tip.
- Connect the RHV to a three-way stopcock that is connected to a continuously running flush of heparinized saline.

Table 12.3 Enterprise™ stent lengths and diameters in various vessel widths

Unconstrained stent diameter (mm)	Unconstrained stent length (mm)	Recommended parent vessel diameter (mm)	Length foreshortening (mm)
4.5	14	3–4	1.1
	22	3–4	1.9
	28	3–4	3.2
	37	3–4	4.7

- Ensure the microcatheter (and all catheters introduced into the patient) is free of air bubbles.
- Using fluoroscopy and roadmapping, advance a Prowler Select Plus microcatheter over a microwire and cross the site for stent deployment.
- Select the appropriate Enterprise stent and inspect the package to rule out any damage or breakage in sterility.
- Using sterile precautions, remove the dispenser hoop from the package and place it on the sterile equipment table.
- Free the delivery wire from the clip on the dispenser hoop.
- Grasp the introducer and the delivery wire at the point where it exits from the dispenser hoop. This will prevent stent movement.
- While holding the introducer and delivery wire, remove the system from the dispenser hoop. Make sure the stent is not inadvertently partially deployed.
- Ensure that the wire is not kinked and the introducer is undamaged.
- Do not attempt to shape the distal end of the delivery wire.
- Loosen the RHV of the microcatheter.
- Insert the distal end of the introducer partially into the RHV.
- Tighten the RHV around the introducer.
- Press the wings (or pull the tab, utilize whatever the provided mechanism) of the pediatric transducer on the tubing leading to the microcatheter, which will result in increased flow. Confirm that the fluid is exiting from the proximal end of the introducer. Purge the device until you are certain that the saline flush has evacuated out any air from the system.
- Slightly loosen the RHV, and grasping the introducer and wire together, advance the introducer until it completely engages the hub of the microcatheter.
- Advance the delivery wire to transfer the stent from the introducer into the microcatheter. Do not torque the wire at any point.
- Continue to advance the wire until the marker at 150 cm (from the distal wire tip) enters the RHV.
- Loosen the RHV and slide the introducer off the wire.
- Using fluoroscopy, observe the stent as it is advanced toward the microcatheter tip.
- Align the stent positioning marker on the wire across the neck of the aneurysm.
- Once positioned, confirm the following markers are visible on fluoroscopy in the following sequence distal to proximal.

    a. Distal tip of catheter.
    b. Distal marker on delivery wire.
    c. Distal stent markers (appear as a single marker, until stent is deployed).
    d. Stent positioning marker on delivery wire (this is in the mid-region of the stent.
    e. Small marker indicating the extent to which the stent can be partially deployed and still recaptured (recommended by the manufacturer to be performed only once).
    f. Proximal stent markers (appear as a single marker, until stent is deployed).

g. Proximal marker on delivery wire.

h. Proximal marker on the catheter (the position of this marker is not crucial, provided the above are positioned adequately).

- Also ensure the distal tip of the guide catheter is visible and the catheter is stable, so it will not inadvertently collapse during stent deployment.
- Remove all slack from the system.
- Ensure the microcatheter RHV has been loosened.
- Slowly retract the microcatheter under live fluoroscopy while holding the delivery wire stable, so that it does not move. The marker on the microcatheter tip will be noted to move proximally toward the markers on the delivery wire.
- As the microcatheter is retracted further, the distal stent markers will separate indicating the deployment of distal stent.
- Continue to retract the microcatheter as it passes over the stent positioning marker.
- When the catheter reaches the small marker proximal to the positioning marker, the stent can still be re-sheathed by advancing the microcatheter over the wire. However, once the microcatheter is pulled proximal to this marker, the stent can no longer be recaptured.
- Up to this point, if stent needs to be repositioned, re-sheath the stent by maintaining tension on the wire and gently advancing the microcatheter over the stent. The distal stent markers will be noted to collapse into a single marker as before. If any resistance is encountered during microcatheter advancement, do not continue to push the catheter. Gently, retract the catheter a bit (without crossing the 'recapture limit' marker) and then re-advance.
- Retract the microcatheter over the proximal stent markers, which will result in the separation of the marker into four distinct markers, indicating the complete deployment of the stent.
- Once the microcatheter is well proximal to the stent, if needed re-advance it over the delivery wire. It will cause the microcatheter to advance within the stent, and in order to maintain vascular access, the catheter tip may be positioned distal to the stent.
- Retract and discard the delivery wire.
- At this point, another microwire may be used, e.g., Transend 0.010 or 0.014 to redirect the microcatheter through the stent tines into aneurysm. To use a different microcatheter for coiling the aneurysm, use an exchange length microwire.
- Following placement of the stent, the option is to perform coiling in the same sitting, or do so once the stent has endothelialized.
- In elective cases, we prefer performing stent placement and coil embolization in a staged fashion. Therefore, after stent placement we wait a month while the patient is on ASA + Plavix. Waiting until the stent has endothelialized decreases the likelihood of stent dislodgment during manipulation.

Fusiform Aneurysms

- The deployment of stent is as described above.
- The stent coverage should extend beyond the fusiform segment on either side.
- A decision is made whether stenting alone (including deploying two or more stents within each other) will suffice. If feasible, after stenting the patient undergoes angiography in a month. If the vessel morphology is stable or the fusiform aneurysm has attenuated, no further action may be required. Otherwise, stenting followed by coiling is performed.
- In addition to Enterprise stent as described above, another option is Pipeline Vascular reconstruction device (See, Pipeline Embolization Device section below).

Other Stents

- We most frequently use Enterprise™ stent due to its ease of deployment. Other stents, e.g., Neuroform EZ™ (Stryker Neurovascular) and Wingspan™ (Stryker Neurovascular), are also available in market. Unlike Enterprise™, these stents offer a range of diameters. Table 12.4 presents the specifications of Wingspan stent.

Table 12.4 Wingspan stent, guide catheter, and wire dimensions for various caliber vessels

Sizing guidelines for Wingspan stent system						
Labeled stent diameter (mm)	Labeled stent length (mm)	Maximum diameter of expansion (mm)	Vessel diameter (mm)	Useable length of delivery system (cm)	Maximum guidewire diameter	Minimum guide catheter internal diameter
2.5	9	2.8	>2.0 and ≤2.5	135	0.36 mm (0.014 in.)	1.63 mm (0.064 in.)
	15					
	20					
3.0	9	3.4	>2.5 and ≤3.0			
	15					
	20					
3.5	9	3.9	>3.0 and ≤3.5			
	15					
	20					
4.0	9	4.4	>3.5 and ≤4.0			
	15					
	20					
4.5	9	4.9	>4.0 and ≤4.5			
	15					
	20					

Postoperative Management and Follow-up

- Admit to NSICU for overnight observation.
- 0.9% NS + 20 meq KCl @ 150 cc/h X 2 h, then decrease to 100 cc/h if patient is NPO.
- Keep right/left leg (whichever side was used for procedure) straight X 2 h, with head of bed (HOB) elevated 15°.
- Check groins, DP's, vitals and neurochecks q 15 min X 4, q 30 min X 2, then q h.
- Plavix 75 mg PO daily X 4 weeks.
- ASA 81–325 mg PO daily indefinitely.
- Advance diet as tolerated.
- Review/Resume pre-procedure medications, except oral hypoglycemics, which are resumed 48 h after procedure and when good oral intake is established.
- Any inexplicable change in neurological examination should lead to thorough investigation including CT head and if indicated repeat angiography.
- Also monitor the access site for pseudo-aneurysm, vessel occlusion, etc.
- Discharge (D/C) next morning after mobilizing (if no complications/other ongoing medical concerns requiring hospitalization).
- The patient should be ambulant, able to void, and back to pre-procedure status at time of discharge.
- Follow up (F/u) on outpatient basis in 4 weeks.
- May plan placing coils at 1 month if not done along with stenting.
- F/u angiography at 3 months, 6 months, and 1 and 2 years.
- If the aneurysm is noted to recur requiring treatment, the surveillance restarts as for a newly coiled aneurysm.

Problems Encountered During Enterprise Stent Deployment and Solutions

- Table 12.5 shows some possible problems/solutions.

Balloon-Assisted Coiling

- We use balloon-assisted coiling infrequently. However, when required, one option is Hyperform™ balloon occlusion system (Covidien, Plymouth, MN). It is performed as follows.

Table 12.5 Problems/solutions during Enterprise stent deployment

Problem	Solution
Difficulty passing the microcatheter between the stent tines into the aneurysm	• If an elective coiling is being performed, consider staging the procedure to allow the stent to endothelialize. We have found that returning after a month, we have been able to pass the microcatheter into the aneurysm without any difficulty
	• Consider using a different catheter that has a tapered end, e.g., Headway 17 (Microvention, Aliso Viejo, CA). It frequently proves better at getting though stent tines
Difficulty passing the microcatheter through the much smaller space between tines of 2 or more overlapping stents	• Navigation in such a situation is challenging. A tapered microcatheter such as Headway 17 (Microvention, Aliso Viejo, CA) frequently proves better at getting through the stent tines
	• Additionally, try a smaller caliber microwire and also vary the stiffness, e.g., floppy, if standard or firm do not work
Stent moved during deployment	• The stent can be re-sheathed and repositioned provided it has not been unsheathed beyond the 'recapture limit' (identified by the small marker proximal to the stent positioning marker). Re-sheath the stent by maintaining tension on the microwire while gently advancing the microcatheter over the stent. If resistance is encountered, retract the microcatheter slightly and then re-advance. Do not attempt to push the stent forward. If it has already been deployed beyond the recapture limit, do not attempt to re-sheath and complete the deployment. If needed, advance and deploy additional stent/s to address any uncovered areas of the neck. However, first assess if that is necessary at all, e.g., even partial coverage may have converted the aneurysm from a broad-necked to narrow-necked lesion and hence able to maintain deployed coils within the aneurysm sac

Additional Equipment Needed

- Microcatheter for coiling aneurysm (we most commonly use Excelsior SL-10).
- Microwire (consider using a 0.010 or 0.014 wire, e.g., Transend microwire, which can then be reused for the balloon catheter).
- Hyperform balloon catheter (Covidien, Plymouth, MN).

Indications

- Broad-necked saccular aneurysms where coils cannot be kept within an aneurysm.
- H/o difficulties with stents, e.g., in-stent stenosis consequent to intimal hyperplasia.
- Broad-necked saccular aneurysms where the use of stent may be contraindicated, e.g., recent SAH making the use of ASA + Plavix risky, known resistance to ASA/Plavix, or metal allergy.

Technique

- Administer 5000 IU of heparin bolus once the guide catheter is in place, for an unruptured aneurysm. In case of ruptured aneurysm, heparin bolus is delayed until the first coil has been placed in the aneurysm.
- Perform ACT 15–20 min and then an hour after the bolus. Thereafter, hourly ACTs are performed through the intervention.
- Additional heparin is administered based on results of ACT. The goal is to maintain ACT between 250 and ≤ 300.
- Advance the microcatheter connected to a continuously running flush of heparinized saline over the microwire and position the tip of the microcatheter within the aneurysm, as described above.
- Retract and remove the microwire after ensuring the microcatheter is stable within the aneurysm.
- Wipe the wire with a piece of moist telfa, as it is removed from the microcatheter and place it in a bowl containing heparinized saline.
- Tighten the microcatheter RHV.
- Remove the balloon catheter system from its package in a sterile fashion.
- Attach an RHV to the balloon catheter.
- Draw contrast solution in 2/3 1/3 strength into a 3-ml syringe (manufacturer recommendation is a 50:50 dilution. However, we use 2/3 contrast dilution for better visualization and have had no problems with it).
- Attach the 3-ml syringe and a 1-ml cadence syringe to a three-way stopcock.
- Draw some of the contrast into the cadence syringe.
- Attach this system to the RHV on the balloon catheter using the remaining free port of the stopcock.
- Purge all air out of the catheter by injecting it with the contrast solution from the 3-ml syringe.
- Introduce the 0.010 microwire into the RHV and advance it through the catheter until it almost reaches the tip of the catheter.
- Flush the catheter lumen again to ensure all air has been removed from the system.
- Advance the microwire past the tip of the catheter.

- Turn the stopcock such that it is open to the cadence syringe.
- Inflate the balloon to ensure that it is functional. It will 'stick' when inflated for the first time.
- Check for air bubbles.
- If bubbles are present, withdraw the wire and flush the catheter again, as described above.
- Place the system in basin with sterile saline, until ready for use.
- Advance the balloon catheter and wire through the RHV of the guide catheter and continue advancing such that the balloon catheter and wire reach the tip of the guide catheter.
- Using fluoroscopy and roadmap in working view, advance the balloon catheter over the microwire to position the markings on the proximal and distal aspect of the balloon across the aneurysm neck.
- It is imperative that the tip of the microcatheter within the aneurysm is observed at all times so it does not inadvertently slip out of the aneurysm or worse still, move forward risking aneurysm rupture.
- After positioning the balloon catheter, ensure the tip of the microwire is distal to the tip of the balloon catheter, as the distal inflation holes on the catheter must be occluded.
- When satisfied with balloon positioning, commence balloon inflation by using the 1-ml cadence syringe attached to the RHV of the balloon catheter and the compliance chart provided with the balloon catheter.
- The inflation should be performed gently.
- When the inflation is complete, commence deploying the framing coil in the aneurysm.
- When coil deployment is complete, deflate the balloon to verify that the coil will stay within the aneurysm and is not at risk of herniating out into the blood vessel. If the coil is noticeably moving with arterial pulsations, it is at risk of herniating out of the aneurysm after detachment. Retract and remove the coil and place another with a larger diameter.
- Detach the coil after ensuring that the coil is stable.
- Deflate the balloon by gently retracting the syringe plunger and not by retracting the microwire.
- If needed, re-inflate the balloon again when deploying the next coil.
- Subsequently, if deployed coils are staying within the aneurysm or framing coil, the balloon may not require to be re-inflated. Otherwise, continue the steps as described above, until the aneurysm is satisfactorily coiled.
- Do not detach the coil before ensuring that it remains stable within the aneurysm when the balloon is deflated.
- After completion of coiling, perform angiography in standard AP and lateral views, prior to removal of the microcatheter.
- Ensure that there is no unanticipated finding such as a vessel occlusion or 'cutoff' by emboli, when compared to pre-coiling angiogram.
- If embolic occlusion is present, use the microcatheter to administer Reopro or TPA.

- If angiogram is unremarkable, remove the microcatheter.
- Retract the guide catheter into the femoral vessels.
- Position the fluoroscopy tube at 33–45° ipsilaterally over the femoral region.
- Perform a femoral angiogram.
- If femoral angiography is unremarkable and the vessel is ≥ 4 mm, close the arteriotomy site by exchanging the sheath for an angioseal, or other closure device of choice. Manual compression may also be used.
- If it is anticipated that the patient may undergo another angiogram/intervention in 72 h, then the sheath may be left in the artery.

Problems Encountered During Balloon-Assisted Coiling and Solutions

- Table 12.6 shows some possible problems/solutions.

Table 12.6 Problems/solutions during balloon-assisted coiling

Problem	Solution
Coil noted to be moving within the aneurysm with arterial pulsations when balloon is deflated	• The coil is smaller than the diameter of the aneurysm and therefore, in danger of herniating out of the aneurysm after detachment. Consider removing and re-sheathing the coil and replacing it with a larger diameter coil. The removed coil may be used later during coil embolization when a coil with smaller diameter is required, provided it can be deployed smoothly
	• Alternatively, if it is not desirable to remove the coil, or it cannot be removed, or it has already been detached, Then, an option is to rapidly deploy and detach additional coils that may trap the coil at risk of herniating. However, this is a risky strategy as the coil may herniate out of the aneurysm before additional coils can be placed. Or, the coil being deployed to trap the coil at risk may inadvertently push out the unstable coil. To avert this, if the balloon is in position, inflate it and rapidly deploy another coil to secure the one at risk

Pipeline® Embolization Device (PED)

- FDA has approved a new stent more recently: 'Pipeline Embolization Device' (PED, EV3, Irvine, CA). The woven design is believed to allow less blood to enter the aneurysm and therefore encourages stasis. Two or more of these may need to be deployed within each other to causes adequate flow stasis in the aneurysm. Adjunctive coil placement in the aneurysm may also be undertaken to encourage aneurysm thrombosis.

Indications and Case Selection

- Large or giant wide-necked ICA aneurysms, from petrous to the superior hypophyseal segments (Fig. 12.7a, b), although it has been used in the BA.
- Presently, patients must be 22 years of age or older.
- Its efficacy for usage in bifurcation aneurysms has not been studied.

Contraindications

- Ruptured aneurysm (due to requirement of pre-embolization dual antiplatelet therapy).
- Patients in whom dual antiplatelet therapy is contraindicated.
- Patients who have not received dual antiplatelet therapy (ASA and clopidogrel) prior to procedure.
- Active bacterial infection.
- Metal allergy to cobalt, chromium, platinum, or tungsten.
- Patients who have preexisting stent in the parent artery at the target aneurysm location (relative contraindication).

Preoperative Management

- Load patient with 300 mg Plavix®, followed by ASA 325 and Plavix 75 mg daily for 1 week. This preloading is important.

Equipment

- Rotating hemostatic valves (two).
- Fluid delivery system (for sheath, catheter, and microcatheter).
- Pressure tubing 12″ (for connection between injector and diagnostic/guide catheter).
- Low pressure tubing (3, i.e., for sheath, guide catheter and microcatheter).
- Injector syringe 150 ml.
- Syringes (20 ml, 3; 10 ml, 3).
- Fluoroscope band bag.
- Transducer 30 ml/min (for each heparinized saline flush system, usually 3, i.e., for sheath, diagnostic/guide catheter, and microcatheter).
- 1% Lidocaine + syringe with 18G and 22G needles (for local anesthesia. Anesthetic is drawn from the bottle with 18G needle and skin is anesthetized using 22G needle).
- Single-wall needle 18G or micropuncture kit sheath, e.g., Terumo 6 Fr 10 cm
- 2-0 Silk suture.
- 8-Fr short sheath.
- Guidewire, e.g., Terumo® angled glidewire 0.035 150 cm.
- 6-Fr shuttle sheath 90 cm, with 5-Fr H1 slip catheter 125 cm (Cook Medical, Bloomington, IN) **or** 6-Fr Neuron Max sheath 90 cm, with 5-Fr H1 Neuron Select catheter, 125 cm (Penumbra, Almeda, CA), or 5-Fr H1 slip catheter 125 cm.
- Microguidewire Transend SL 150 cm or Transend Ex 182 cm or
- Synchro2 microwire 200 cm standard or soft.
- 5-Fr Navien intracranial support catheter (Covidien Vascular Therapies, Mansfield, MA). The 115 cm length is commonly used.
- Pipeline® Embolization Device—Classic (Covidien Vascular Therapies, Mansfield, MA), or the more recently available
- Pipeline® Embolization Device—Flex.
- The difference between the two is the deployment system. The latter being simpler.
- Table 12.7 shows diameter of vessel and lengths of PED available
- 0.027″ I.D. catheter, e.g.,

  - Marksman™ 2.8 Fr (ev3, Irvine, CA); distal flexible length 10 cm available in working lengths of 105, 135, and 150 cm. This is our preferred micro-catheter, or
  - Mass Transit™ (Cordis Neurovascular, Warren NJ), or
  - Renegade™ Hi-Flo (Stryker Neurovascular, Fremont, CA).

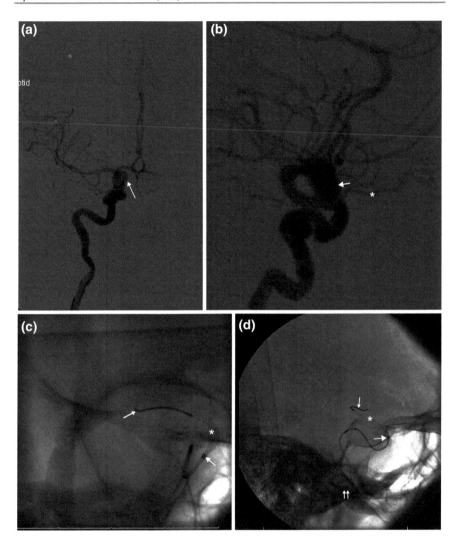

(images continued on pages 191 and 193)

Fig. 12.7 A large ophthalmic aneurysm (*arrow*, **a** and **b**). The ophthalmic artery is well appreciated (*asterisk*, **b**). Single shot images taken during pipeline device placement (**c–h**). The half Towne's view (**c**) demonstrates the radiopaque end of the delivery wire (*slender arrow*) in MCA. The partially deployed stent is appreciated (*asterisk*). The radiopaque marker indicating the tip of the Marksman microcatheter (*thick arrow*) has been partially retracted over the PED. The lateral view demonstrates the same (**d**).

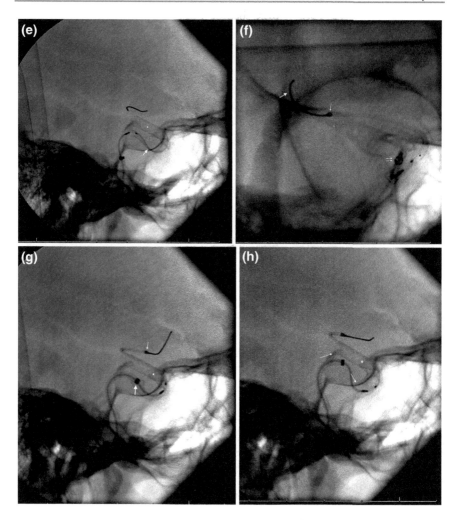

(images continued on next page)

Fig. 12.7 The tip of Navien catheter is seen further proximally (*double arrows*). The PED has been completely deployed (**e**). This lateral view demonstrates the maintenance of wire access distal to PED. The PED is fully deployed and well opposes the ICA walls distally (*asterisk*). However, the device has not expanded further proximally (*arrow*). In order to expand the proximal aspect of PED, maneuvers are undertaken. The Marksman microcatheter has been advanced over the wire through the stent (**f**). The tip of microcatheter (*slender arrow*) is seen at the proximal aspect of the radiopaque end of delivery wire (*thick arrow*). The distal tip of wire end is well within the M2. The tip of Navien (*double arrows*) is proximal to the PED (*asterisk*). When compared to (**e**), the lateral view (**g**) demonstrates some expansion of the PED (*asterisk*). The tip of Marksman catheter (*slender arrow*) is in the MCA, well distal to distal end of PED. The tip of Navien catheter (*thick arrow*) is adjacent to the proximal end of PED. Complete expansion of the PED (**h**).

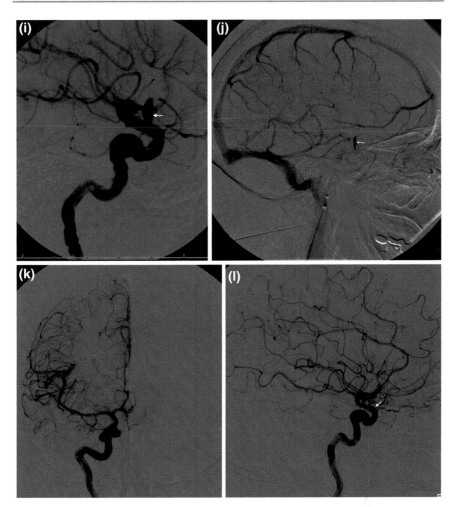

Fig. 12.7 The proximal and distal ends (*slender arrows*) of the PED (*asterisk*) are of similar caliber. The immediate post-intervention angiography in lateral view demonstrates the aneurysm partially (**i**, *arrow*). Unlike coiling, this is an anticipated outcome. Due to contrast stasis, the aneurysm can be appreciated well into the venous phase (**j**, *arrow*). Angiography at 6 months (**k, l**) demonstrates complete resolution of aneurysm (compare to **a** and **b**). The *arrow* (**l**) points to the region of origin of obliterated aneurysm

Table 12.7 Diameter of vessel and lengths of PED available

Vessel diameter (mm)	PED length (mm)
2.50, 2.75	10, 12, 14, 16, 18, 20
3.00, 3.25, 3.50, 3.75, 4.00, 4.25, 4.50, 4.75, 5.00	10, 12, 14, 16, 18, 20, 25, 30, 35

Technique

- As this is a relatively recent technology, the authors presently do not have an extensive experience with it. It is worth noting that in the USA, in order to attain certification for device usage, FDA mandates that the first five cases are performed proctored by a physician with expertise in Pipeline® Usage. Additional five cases are done with support of certified ev3 representative.
- Gain access to femoral artery using modified Seldinger technique.
- Insert 8-Fr short sheath over J-wire. The advantage of interposing an 8-Fr short sheath between the vessel wall and the shuttle or Neuron Max sheath is that the vessel is not traumatized by movement of the longer sheath being navigated to its position, also eliminating consequent patient discomfort. Additionally, the short sheath enables easier control during vascular access closure at the end of procedure.
- The short sheath is connected to a continuously running flush of heparinized saline.
- Ensure all flush systems are free of air bubbles and other foreign bodies.
- Secure the sheath to the patient's skin using 2-0 silk suture.
- Prepare a 6-Fr long sheath (shuttle or Neuron Max), connect it to continuously running flush of heparinized saline, and ensure that it is free of air bubbles.
- Insert a 5-Fr H1 catheter and connect it to continuously running flush of heparinized saline into the sheath.
- Advance a 0.035 angled glidewire into the catheter.
- Insert this coaxial system through the short sheath into the patients' vasculature.
- With the guidewire leading, catheterize the intended vessel (e.g., ICA).
- Advance the guide sheath over the wire and H1 catheter into the ICA. When suitably positioned, retract and remove the glidewire and H1 catheter.
- Perform baseline angiography and angiography in working views.
- Administer heparin 5000 IU IV after the sheath has been positioned.
- Send an ACT approximately 15 min after administration of heparin, and repeat ACT hourly. Aim to maintain ACT between 300 and 350 s throughout the procedure by administering additional heparin as needed. Alternatively, after administration of 5000 IU heparin bolus, 1000 IU is administered hourly throughout the procedure without performing ACTs.
- The angiographic views should enable good visualization of the neck of the aneurysm, as well as adjacent vessels to enable safe PED placement.
- Additionally, the views should also enable the visualization of the tip of the guide catheter, so that the surgeon remains cognizant of its location.
- Connect a 5-Fr Navien catheter to a continuously running flush of heparinized saline.
- Attach the Marksman™ microcatheter to a continuously running flush of heparinized saline.
- Introduce the Marksman catheter into the Navien.
- Insert a microguidewire (e.g., Synchro2 microguidewire) into the microcatheter.

- Advance the microwire tip beyond the catheter tip.
- Shape the tip of wire using the provided mandrel. Then, withdraw the tip back into microcatheter. The shape of the tip will depend upon the location of the aneurysm. The most common tip shape is 45°.
- (For efficiency, we prepare the long guide sheath-H1 and Navien–Marksman systems concurrently, prior to introducing and positioning the guide sheath in ICA. This results in the guide sheath not remaining in the vasculature unnecessarily. The Navien–Marksman system is set aside immersed in a large bowl of heparinized saline, while the shuttle sheath is being navigated into position).
- Advance the Naviencatheter, Marksman microcatheter and microguidewire through the guide sheath.
- Perform roadmapping through the sheath while the microcatheter is proximal to sheath tip in the working view.
- Navigate the Navien–Marksman system over the microwire utilizing both planes.
- Position the Navien in cavernous ICA.
- Advance the tip of microcatheter at least 20 mm distal to the aneurysm. Commonly, our final position of the microcatheter tip is near the M1–M2 junction of MCA, or even in the proximal M2.
- If needed, the Navien may be advanced further over the microcatheter–microwire to bring it close to the aneurysm.
- Advance the guide sheath over the Navien for further stability. If needed, it may be positioned intracranially as well.
- Remove the microwire completely, once appropriate positioning has been achieved.
- In effect, a triaxial system has been created that provides good stability for pipeline deployment.
- Remove all slack from the system.
- Measure the ICA proximal and distal to the neck of the aneurysm and the intervening length between these points, to select the size of PED.
- Select the PED of appropriate size. Bear in mind, the PED is elongated 2.5 times its maximally expanded deployed configuration when it is constrained within the microcatheter.
- The PED comes mounted on a delivery wire and constrained in a sheath.
- Loosen the RHV of the microcatheter.
- Hold the sheath and wire together, so that the PED is not inadvertently dislodged. The sheath is inserted halfway into the RHV and the RHV tightened around it.
- Irrigate the system using the neonatal transducer, until fluid droplets are noted to emanate from the proximal tip of the sheath.
- Now loosen the RHV and advance the sheath until it is securely appositioned to the hub. Re-tighten the RHV.
- Advance the PED through the sheath into the microcatheter by firmly pushing in the delivery wire. The sheath is removed and discarded.

- Once the markers on the wire reach the RHV, further advancement is performed under fluoroscopy.
- Advance the PED through the extent of microcatheter by firmly pushing in the delivery wire and position the PED across the neck of the aneurysm. During this advancement, do not pull back or torque the wire. Another option is to position the microcatheter and advance the PED beyond the intended position and then later simultaneously pull back microcatheter and delivery wire to properly position the device, after partial deployment. Usually, we continue to advance until the tip of the delivery wire is at the tip of the microcatheter, in an M2 branch.
- A single shot is taken to confirm all the markings.
- Partially, unsheath the PED by withdrawing the microcatheter backwards, while holding the delivery wire and therefore the PED stationary. The withdrawal brings the tip of the microcatheter just proximal to the radiopaque distal delivery wire, in the mid- to proximal M1 segment.
- The wire is then firmly pushed to push out the distal end of PED from the microcatheter (for PED—Flex).
- (PED Classic: Open the PED by rotating the wire clockwise. Do not make more than ten rotations, or the wire may break. These rotations are not needed or performed for PED—Flex).
- The distal marker will separate into multiple markers, indicating opening up of distal aspect of pipeline (the same effect that is achieved in PED Classic by clockwise rotation).
- Now both the microcatheter and delivery wire are simultaneously and carefully retracted to position the PED across the neck of the aneurysm (Fig. 12.7c, d).
- All slack is removed, and if needed the Navien and guide sheath are advanced over the microcatheter for more support.
- Again, small robust wire pushing is performed to unsheath further PED.
- The microcatheter is pulled back while the wire is maintained stationary, when the microcatheter is noted to hug a wall of ICA, until it is re-centered.
- Further unsheathing is performed using this 'push-pull' technique.
- Deliberately, deploy the remainder of the PED by pulling back the microcatheter over the delivery wire. This is an unhurried process, with the objective of well aligning the device to the walls of the vessel. When the width of the artery appears wider than the device, gently push the microwire forward slightly to foreshorten the device, which makes the PED wider in diameter. When the width of the vessel is narrow, pull the microcatheter and hence device slightly to lengthen it. The entire device is gradually unsheathed and deployed in this 'push' 'pull' fashion (Fig. 12.7e, f).
- Pulling back on the delivery wire can also cause the microcatheter to advance forward over the PED.
- During deployment, the assistant keeps a constant eye on wire tip, which will advance forward as the pipeline is unsheathed.
- Once the deployment is complete, and the microcatheter is proximal to the device, advance the microcatheter over the wire through the PED and position it

distally. This is done by pulling on the wire, which causes the microcatheter to climb up the wire Fig. 12.7g, h).
- Perform angiography to confirm satisfactory deployment of PED (Fig. 12.7i, j).
- Retract the wire through the microcatheter while gently rotating it clockwise. Remove the microcatheter and microwire concurrently.
- Remove the RHV from the Navien and allow it to backbleed. Then, flush it with heparinized normal saline.
- Perform post-procedure angiography. *Expect* to find residual filling of aneurysm in PED deployment. In majority of the cases, this will usually attenuate and resolve completely over next few weeks to months (Fig. 12.7i, j).
- If the angiogram does not show any problems, e.g., vessel cutoff or dissection. Retract and withdraw the Navien and guide sheath.

Caution

- Prior to deploying the PED, ensure that the guide sheath remains stable during manipulation. If it is displaced downwards during procedure, it may require to be re-advanced to its original position, to provide stability. To do this, remove all slack from the system. If already positioned, tighten the RHV of the microcatheter. Loosen the RHV of the guide sheath, and visualizing under fluoroscopy, advance the guide catheter forward over wire/microcatheter.

Caution

- Do not pull back or torque the wire when advancing the PED in the micro-catheter. Such maneuvers many interfere with or prevent PED release.
- PED Classic: During initiating deployment, do not rotate the delivery wire more than ten full turns, as over rotation may result in wire breakage.
- Perform femoral angiography, and if arteriotomy is proximal to femoral bifur-cation, exchange 8-Fr short sheath for 8-Fr angioseal.

Postoperative Management and Follow-up

- Admit to NSICU for overnight observation.
- 0.9% NS + 20 meq KCl @ 150 cc/h X 2 h.
- Keep right/left leg (whichever side was used for catheterization during the procedure) straight X 2 h, with HOB elevated 15° (e.g., with a single pillow).

- Check groins, DP's, vitals, and neurochecks q 15 min X 4, q 30 min X 2, then q hr.
- Plavix 75 mg PO daily X 3–6 months.
- ASA 81–325 mg PO daily indefinitely.
- Advance diet as tolerated.
- Review/Resume pre-procedure medications (except oral hypoglycemics, which are resumed when oral intake is established).
- Any inexplicable change in neurological examination should lead to thorough investigation including CT head and if indicated repeat angiography.
- Also monitor the access site for potential complications, e.g., pseudo-aneurysm, vessel occlusion.
- D/C patient next morning after mobilizing (if no complications/other ongoing medical concerns requiring hospitalization).
- The patient should be ambulant, able to void, and back to pre-procedure status at time of discharge.
- F/u on outpatient basis in 2–4 weeks.
- F/u angiography at 6 months (Fig. 12.7k, l).

Problems Encountered During PED Deployment and Solutions

- Table 12.8 shows some possible problems/solutions.

Table 12.8 Problems/solutions during PED deployment

Problem	Solution
PED does not release	• PED Classic: The delivery wire should be rotated clockwise to open the PED. If the device does not open after ten full turns (do not turn any further), remove the entire system (microcatheter and PED delivery system) simultaneously and use a new PED
Delivery wire breaks	• Attempt to remove the fractured piece using a retrieval device such as Alligator™ retrieval device (Covidien, Plymouth, MN). If the fractured component is appositioned by PED against the vessel wall and appears stable, consider leaving it in situ
Wire tip of the delivery system gets stuck in the mesh of delivered PED	• Rotate the wire clockwise while advancing the wire to try to release it. Then, slowly pull back on the delivery wire
PED inadvertently partially deployed into the aneurysm	• Attempt to retrieve and reposition the PED across the aneurysm neck. To this end, successful use of an Alligator™ retrieval device (Covidien, Plymouth, MN) has been reported

(continued)

Table 12.8 (continued)

Problem	Solution
Proximal end of pipeline does not fully expand/apposition vessel wall	• If the proximal end of the pipeline is still within the microcatheter, push the wire forward to foreshorten the device (hence, increasing its diameter), then pull back on microcatheter. Use the 'push-pull' technique to suitably deposit the pipeline device • If the proximal end of the pipeline is no longer within the microcatheter, i.e., the device has been completely deployed, advance the microcatheter over the wire through the pipeline. Advance the Navien closer to the proximal end of pipeline. Retract the microcatheter back and forth, performing 'wagging' maneuvers. The manipulation may result in complete opening of the proximal end (Fig. 12.7g–h) • If multiple attempts at manipulation are unsuccessful, then advance the Marksman distal to the pipeline. Remove the delivery wire while rotating it. Advance an exchange length microwire through the Marksman, then retract, and remove the Marksman microcatheter, while maintaining the wire in position • Prepare a Gateway balloon dilatation catheter (Stryker Neurovascular; see intracranial angioplasty and stenting for technique) and advance it over the wire positioning it in the unexpanded PED. Inflate the balloon while using fluoroscopic visualization. This will cause the PED to expand. Deflate and remove the balloon catheter

Location-Specific Considerations

- For ICA and its branches, the stent options include Enterprise and PED. Other options are Wingspan™ and Neuroform.
- In case of vertebrobasilar system, Enterprise, Neuroform, and Wingspan remain an option. PED presently is indicated for ICA (from petrous to superior hypophyseal segment). However, it has been used in cervical ICA, MCA, and vertebrobasilar system.
- Presently, our preferred stent during coiling remains Enterprise, because of its ease of deployment.

Suggested Readings

1. Instructions for use, Codman Enterprise™ Vascular Reconstruction Device and Delivery System. Codman Neurovascular Inc.
2. Khan SH, Nichols C, Depowell JJ, et al. Comparison of coil types in aneurysm recurrence. Clin Neurol Neurosurg 2012;114(1):12–6.
3. Lylyk P, Miranda C, Ceratto R, et al. Curative endovascular reconstruction of cerebral aneurysms with the pipeline embolization device: The Buenos Aires experience. Neurosurgery 2009;64(4):632–42.

Vasospasm

13

Indications for Treatment and Case Selection

- Symptomatic vasospasm secondary to SAH from ruptured aneurysm that is not responsive to a 2–4 h trial of maximal pharmacological therapy (Fig. 13.1).
- Vasospasm secondary to mechanical manipulation.

Preoperative Management

- The aneurysm should be secured by clipping or coiling prior to pharmacological or endovascular management of vasospasm.
- Ensure the MAP is ≥ 70 mmHg.
- Preoperative intubation, if there are any concerns about the patient's ability to protect airway.
- Verify laboratory values including platelet count, BUN, CR, APTT, PT/INR, and ß-HCG for females of reproductive age group.
- In case of renal insufficiency, diabetes, CHF, etc., ensure usage of diluted non-ionic contrast agent and carefully pre-plan to maintain contrast load to minimum.
- NPO (for ≈6 h) when procedure is to be performed under general anesthesia.
- Obtain informed consent for angiography and angioplasty.
- Ensure two IV lines inserted.
- Insert Foley. Patient will be more comfortable and cooperative with an empty bladder in case the procedure becomes prolonged.
- Position patient on neuroangiography table.
- Attach patient to pulse oximetry and ECG leads for monitoring O_2 saturation, HR, cardiac rhythm respiratory rate, and BP.

© Springer International Publishing AG 2017
S.H. Khan and A.J. Ringer, *Handbook of Neuroendovascular Techniques*,
DOI 10.1007/978-3-319-52936-3_13

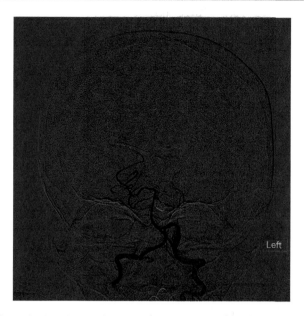

Fig. 13.1 Left vertebral angiogram demonstrating vasospasm of basilar artery. Flow restriction because of the vasospasm is demonstrated by the significant contrast reflux into the right vertebral artery (VA). The spasm of the basilar artery has resulted in the caliber of this vessel appearing smaller than that of the VAs. In addition to caliber, vasospasm is also diagnosed by observing the caliber of the affected vessel at termination, i.e., where it branches. A vessel in vasospasm will appear bulbous or of a larger caliber at termination. By contrast, a congenitally hypoplastic or stenosed vessel does not demonstrate this bulbosity

Technique

- After the groin region is appropriately prepped and draped, palpate the femoral artery.
- Immobilize a segment of the artery between the index and middle fingers.
- Infiltrate the skin overlying the immobilized segment with local anesthesia using 1% lidocaine with epinephrine.
- Make a small, superficial stab incision in the anesthetized skin.
- Using modified Seldinger technique, perform an arteriotomy (see Chap. 2 for technique for arteriotomy and sheath placement) and make an exchange over wires to place a sheath in the femoral artery.
- The sheath should be ≥ 6 Fr, just in case a procedure such as angioplasty needs to be performed.
- The sheath is connected to a continuously running flush of heparinized saline.
- Connect a diagnostic catheter (e.g., 5 Fr Glidecath) to a continuously running flush of heparinized saline.
- Introduce a 0.035 glidewire into the catheter.

- Ensure that sheath and catheter systems are free of air, or any other foreign bodies.
- Once the catheter is in the sheath, advance it over the wire using fluoroscopy.
- If the patient's vasculature is anticipated to be non-tortuous, consider using a Guide catheter, e.g., 6 Fr Envoy instead of the diagnostic catheter. It will save the time required for exchanging the diagnostic catheter for a guide catheter, in case intervention is decided upon.
- During diagnostic angiography esp. when using a guide catheter, when a vasospastic segment is identified, it is best to treat it at least chemically before proceeding to the next vessel. It may save some time by eliminating the need to catheterize the same artery more than twice.
- Study the vasculature most at risk of vasospasm first based on history (i.e., if location of an aneurysm is known), symptomatology and studies such as TCD's. We usually also perform a CT perfusion study to assess whether or not angiography or intervention is warranted.

Selective Intra-arterial Pharmacological Intervention

- The guide catheter is securely positioned in the pertinent artery of the neck (Carotid or vertebral depending upon the intracranial vessel being treated).
- A microcatheter (e.g., Excelsior SL 10 with transcend 0.010 or 0.014 guidewire) is prepared.
- The microcatheter is connected to a continuously running flush of heparinized saline.
- It is ensured that the entire system is free of air or any other foreign matter.
- Advance the microcatheter with contained microwire into the RHV of the guide catheter.
- Advance the microcatheter over the microwire until both reach the distal tip of the guide catheter.
- Perform a roadmap.
- With the help of roadmap guidance, advance the microcatheter over the microwire to position the catheter tip just distal to the segment in spasm.
- Remove the microwire.

Verapamil

- Indicated for mild non-flow limiting vasospasm that does not warrant angioplasty or moderate vasospasm that cannot be safely treated with angioplasty.
- It may also be indicated in those who have vasospasm consequent to manipulation during endovascular intervention.

- We also use it prior to performing angioplasty, so that the dilatation is performed on the relaxed dilated artery rather than a relatively rigid vasoconstricted artery.
- Verapamil is our agent of first choice. We have found it to be safe and effective to the extent that, we use it almost exclusively.

**Dose:** 5–10 mg is injected gradually (over 2–10 min) as the microcatheter is withdrawn through the spasmodic segment. Up to 20 mg may be given into each arterial tree. Inject gradually to ensure there is no significant drop in BP or bradycardia.

Alternatively, verapamil injection is frequently performed through the diagnostic or guide catheter positioned further proximally in internal carotid artery (ICA), or VA. This approach has the significant advantage of being quicker and bypasses the complexities of using a microcatheter. However, the amount of verapamil reaching the spastic segment may be less.

Contraindications

- Acute MI, severe CHF, cardiogenic shock, severe hypotension, second or third degree AV block, sick sinus syndrome, marked bradycardia, hypersensitivity to the drug, Wolff–Parkinson–White syndrome, Lown–Ganong–Levine syndrome.

Nicardipine

- Nicardipine is diluted with normal saline to a concentration of 0.1 mg/ml and administered in 1-ml aliquots to a maximum dose of 5 mg per vessel.
- Similar to verapamil administration above, administer gradually as the catheter is withdrawn through the spastic segment of the vessel. Gradual administration will also attenuate the likelihood of untoward side effects, e.g., transient tachycardia, hypotension or, increased intracranial pressure (ICP).

Contraindications

- Hypersensitivity to the drug.
- Aortic stenosis.

Papavarine

- It is a short acting, with a half life of less than 1 h.
- It may be used for cerebral vasospasm. However, due to the short duration of action other agents, e.g., verapamil are preferable.
- Papavarine may be used for angioplasty pre-treatment to enable placement of balloon catheter by causing vasodilatation.

Dose: Available in 3% concentration (30 mg/ml) at pH 3.3. 300 mg of Papaverine is diluted in 100 ml of normal saline to obtain a 0.3% concentration.

- Papavarine is administered intra-arterially through the microcatheter, which is positioned just proximal to the segment in vasospasm.
- The 300-mg dose is administered at a rate of 3 ml/minute.
- Do not mix Papaverine with contrast agents or heparin. That may result in precipitation of crystals.
- Side effects include, rapid increase in ICP, thrombocytopenia, hypotension, seizures, etc. (see 'Papavarine' in Chap. 18 'Pharmacological Agents' for details).

Contraindications

- Increased ICP; glaucoma; hypersensitivity to Papaverine; atrioventricular block; acute myocardial infarction; recent stroke and, liver function disorders.

Nitroglycerine

- It is used more in case of vessel spasm during catheterization rather than SAH-induced vasospasm.

  Dose: 100–300 µg through the catheter.

- Side effects include headache, orthostatic hypotension and tachycardia, paradoxical bradycardia and anaphylactoid reactions.

Contraindications

- Hypersensitivity to drug, severe anemia, increased ICP and methemoglobinemia.

Angioplasty

- Is indicated in refractory vasospasm that does not respond to pharmacological and hemodynamic interventions.

Devices

- An Envoy guide catheter is deployed as indicated above, which should be at least 6 Fr.

- However, if the patient has a tortuous vasculature, then use a 6 Fr shuttle sheath (80 cm; a longer sheath may be used if the patient is tall), which may be advanced initially over dilator into the descending aorta and then into the cervical carotid, or subclavian artery over 6 Fr H1 slip catheter. A shuttle sheath is preferable in tortuous vasculature because it will provide greater support and significantly decrease the likelihood of the apparatus collapsing into the aortic arch at critical time points, e.g., during stent deployment.
- 6 Fr H1 slip catheter.
- Rotating hemostatic valves (2). Ensure the RHV attached to the guide catheter is $\geq 0.096''$ or 2.44 mm.
- Pediatric transducers (30 ml/hr; 2).
- Diagnostic catheter: Terumo® front angled glidecath 5 Fr (for diagnostics).
- Front angled glidewire (0.035; Terumo).
- Balloon dilatation catheter (non-compliant or semi-compliant).
- For treatment of vasospasm, we recommend usage of a non-compliant/semi-compliant balloon catheter. We have found that compliant catheters expand much more in the non-stenosed segment before they affect the stenosed segment (the stenosed segment will appear as a 'waist'). It may result in arterial rupture at the overinflated non-stenosed segment, while attempting to dilate the stenosed segment to the desired diameter. This is not a problem with non-compliant/semi-compliant catheters.
- The size and type of balloon dilatation catheter will depend upon the location of spasm in the arterial tree. Table 13.1 below contains examples of balloon dilatation catheters for various locations.
- The size of the balloon dilatation catheter is based on the vessel size, as explained later in the 'procedure' section. For safety reasons, the balloon diameter should be equal to or less than the caliber of the normal vessel.
- Inflation device with manometer.
- Syringes 20 cc, 10 cc (at least 3), 20 cc (at least 4), 3 cc (for ACT).
- Three-way stopcock: 3.
- Torque device.
- Telfa strip.
- Mandrel for shaping microwire tip.
- Angioseal™ closure device (6 Fr). Use larger size if a larger sheath is inserted.
- Angioplasty using a Gateway™ balloon dilatation catheter is described below. The technique remains the same with other dilatation catheters.
- Remove the contents of the Gateway™ dilatation catheter from its package and transfer them onto the table, maintaining sterile precautions.
- Remove the catheter from the protective hoop.
- Ensure the catheter is not kinked, bent, or otherwise damaged.
- Hold the catheter proximal to its balloon segment and with the other hand, gently remove the stylet from the distal tip of the catheter.
- Slide the protective sheath off the balloon.
- Note that the balloon has radiopaque markers to aid in its positioning in the stenosed segment.

Table 13.1 Examples of semi-compliant balloon dilatation catheters that may be used for overcoming vasospasm

Artery	Balloon catheter type	Balloon diameter (mm)	Balloon length	Guidewire
CCA and ICA (cervical), Subclavian, VA	Voyager RX/OTW (Abbott Vascular)	2.0, 2.5, 2.75, 3.0, 3.25, 3.50, 3.75, 4.0, 4.5, 4.75	6, 8, 12, 15, 20, 25 (mm)	0.014 (The RX type can also be navigated over the guidewire attached to Accunet)
	Viatrac RX/OTW (Abbott Vascular)	4.0, 4.5, 5.0, 5.5, 6.0, 6.5, 7.0	15, 20, 30, 40 (mm)	
	Aviator® Plus RX (Cordis Endovascular)	4.0, 4.5, 5.0, 5.5, 6.0, 6.5, 7.0	1.5, 2.0, 3.0, 4.0 (cm)	
	FoxCross (Abbott Vascular)	3–14	20–120 (mm)	0.035
ICA, MCA and VA	Gateway (Boston Scientific, Natick MA)	1.5, 2.0, 2.25. 2.5, 2.75, 3.0, 3.25, 3.5, 3.75, 4.0	9, 15, 20 (mm)	0.014 (use soft guidewire with floppy part within the stent, in particularly tortuous vessels)
	Voyager RX (Abbott Vascular)	2.0, 2.5, 2.75, 3.0, 3.25, 3.50, 3.75, 4.0, 4.5, 4.75	6, 8, 12, 15, 20, 25 (mm)	0.014 (The RX type can also be navigated over the guidewire attached to Accunet)
Subclavian artery	Ultra-thin Diamond™ (Boston Scientific, Natick, MA)	3, 4, 5, 6, 7, 8, 9 10, 12	1.5, 2, 3, 4, 6, 8, 10 (cm)	0.035

- We prep the catheter in vivo. However, below is the ex vivo technique as described by the manufacturer.
- Fill a luer-lock syringe with 3 ml of contrast medium.
- Connect a three-way stopcock to the provided port on the balloon catheter. Flush through the stopcock using heparinized saline.
- Connect the syringe with contrast to the stopcock.
- Hold the syringe with nozzle pointing downward and aspirate for 5 sec. Then, release the plunger.
- Remove the syringe and evacuate all air from the barrel.
- Reconnect the syringe and aspirate until bubbles no longer appear during aspiration. If air bubbles persist, do not use the device.
- Disconnect the syringe.
- Wet the hydrophilic outer shaft of the balloon catheter.
- Fill a 20-cc syringe with 15 cc contrast and 5 cc heparinized NS (2/3:1/3 concentration).
- Attach a three-way stopcock to the inflation device and connect the 20-cc syringe containing contrast medium to the sideport of the stopcock.

- Aspirate the contrast into the inflation device, leaving only 1–2 cc within the syringe.
- Purge any air out of the barrel and tubing of the inflation device, all the way to the distal portal of the stopcock.
- Leave inflation device on table, until needed.

Deployment

- Attach the balloon catheter to a continuously running flush of heparinized saline via the provided portal using a three-way stopcock. Carefully advance the guidewire through the hub of the balloon catheter.
- Advance the over-the-wire (OTW) balloon catheter using fluoroscopy and road mapping.
- In case a microcatheter is already in the desired location, an exchange length microwire may be advanced through it and the microcatheter retracted and removed. The OTW balloon catheter can then be advanced over the wire.
- Loosen the RHV of the guide catheter and advance the balloon catheter, over the wire, into it.
- In case of RX balloon catheter, ensure that the guidewire exits the notch 25 cm proximal to the RX balloon catheter tip.
- Then tighten the RHV just enough to prevent excessive blood loss, while not causing a hindrance in advancing the balloon catheter.
- Advance the balloon catheter over the wire into the guide catheter.
- Take care that the position of the guidewire is maintained during this maneuvering. Occasionally, confirm the same by fluoroscopy.
- Continue to advance the dilatation catheter over the guidewire until the proximal marker on the balloon catheter aligns with the hemostatic valve. This indicates that the balloon catheter tip has reached the tip of guide catheter. Doing so also spares the patient unnecessary irradiation.
- Perform roadmapping for further navigation and appropriate deployment of the balloon catheter system.
- Using fluoroscopy and roadmapping, continue to advance the balloon catheter over the guidewire until it is appropriately positioned in the stenosed segment (Fig. 13.2a).

Angioplasty

- Recover the inflation device from the table.
- Use the distal free port of the stopcock attached to the inflation device (which is in line with the inflation device) to make a wet (meniscus to meniscus) connection with the balloon port of the catheter.

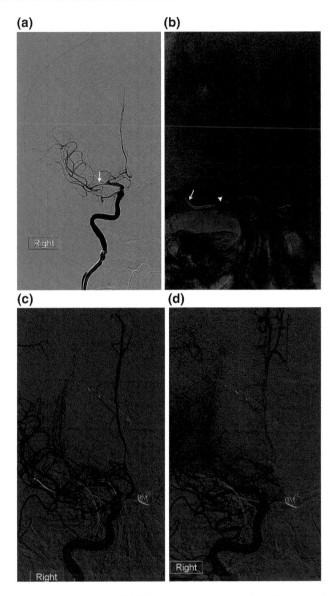

Fig. 13.2 a Severe vasospasm of RMCA (*arrow*) in a patient with a coiled left PComm aneurysm. She was administered 20 mg of verapamil infiltrated into the middle cerebral artery (MCA) as the microcatheter was retracted. This resulted in attenuation of the spasm on angiography performed 20 min later. At this point, a Gateway™ 2 × 9 mm balloon catheter was advanced over microwire into the affected MCA segment. Angioplasty was performed for sustained results. **b** is a fluoroscopy image during angioplasty, demonstrating the tip of the microwire beyond the MCA bifurcation (*arrow*). The dilated proximal aspect of the balloon can be appreciated (*arrowhead*). Repeat angiography with balloon catheter still in MCA (**c**) and following retraction of catheter (**d**), demonstrates significant attenuation of the vasospasm esp. if compared to pre-treatment angiogram (**a**). Note that the ACA, which was not treated, continues to manifest vasospasm through all the images

- Ensure that this connection is secure so that it will not disconnect during angioplasty.
- Close the stopcock to the inflation device.
- To perform in vivo balloon preparation, aspirate the syringe (with nozzle pointing down) attached to the sideport of the stopcock to purge air out of the balloon catheter system.
- Slowly release the plunger of the syringe, so that the air in the catheter is replaced with contrast left in syringe for purpose. Repeat this step once or twice.
- Close the stopcock to syringe and open it to the inflation device.
- Place the compliance card in front of you in the operating field, where you can easily look at it while performing angioplasty.
- Initially, inflate the balloon to a very low pressure (1 atm) and again confirm that it is appropriately positioned across the stenosed segment. Also look at the radiopaque markers for confirmation of balloon position. These markers are more easily visualized on the native image. While viewing the compliance card periodically, begin inflating the angioplasty balloon using the balloon inflation device.
- Inflate slowly by turning the screw provided on the inflation device at a rate ≤ 1 atm/15 s (to 'stretch' not 'crack' the vessel).
- Keep track of and document the inflation time (during which the blood flow will be interrupted by the balloon).
- Step on fluoroscopy pedal frequently to visualize progression of angioplasty (Fig. 13.2b).
- During inflation, the balloon may acquire a 'waist' due to the stenosis. It resolves with the progression of angioplasty.
- Once the goal pressure is reached, deflate the device.
- Confirm complete balloon deflation fluoroscopically.
- In order to achieve complete deflation, one may need to open the stopcock to the syringe and vigorously aspirate. Close the stopcock to syringe while the aspiration is fully applied.
- Confirm complete balloon deflation fluoroscopically.
- Perform follow-up (f/u) angiography to evaluate results of angioplasty (Fig. 13.2c). If needed, repeat the angioplasty.
- Do not exceed the recommended balloon pressures indicated on the compliance card.
- Once angioplasty is completed and balloon completely deflated, withdraw the balloon catheter over guidewire partially. Use fluoroscopy to ensure the guidewire does not move down as well and continues to cross the lesion.
- Perform angiography to assess results angioplasty (Fig. 13.2d).
- Following completion of procedure, perform post-interventional angiography in standard half Townes (Townes in case of VA) and lateral views to rule out any complication such as vessel cut off due to embolism, prior to giving up access.
- At this point, if no further intervention is planned both catheter and wire may be retracted.

- Once the balloon catheter exits from the hemostatic valve of the guide catheter, wipe it clean with Moist Telfa and store it by keeping it submerged in a basin with heparinized saline.
- If the guide catheter has a RHV, ensure it is tightened adequately following balloon catheter withdrawal.

Postoperative Management and Follow Up

- Admit patient to NSICU for at least overnight observation. Further ICU stay will depend upon the patient's clinical condition.
- Generally, 0.9% NS + 20 meq KCl @ 150 cc/hr × 2 h, then decrease to 100 cc/hr while patient is NPO.
- Keep right/left leg (whichever side was used for arteriotomy) straight × 2 h (in case of angioseal closure) or 6–8 h (in case manual compression was applied), with HOB elevated 15°.
- Check groins, DP's, vitals and neuro checks q 15 min × 4, q 30 min × 2, then q hr.
- After arteriotomy closure, initiate IV heparin for 12 h, if there are no contraindications. We usually administer 900 IU/hr for 12 h in patients <70 kg and 1300 IU/hr for those >70 kg. Some oozing from arteriotomy side may occur while patient is receiving heparin and usually is of no concern.
- Advance diet as tolerated.
- Review/Resume preprocedure medications (except oral hypoglycemics, which are initiated 48 h post-intervention and if good PO intake is established).

Suggested Reading

Ringer AJ, Nichols C, Khan SH, Abruzzo TA, Angioplasty and stenting for management of intracranial arterial stenosis. in Hemorrhagic and Ischemic Stroke (Eds. Bendok RB, Naidech AM, Walker MT, Batjer HH) 402–412 (Thieme, New York, 2011).

Vascular Malformations

14

Arteriovenous Malformations (AVM)

Indications and Case Selection

- A surgically inaccessible AVM or the surgical approach carries a high risk of morbidity and mortality.
- As a 'combined' approach where embolization is performed to downsize the AVM to make it amenable to surgical or radiosurgical (or both) intervention.
- Presence of associated lesions, e.g., aneurysm or pseudoaneurysm on the feeding pedicle or nidus, venous thrombosis, venous outflow restriction, venous pouches or dilatations.
- Symptoms from AVM that interfere significantly with the patient's activities and lifestyle.
- As a palliative treatment in an AVM that is not completely treatable by any approach due to location and/or diffuse morphology, but is symptomatic.

Contraindications

- The contraindications below are relative:

  - An asymptomatic AVM where the risk of treatment is higher than not treating.
  - If the deficits following treatment would result in significant limitation of activity, lifestyle or untoward impact on occupation.
  - A less than 3 cm superficial AVM that is completely amenable to surgical resection.
  - Provocative tests demonstrating intolerance to embolic occlusion.
  - Recent major surgery.
  - Pregnancy.

© Springer International Publishing AG 2017
S.H. Khan and A.J. Ringer, *Handbook of Neuroendovascular Techniques*,
DOI 10.1007/978-3-319-52936-3_14

- – Contraindication to anticoagulants and/or thrombolytics.
- – *NBCA* should not be used in those with allergy to cyanoacrylates, ethiodol, or iodine. Premedication in those with iodine allergies is a consideration.
- – *PVA* should not be used as a therapeutic option (other than in cases such as epistaxis). It is usually indicated to effect pre-surgical devascularization of a lesion.

Preoperative Management

- • ASA 325 mg on morning of procedure.
- • Verify laboratory values including Platelet count, BUN, CR, APTT, PT/INR, and ß-HCG (in premenopausal females).
- • Liquids only on morning of procedure.
- • NPO (for ≈6 h) when the procedure is performed under GA.
- • Continue prescribed medications (including ASA and antihypertensives).
- • Insert 2 IV lines.
- • Insert Foley catheter

Technique

- • Secure access to femoral artery (usually) using modified Seldinger technique.
- • Depending on your treatment plan, the sheath should be 6 Fr or larger (see Chaps. 1 and 2 for details and technique of gaining vascular access).
- • Consider using a longer sheath, if the patient has a tortuous vasculature.
- • Prepare a 6 Fr or larger guide catheter, attached to a continuously running flush of heparinized saline. Ensure there are no microbubbles or foreign bodies in the system.
- • Advance the guide catheter over a wire through the sheath.
- • Position in the pertinent vessel using fluoroscopy and road mapping.
- • Prepare a microcatheter and attach it to a continuously running heparinized saline solution.
- • When selecting a microcatheter, take into consideration the type and size of embolic agent to be used to treat the AVM, e.g., if Onyx® (Micro Therapeutics Inc., Irvine, CA) is to be used, then the microcatheter must be dimethyl sulfoxide (DMSO) compatible, e.g., Marathon® (Micro Therapeutics Inc., Irvine, CA) microcatheter. Similarly, when anticipating using thicker coils, e.g., GDC 18 (0.018″ thick), then use an Excelsior 1018 (Boston Scientific, Fremont, CA), instead of Excelsior SL-10.
- • If needed, perform 3-D angiography to better study the morphology, feeding arteries and venous drainage of the AVM. The 3-D angiogram will also enable selection of appropriate working views.
- • If there is a difficulty visualizing the lesion satisfactorily because of high flow, consider increasing the number of frames in a second from the usual 4 FPS to 7.5.

- Administer 5000 units of heparin, check ACT in 20 min. Thereafter, check ACT hourly and giver further doses of heparin as needed to maintain ACT between 250 and 300.
- Advance the microcatheter over a microwire, through the guide catheter, to its target position using fluoroscopy and roadmapping as needed.
- If performing endovascular embolization via the transarterial route using liquid embolic agents, wedge the catheter as close as possible to the fistula.
- In case the AVM derives its feeding arteries from more than one main artery, e.g., feeders from anterior cerebral artery (ACA) and middle cerebral artery (MCA), or contralateral arteries, then embolize only one arterial tree in a given session. Allow the AVM to acclimatize before proceeding with the next stage.
- Below follows a description of technique taking into account specific embolic agents.

Embolic Agents

Coils

- Measure the maximum width of the vessel or AVM pouch to be embolized and select the appropriate sized coils.
- Based on the selected coils, choose a microcatheter size that will enable deposition of the thickest coil selected (see Table 14.1)
- Ensure the microcatheter has two radiopaque markers: one indicating the distal tip of the catheter and the second (proximal) marker indicative of the coil being out of the catheter and in the vessel/aneurysm lumen, when the proximal marker is just crossed by the radiopaque marker on the coil pusher forming a perfect 'T'.
- 'Unlock' the coil. This maneuver involves counter clockwise twisting of the distal sheath at crimped site in case of GDC coils. In case of hydrocoils, slip the tubular black plastic piece off the sheath.
- Using the pusher, advance the coil out of sheath to soften it in warm Ringers lactate (in case of GDC), or sterile steam (for hydrocoils). Then retract it back into the sheath.
- Loosen the RHV of microcatheter and introduce the sheath until it touches and is in continuity with the hub of microcatheter. The RHV should be just tight enough that the coil can be easily advanced and retracted, without causing blackflow.
- Prevention of backflow is particularly important in case of hydrocoils. To prevent it, a small tubing and one way stopcock are interposed between the RHV and microcatheter hub.

Table 14.1 Coil thickness and Microcatheter

Coil/guidewire diameter/thickness (inches)	Microcatheter
0.010–0.012	Excelsior SL-10®; Prowler 10®
0.014	Prowler 14®
0.018	Excelsior 1018®; Prowler Plus®

- Prior to opening the RHV, the stopcock is turned so that the microcatheter is closed to the RHV, preventing backflow. Once the coil sheath is advanced through the RHV, tighten the RHV around the sheath (just enough to still enable smooth movement of sheath) and then open the one way stopcock to access the microcatheter. Advance the sheath all the way to microcatheter hub and then tighten the RHV more. However, one should still be able to move coil within the sheath without any difficulty.
- Deploy the coil using fluoroscopy and roadmapping.
- Once satisfied with the coil placement, detach the coil from the pusher by using the device provided for purpose, which passes an electrolytic current through the soldered joint between the coil and the pusher.
- We preferentially use GDC coils. However, if hydrocoils are used, bear in mind that they expand on exposure to blood. Therefore, the time available for manipulation/deposition is limited (approx. 5 min). Taking too much time will cause the coil to expand causing inability to withdraw, or properly place them. Conversely, they may expand within the microcatheter causing occlusion and requiring the microcatheter to be replaced. For the same reason, ensure the microcatheter remains free of blood.
- Deposit as many coils as necessary to affect obliteration of the lesion.
- Sometimes a 'combined' strategy may be used, in which case coils are initially deposited to slow the rapid blood flow through the AVM, followed by occlusion using liquid embolic agent. If this strategy is used, ensure that the microcatheter is exchanged for one compatible with the liquid embolic agent.

Onyx

Additional Equipment/Devices

- Onyx® 18, or Onyx® 34 (consider 34 for cases with brisk blood flow across fistula).
- A DMSO-compatible microcatheter, e.g.,:

  - Marathon™ (ev3 Neurovascular, Irvine CA).
  - Echelon™ (ev3 Neurovascular, Irvine CA).
  - Rebar™ (ev3 Neurovascular, Irvine CA).
  - Ultraflow™ (ev3 Neurovascular, Irvine CA).

- Onyx mixer.

  - (See Chaps. 1 and 2 for equipment/devices for vascular access and navigation).

Procedure

- Select a DMSO-compatible microcatheter and connect it to a continuously running flush of heparinized saline. We use Marathon™ microcatheter most frequently for the purpose.
- Advance the microcatheter over a microwire, e.g., (Transend 0.010) using fluoroscopy and roadmapping as indicated. Other microwire options available for a marathon catheter include Mirage™ (ev3, 0.008) or X-Pedion™ (ev3, 0.010).
- If a non-DMSO-compatible microcatheter is already in position (e.g., coiling was performed) and the vasculature had proven challenging to navigate, exchange the microcatheters over an exchange length wire (300 cm, see Chap. 5 for details on microwires).
- When withdrawing the microcatheter to be discarded, or advancing the new microcatheter, keep an eye on the tip of microwire to ensure it does not advance inadvertently, or fall back.
- For Satisfactory Onyx administration, 'wedge' the tip of microcatheter. This means placing or 'wedging' the catheter tip against the vessel wall where it branches.
- Angiographically, confirm the correct position of the microcatheter tip and then clean the contrast out of the catheter by flushing with saline. This can be easily done with the pediatric transducer (depending upon its mechanism, press the wings of the transducer together, or pull the provided tab, to increase the flush rate and when done, 'release' the mechanism).
- When ready to perform embolization, perform a blank roadmap, i.e., step upon the pedal as if performing a roadmap, but do not actually inject contrast.
- Ensure the entire microcatheter system is free of blood.
- Draw up the DMSO into the provided yellow colored syringe.
- Disconnect the RHV from the microcatheter and attach the syringe with DMSO to the microcatheter. Make a meniscus to meniscus connection, ensuring there are no air bubbles or blood in the microcatheter. If needed, fill the hub of microcatheter with saline to ensure a proper connection.
- Forewarn the patient that s/he may experience a 'garlic like taste' in the back of the throat with DMSO injection. Additionally, during injection and for a day or two thereafter, the patient's breath and skin may carry the peculiar odor of DMSO.
- Very slowly, inject 0.3–0.8 ml of DMSO depending on the deadspace of the microcatheter, such that the entire catheter is primed with it.
- While undertaking the placement of the microcatheter and its priming, Onyx 18 or 34 is prepared concurrently, bearing in mind the following:

  - Onyx 18 (the numbers 18 or 34 are indicative of viscosity at 40 °C) penetrates deeper into the nidus because of its lower viscosity.
  - Onyx 34 should be used in high flow malformations, as it is less likely than Onyx 18 to flow into the venous sinus when injected from the arterial side.

- Onyx solidifies in 5 min after exposure to blood or saline. To prevent this solidification within the microcatheter itself, ensure that it is free of contrast, saline and blood during Onyx injection.
- The temperature of Onyx should be between 19 and 24 °C when used. If it is frozen because it was stored at a cooler temperature, take the bottles out at the outset of procedure and allow them to thaw at room temperature.
- Place the bottle of Onyx on the Onyx mixer and set the mixer at 8. The mixer can concurrently shake 4 bottles at a time. Shake the Onyx bottle using the mixer for at least 20 min. The mixing should continue until you are just ready to inject Onyx. This will cause a thorough mixing of Onyx and tantalum powder, which assists in satisfactory visualization of the deposited Onyx.
- Immediately prior to injection, draw up Onyx in the provided white 1-ml syringes. To do so, hold the bottle upright (in contrast to when drawing up other low viscosity fluids into a syringe, e.g., 1% Lidocaine) and aspirate using an 18G or 20G needle. If any air is noted in the syringe, turn the bottle over such that the bottle is superior and the syringe is below it. Inject the air into the bottle. Turn the bottle upright again, such that the syringe is again on top and continue to draw up Onyx. Draw a total of 1 ml of air-free Onyx into the syringe.
- Detach the yellow DMSO syringe from the hub of the microcatheter.
- Hold the catheter hub vertically and overfill the hub with DMSO.
- Holding the Onyx syringe upright, make a meniscus to meniscus connection, ensuring that no air is introduced into the system.
- Maintain the syringe containing Onyx in a vertical position. Maintain this position until the Onyx passes beyond the hub of the microcatheter. After that, the syringe can be held in a more comfortable position.
- Inject Onyx slowly at a rate of 0.16 ml/min and not to exceed 0.3 ml/min. The injection should be slow and deliberate, using gentle thumb pressure.
- After injecting approximately 0.3 ml (the volume of the microcatheter), track the Onyx under live fluoroscopy.
- Visually ensure that none is going into a venous sinus, or the non-feeding arteries.
- If there is reflux of Onyx over the microcatheter, wait for a couple of minutes to allow the Onyx to solidify. The solid Onyx plug may prevent further reflux. However, the reflux over the microcatheter should be no greater than 1 cm. Otherwise, it may become difficult to extract the catheter and lead to complications.
- Once the contents of the syringe are completely injected, disconnect the syringe and replace with the next Onyx syringe making a 'meniscus to meniscus' connection. Again, ensure that no air or other substances such as, blood and contrast gain entrance into the microcatheter.
- After the treatment is complete, wait a few seconds, slightly aspirate the syringe and gently pull the microcatheter to separate it from the cast.

- If a resistance is encountered because the tip of microcatheter is strongly adherent to the Onyx plug, maintain a constant, gentle but firm pull upon it, until a sensation of 'giveaway' is felt when the tip of microcatheter. breaks free from Onyx.

Double-Injection Technique

The technique first described by Dr. Robert Mericle enables better image interpretation during embolization, resulting in safer, more confident and usually a much greater volume of Onyx deposition. The operator can confidently determine that the Onyx deposition is entirely within the nidus perimeter and is not entering the draining vein prematurely, or refluxing excessively on to the catheter. This information is crucial as the angioarchitecture of the AVM may not be completely clear during embolization, leading to difficulties in determining whether to stop or continue, or alter the force or speed of injection.

- Selectively catheterize an arterial branch directly supplying the AVM nidus as described above.
- Use the best angiographic projections in two orthogonal planes to demonstrate the feeding arteries and draining veins distinctly from the nidus (Fig. 14.1a–o). If needed, use 3D angiography to select the appropriate working views.
- Ensure that only the AVM is being supplied through the selected branch and not the normal cortical vasculature.
- Gently perform microangiography through the microcatheter and allow the contrast to washout.
- Then during the same run, repeat angiography through the guide catheter. Both injections are done as a single run. (*Do not step off the pedal in between the injections.*)
- Scroll through the completed run to select the frame where the microcatheter DSA run is at its peak opacification.
- 'Rcmask' the selected frame.
- The inverted 'remasked' microangiography run will appear white when played through the (black) Guide catheter run, i.e., the two runs are superimposed.
- Using erasable markers or surgical marking pens, draw the following on the biplane DSA monitors.

  (i)   The perimeter around the nidus.
  (ii)   Perimeter of the nidus component visualized via the microcatheter. injection.
  (iii) Location of draining veins.
  (iv)   Position of microcatheter tip and course of the microcatheter.
  (v)   Possibly, other adjacent feeding pedicles.

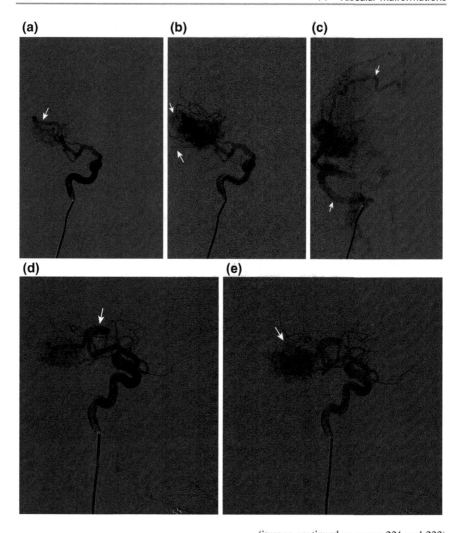

(a)   **(b)**   **(c)**

(d)   **(e)**

(images continued on pages 221 and 222)

Fig. 14.1 A right internal carotid artery injection demonstrating temporal AVM in AP (**a**) and lateral (**d**) views. The main feeding trunk of the MCA has hypertrophied (*arrow*) and is of the same caliber as the proximal M1 segment. (**b** and **e**) Due to the brisk flow, the venous drainage can be seen (*arrows*) in arterial phase. (**c** and **f**) The venous drainage (arrows) from the AVM is via cortical veins to the SSS and via vein of Labbé to right transverse sinus (**f**, *thick arrow*). (**g**) Angiography performed by injecting contrast through the microcatheter (*thin arrow*) rather than the guide catheter (*thicker arrow*). Therefore, only the AVM nidus (*) supplied by the catheterized branch is seen. The embolic agent, e.g., Onyx injected through the microcatheter will deposit largely in this part of the AVM. The microangiographic run has been 'remasked' and hence the appearance of the contrast as *white* rather than the characteristic *black*. Using double injection technique, the contrast from microangiography is allowed to wash out and then additional contrast is injected through the Guide catheter in the same run (Don't step off the pedal in between the two runs). In the microangiography run, where the nidus is most obvious, it is remasked, and will appear as it does in (**h**), superimposed on the Guide catheter (**h**) run.

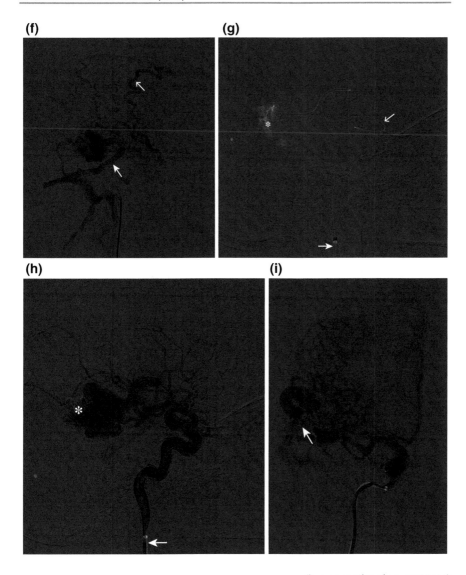

(images continued on next page)

Fig. 14.1 The arrow in the lateral view (**m**) overlies the vein of Labbé and point to the Onyx casted MCA branch that was the largest feeder to the AVM. The asterisk (*) demonstrates the part of the nidus supplied by the catheterized branch compared to the rest. We demarcate on the monitor, the outline of the catheterized nidus, the perimeter of the entire AVM, the draining veins and the course of microcatheter, using different colored erasable markers. As long as the table or patient are not moved, these demarcations remain reliable. If the embolization is undertaken visualizing these perimeters, it is safer. (**i**) The Onyx cast (*arrow*) consequent to embolization via microcatheter is well visualized. Arterial phases in AP (**j**) and lateral (**k**) views from post-embolization angiography. There appears to be a complete embolization of the AVM with only the Onyx cast (*arrow*) demonstrating the AVM. Due to the redistribution of blood flow, the normal vasculature including the lenticulostriate arteries (*arrowhead*) are much better visualized when compared to pre-embolization images (see **b** and **e**). Venous phase of angiography in AP (**l**) and lateral (**m**) views better demonstrate the normal cortical veins and sinuses. There is attenuation in the size of the vein of Labbé.

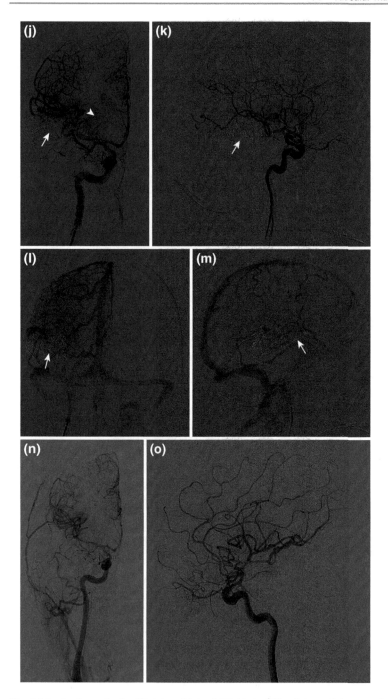

Fig. 14.1 Angiography in AP (**n**) and lateral (**o**) views following craniotomy and resection of embolized AVM. The Onyx cast is gone and normal vasculature persistsThe arrow in the lateral view (**m**) overlies the vein of Labbé and point to the Onyx casted MCA branch that was the largest feeder to the AVM. Angiography in AP (**n**) and lateral (**o**) views following craniotomy and resection of embolized AVM. The Onyx cast is gone and normal vasculature persists

- Draw each of the above in a different color, e.g., nidus visualized through microcatheter: red; veins: blue; microcatheter: green; perimeter of nidus through guide catheter: black.
- As long as the patient, table and biplanar image intensifiers remain unchanged in position, these landmarks remain reliable, throughout prolonged injections.
- As described above, treat the microcatheter with DMSO prior to embolization.
- Perform blank roadmaps and commence onyx embolization.
- When the amount of Onyx equal to the volume of the catheter has been injected (approx. 0.3 ml), commence checking the progress of Onyx deposition into the nidus in both planes, by transiently stepping on the pedal frequently to obtain fluoroscopic images.
- Perform new roadmaps when the previously deposited Onyx needs to be subtracted to better visualize new deposition.
- As long as the Onyx deposition is within the perimeter of AVM (obtained through the Guide catheter), it is safe to continue even if the deposition is in area not delineated by the microangiography run.
- Once the treatment is complete, wait a few seconds, slightly aspirate the syringe and gently pull the microcatheter to separate it from the cast.
- In case resistance is encountered because the tip of microcatheter is adherent in the Onyx plug, maintain a constant, gentle but firm pull upon it, until a sensation of 'give way' happens when the tip of microcatheter breaks free from Onyx. Occasionally, a quick 'wrist flick' is required to achieve separation of the microcatheter tip from the Onyx cast.

NBCA

Additional Equipment/Devices

- Trufill kit comprising of NBCA/ethiodol/tantalum (Trufill, Cordis Endovascular).
- A small (1.5–1.8 Fr) flow directed, non-reinforced catheter, e.g.:

  - Regatta (Cordis, Miami, FL).
  - Spinnaker Elite (Boston Scientific, Fremont, CA).
  - Ultraflow (ev3).
  - (See Chaps. 1 and 2 for additional equipment/devices for vascular access and navigation).

Procedure

- Advance the microcatheter attached to a continuously running flush of heparinized saline, over a microwire, placing its tip in the distal aspect of the feeding artery, using standard techniques. Depending on operator preference and nidal anatomy, the catheter tip may be wedged or positioned free.

Table 14.2 NBCA Manufacturer Recommended Concentrations

Condition	Ethiodol: NBCA ratio	Ethiodol volume (cc)	NBCA volume (cc)
For deep penetration of the nidus, in the absence of AV fistula or high flow rates	3:1 75% Ethiodol:25% NBCA	0.75	0.25
	2:1 67% Ethiodol:33% NBCA	0.67	0.33
Feeding pedicle injections close to the nidus at high flow rates where venous opacification occurs within 0.5 sec on contrast injection	1:1 50% Ethiodol:50% NBCA	0.50	0.50
	1:2 33% Ethiodol:67% NBCA	0.33	0.67

- Prepare the NBCA mixture on a separate table using clean gloves. This is to prevent any contamination with ionic catalysts.
- Add the vial of tantalum powder to above mixture to enhance its radiopacity.
- For a wedged injection: a comparatively dilute (25–33%) concentration is prepared by mixing 1 cc of NBCA with 2–3 cc of ethiodol in a shot glass.
- Table 14.2 shows various concentrations recommended by manufacturer.
- Induce relative hypotension (20–30% decrease in MAP).
- Perform test injections using subtracted fluoroscopic observation (blank road map) to assess catheter position and optimal rate of injection.
- Ensure catheter lumen is devoid of ionic catalysts by irrigating with 5% dextrose.
- Obtain a blank road map, then commence injecting NBCA slowly, under continuous visualization, over 15–60 sec.
- Adjust the injection rate in order to obtain a solid nidal caste without reflux.
- Stop immediately, if the NBCA enters a draining vein or sinus.
- Resume after a few seconds and continue if satisfactory nidal filling is visualized. If the NBCA enters the vein again or there is proximal reflux, terminate the injection.
- For a non-wedged injection: the NBCA should be more concentrated because of the more rapid flow and shorter arterial-venous transit time through the nidus.
- At higher concentrations (NBCA ≥ 50%) up to 0.5 g of tantalum should be added to the mixture.
- The injection rate is faster and injection time is shorter (1–3 s).
- If there is a large direct fistula, or rapid flow, induce maximal hypotension and a very high concentration of NBCA. Alternatively, coils may be used first to slow down the rate of blood flow, followed by NBCA.

- After completion of procedure, aspirate the microcatheter briskly and remove it quickly.
- Aspirate the guide catheter and examine it fluoroscopically.

PVA

- Polyvinyl alcohol (PVA) is available in sizes ranging from 50 to 1000 μm.
- In the presence of agents like coils, Onyx and NBCA, it is primarily used in devascularization of AVM or tumor prior to surgery. However, Onyx appears to be usurping this role as well.
- A far better indication for PVA is the devascularization of the ECA branches, e.g., in epistaxis or dural supply of meningioma. The explanation below is pertinent to lesions such as AVM, as well as, lesions of ECA, e.g., epistaxis.

Additional Equipment/Devices

- Microcatheter selection should depend upon the size of the PVA particles used, to prevent catheter occlusion by the particles. Preferably use a larger caliber catheter (e.g., 2.3 Fr). If possible, avoid using tapered tip microcatheter, as it is more likely to occlude. We commonly use Marathon (ev3) while treating fistulae in the ECA branches.
- Other microcatheter considerations include Prowler Plus (Codman) and Rapidtransit (Codman).

Procedure

- Advance the microcatheter to its planned location, positioning it as close as possible to the malformation.
- Inspect angiograms carefully for potentially dangerous collaterals that must not be embolized.
- Measure the feeding vessels and lesion to select the appropriate size particles.
- Bear in mind, the smaller the particles, the greater the likelihood of deep penetration into smaller vessels, e.g., precapillaries, resulting in cranial nerve deficits, etc.
- Proceed to prepare the PVA mixture on a separate table/space, taking care that other equipment used during procedure does not get contaminated with the particles. Once the mixture is prepared, change gloves. Take extreme precautions that the PVA particles do not inadvertently contaminate drapes, catheters etc. leading to possibility of embolic complications.
- Inspect the PVA particles for uniformity of size.
- Inject 10 ml of non-ionic contrast into the bottle containing PVA. Conversely, it may be safer to remove the top of the bottle and empty the contents into a shot glass and then add the non-ionic contrast to it.

- Shake to suspend the particles in the contrast.
- Attach a 3-way stopcock to a 20-ml syringe.
- Draw up the suspension into the syringe.
- Attach a 3-ml syringe to the 3 way stopcock. The 3-ml syringe should be attached to the port in line with that which will be attached to the catheter. The larger 20-ml syringe is attached to the port perpendicular to these two.
- Ensure the syringes and stopcock system are free of air bubbles.
- Use the plungers of the small and large syringes to push the suspension back and forth between the syringes, while the stopcock is turned to close off the third (free) port, intended for the microcatheter. The movement will assist in keeping the PVA particles in suspension.
- Draw suspension into the 3-ml syringe from the larger syringe and turn the stopcock, so that the port with the 20-ml syringe is blocked.
- Change gloves and discard any towels etc. contaminated by PVA particles.
- Detach the RHV from the microcatheter and make a meniscus to meniscus connection between the microcatheter and the free portal of the 3 way stopcock. Ensure the system is free of air bubbles.
- Place a towel on the drape under the microcatheter to ensure it catches any PVA particles and the operating field is not inadvertently contaminated by potential emboli.
- Confirm that the microcatheter tip has maintained its position. Perform angiography, if necessary.
- Obtain a blank roadmap.
- Gradually commence injecting the PVA from the 3-ml syringe under direct visualization.
- Monitor carefully to ensure there is no reflux or, that the PVA particles are not flowing into the draining vein/sinus. If this is detected, stop immediately.
- As the feeding vessel or nidus is occluded, resistance is felt during injection.
- Do not attempt to overcome this resistance by using greater force. Such attempts would lead to reflux, or untoward embolization of an unintended vessel.
- As needed, refill the 3-ml syringe from the 20-ml syringe by turning the stopcock to the microcatheter and closing the system to the catheter. Then aspirate the PVA suspension into the 3-ml syringe. To ensure uniform distribution of the PVA particles, agitate the suspension by initially drawing it back and forth between the two syringes. Once a smooth suspension is achieved, fill the 3-ml syringe for administration of PVA via the microcatheter. During the agitation process, ensure that the stopcock is closed to the microcatheter, or the results could be catastrophic.
- After the 3-ml syringe is filled, turn the stopcock to establish continuity between microcatheter and the 3-ml syringe and closing it to the 20-ml syringe.
- Resume injecting PVA under direct vision.
- Once the vessel/nidus is occluded, perform angiography for confirmation of occlusion.
- If the catheter appears obstructed, do not attempt to open it in vivo by a forceful injection or passing microwire through it. Remove the microcatheter completely

from the guide catheter and inspect it. If occluded and unable to re-establish flow by irrigating it, replace it with a new microcatheter.

- When the embolization procedure is complete, withdraw and remove the microcatheter while maintaining gentle suction upon it, so that the PVA particles still contained within it do not inadvertently embolize.
- Discard the microcatheter along with the protective towel placed under it.
- Complete post-procedure angiography.

Location-Specific Considerations

- PVA embolization of ECA branches is relatively safe. However, vigilance should still be exercised, to prevent inadvertent embolization to ICA and its branches.
- Look out for collaterals whereby PVA may inadvertently embolize to ICA circulation.
- The smaller particles may penetrate deep into a nidus, but also are more likely to reach pre-capillary vessels causing cranial nerve palsies and other complications.
- Be extra vigilant when using PVA preoperatively to attenuate the vascular supply to an AVM. As a rule, we do not use PVA in the ICA and its branches and elect to go for other options, e.g., Onyx.

Postoperative Management and Follow-up

- Admit to NSICU for at least overnight observation. Additional ICU stay will depend upon the patient's clinical condition.
- Generally, 0.9% NS + 20 meq KCl @ 150 cc/hr × 2 h, then decrease to 100 cc/hr, if patient is NPO. Discontinue IV fluids once good oral intake is established.
- Keep right/left leg (whichever side was used for procedure) straight for 2 h (in case of angioseal closure) or 6–8 h (in case manual compression was applied), with HOB elevated 15°.
- Check groins, DP's, vitals, and neuro checks q 15 min × 4, q 30 min × 4, then q hr.
- Maintain mild hypotension overnight in case of a smaller AVM.
- In case of obliteration of a significant portion of a larger AVM, or if some embolic agent went into the draining vein/sinus, may maintain hypotension for a longer duration, allowing BP to normalize gradually.
- ASA 81—325 mg PO daily.
- Advance diet as tolerated.
- Review/Resume pre-procedure medications (except oral hypoglycemics which are resumed 48 h after intervention and once oral intake is established).

- Ensure arrangements for postoperative/post-discharge follow-up.
- Discharge after 48–72 h esp. in case of large AVM, monitoring patient for perfusion pressure break through bleeding, seizures and other potential complications.
- F/u on outpatient basis in 4 weeks.
- F/u angiography at 3 months.
- In case an AVM requiring staged embolization, may perform the next procedure in 1–4 weeks time.

Dural Arteriovenous Fistulae (DAVF)

- Angiographically, these will appear as one or more direct, true fistulae between arteries and veins. Unlike AVM, there are no intervening capillaries or nidus.

Indications and Case Selection

- Clinically, DAVF with 'aggressive' features, e.g., ICH, Focal neurological deficit (FND), dementia and papilledema are always considered for treatment. Due to the high annual mortality rate (10.4%) and annual hemorrhage rate (8.1%), the treatment should be expeditious.
- The following angiographic findings warrant strong consideration for treatment:

  - Selective contrast injection into ICA or VA demonstrates delayed cerebral circulation time. The finding is indicative of venous congestive encephalopathy.
  - Pseudophlebitic pattern: Brain surface demonstrating tortuous, dilated collateral veins in the venous phase of the angiogram. This finding is associated with a greater risk of hemorrhage or non-hemorrhagic neurological deficit.
  - Cortical venous reflux (CVR). To ensure that this is not missed, always perform selective (rather than global, non-selective) angiography when assessing for DAVF. Venous stenosis or obstruction is commonly found in patients with CVR.

- If a DAVF is detected, look for additional fistulae, as these are multiple in up to 8%.
- Those with 'benign' features, e.g., pulsatile bruit, orbital congestion, cranial nerve palsy, or chronic headaches, may be considered for treatment if the symptoms are causing considerable discomfort to the patient, or are angiographically progressive. In many cases the treatment is palliative, i.e., the symptoms are reduced, but the fistula is not completely obliterated. Because of the risk of conversion to a more aggressive form, with CVR, the benign type DAVF should continue to be followed, even if treatment is not indicated. This

follow-up may be clinical, with radiological assessment for any change in symptoms. One suggested protocol is to perform MRA with gadolinium annually with follow-up conventional catheter angiography at 3 years. If there is any change in the patient's clinical condition, whether it is worsening, improvement or resolution of the symptoms, perform standard angiography to assess for CVR.

- Asymptomatic DAVF can usually be followed.

Contraindications

- Most contraindications are relative, and a risk benefit assessment is performed on a case by case basis:

    - ICH.
    - Provocative tests demonstrating intolerance to occlusion.
    - Recent major surgery.
    - Pregnancy.
    - Contraindication to anticoagulants and/or thrombolytics.
    - *NBCA* should not be used in those with allergy to cyanoacrylates, ethiodol or iodine. Premedication in those with iodine allergies is a consideration.
    - *PVA* should not be used as a therapeutic option (other than in cases of epistaxis). It is usually indicated for pre-surgical devascularization of lesion.

Preoperative Management

- Verify laboratory values including Platelet count, BUN, CR, APTT, PT/INR, and ß-HCG (in premenopausal females).
- Liquids only on morning of procedure.
- NPO (for ≈ 6 h) when procedure performed under GA.
- Continue prescribed medications (including ASA and antihypertensives).
- Insert 2 IV lines.

Technique

- The approach can be transarterial, transvenous, or a combination. When feasible, the transvenous approach is preferred. The probability of fistula obliteration is greater via the venous route.
- Very infrequently, it is possible to access the venous side via the arterial route because of a large connection between the dural artery and adjacent vein, e.g., in

traumatic DAVF. This is usually not possible in spontaneous DAVF, as the feeding artery is too small.

- Secure access using modified Seldinger technique to femoral artery, femoral vein, or both, depending on your treatment plan (see Chaps. 1 and 2 for detail and technique of gaining vascular access). Preferably, avoid accessing femoral artery and vein on the same side as this leads to the likelihood of arteriovenous fistula at access site.
- Place a 6 Fr or larger sheath and connect it to a continuously running flush of heparinized saline.
- Prepare a 6 Fr or larger guide catheter, attached to a continuously running flush of heparinized saline. Ensure there are no microbubbles or foreign bodies in the system.
- Advance the guide catheter over a wire through the sheath.
- Position in the pertinent vessel using fluoroscopy and road mapping.
- Prepare a microcatheter and attach to continuously running heparinized saline solution.
- When selecting a microcatheter, take into consideration the type and size of embolic agent to be used to treat the DAVF, e.g., if Onyx® (Micro Therapeutics inc., Irvine, CA) is to be used, the catheter must be dimethyl sulfoxide (DMSO) compatible, e.g., Marathon® microcatheter (ev3, 'Irvine, CA). Similarly, when anticipating using larger coils with coil thickness/of 0.018″, use an Excelsior 1018, instead of SL-10 microcatheter. Or, if NBCA is to be used, then a flow directed, non-reinforced microcatheter such as Spinnaker Elite (Boston Scientific) or Regatta (Cordis), should be used.
- If needed, perform 3-D angiography to better study the morphology, feeding arteries and venous drainage of the DAVF. The 3-D angiogram will also enable selection of appropriate working views.
- Administer 5000 units of heparin, check ACT in 20 min. Thereafter, check ACT hourly and give further doses of heparin as needed to maintain ACT between 250 and 300.
- Advance the microcatheter over a microwire, through the guide catheter, to its target position using fluoroscopy and roadmapping as needed.
- If performing endovascular embolization via the transarterial route using liquid embolic agents, wedge the catheter as close as possible to the fistula.
- If using the transvenous route, consider the potential outcome of venous occlusion, e.g., venous infarct if the sinus being occluded is also the main source of drainage for normal veins. In such a situation consider highly selective occlusion that will spare the normal drainage. Alternatively, instead of performing a complete occlusion, consider partial treatment only such that CVR is eliminated, converting the fistula into the benign Borden type I.
- When using the venous route, ascertain that the venous channel is not tenuous (e.g., acute DAVF) rendering it prone to rupture during manipulation. The venous walls become sturdier when the fistula has been present for a while.
- Below follows a description of technique taking into account specific embolic agents.

Embolic Agents

Coils

- Measure the maximum width of the fistulous site to be occluded and select the appropriate sized coils.
- Based on the selection of coils, choose a microcatheter of a size that will enable the deposition of the largest coil selected (See Table 14.1 in 'AVM' section).
- Ensure the microcatheter has two radiopaque markers: one indicating the distal tip of the catheter and the second (proximal) indicative of the coil being out of the catheter and in the vessel/aneurysm lumen, when the proximal marker is just crossed by the radiopaque marker on the coil pusher.
- Soften the selected coil in warm Ringers lactate (in case of GDC) or sterile steam (for Hydrocoils).
- Advance the coil to its target using fluoroscopy and roadmapping.
- Once satisfied with the coil placement, detach the coil from the pusher by using the device provided for the purpose, which passes an electrolytic current through the soldered joint between the coil and the pusher.
- We preferentially use GDC coils. However, if hydrocoils are used, bear in mind that they expand on exposure to blood. Therefore, the time available for manipulation/deposition is limited. Taking too much time will cause a hydrocoil to expand causing inability to withdraw or properly place it. Conversely, it may expand within the microcatheter causing catheter occlusion and requiring catheter replacement. For the same reason, ensure the microcatheter remains free of blood.
- Deposit as many coils as necessary to effect occlusion of the fistula.
- Sometimes a 'combined' strategy may be used, where initially coils are deposited to slow the rapid blood flow through the fistula, followed by occlusion using a liquid embolic agent. If this strategy is used, ensure that the micro-catheter is exchanged for one compatible with the liquid embolic agent.

Onyx

- For additional equipment and technical details, refer to the AVM section above. Also see Fig. 14.2.

NBCA

- For additional equipment and technical details, refer to the AVM section above.
- Remember, if the fistula has a very rapid flow, initially deposition of coils may be in order to attenuate the flow rate.
- NBCA can also be prepared in a more concentrated form.

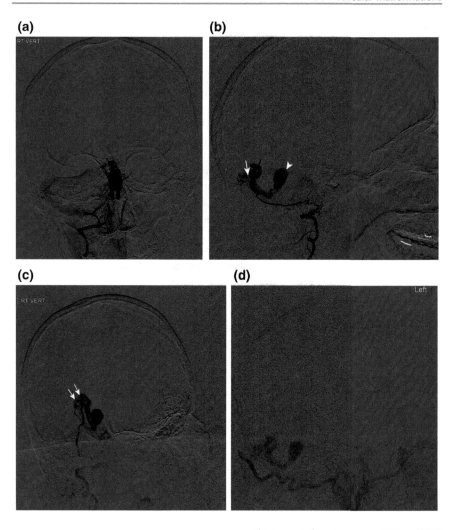

(images continued on pages 233 and 234)

Fig. 14.2 A DAVF with a characteristic extensive blood supply from multiple arterial trees. AP (**a**) and lateral (**b**) views of vertebral angiography demonstrating supply from the dorsal dural branch of the VA. The fistulous connection is apparent (*arrow*), as is a venous aneurysmal sac (*arrowhead*). An oblique view (**c**) demonstrates the arteriovenous fistulous connections even better (*arrows*). The DAVF is also supplied by the occipital artery (**d** and **e**); posterior branches of middle meningeal artery (**f**), where branches advancing to make fistulous connections are obvious (*arrows*); (**g**) 3D reformatted image showing the dural branch of VA supplying the DAVF (compare to **b**). The 3D images can be rotated to select projections suitable for navigation and embolization.

(e)   **(f)**

(g)   **(h)**

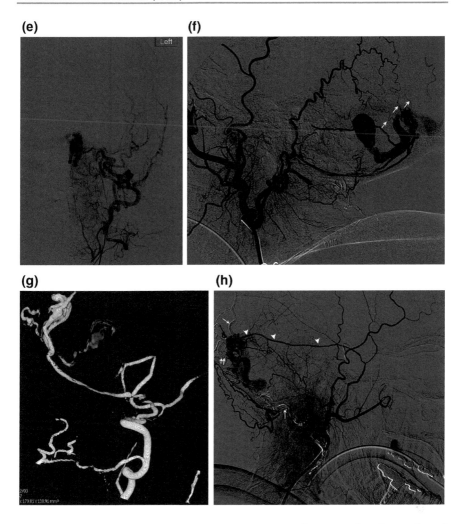

(images continued on next page)

Fig. 14.2 The angiography is then repeated in selected projections for treatment. (**h**) Part of the DAVF has been embolized (*double arrow*) resulting in attenuation of flow through it. An Onyx cast is also noted in the occipital artery (*arrow*). The DAVF continues to be supplied by a posterior branch of the middle meningeal artery (*arrowheads*). (**i**) The posterior branch of middle meningeal artery (*arrows*) participating in supplying the DAVF. The venous channel of the DAVF is obvious (*arrowheads*). (**j**) Embolization has been performed via the meningeal branch and the Onyx cast is appreciated in the venous aneurysmal sac of DAVF as well as the feeding artery (*arrows*). The DAVF including, the associated prominent venous channel, is no longer visible

(i)   **(j)**

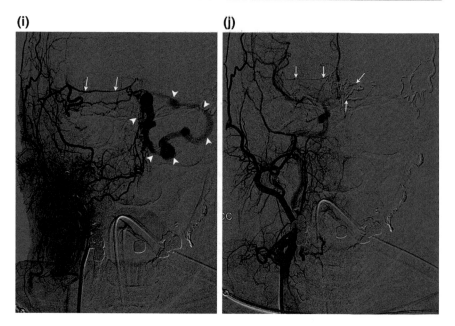

Fig. 14.2

PVA

- For additional equipment and technical details, refer to the AVM section above.

Postoperative Management and Follow-up

- Admit to NSICU for at least overnight observation. Further ICU care will depend upon the patient's clinical condition.
- Refer to AVM section above for details.

Carotid Cavernous Fistulae (CCF)

This section deals with direct (which are usually traumatic) fistulae. DAVF have been addressed in section above. The direct fistula are usually a single shunt between the ICA and carotid sinus

Indications and Case Selection

- Direct fistulae usually require treatment as they frequently do not resolve spontaneously.

- When indicated, treatment usually may be performed within a couple of days of the diagnosis, i.e., treatment does not have to be emergent. As long as the patient is stable, treatment may be provided on an urgent or semi-elective basis.
- Indications for urgent treatment include ICH, epistaxis, increased IOP, decreased visual acuity, rapidly progressive proptosis, cerebral ischemia and enlargement of traumatic aneurysm beyond the cavernous sinus.
- Other indications include corneal exposure, diplopia, proptosis, intolerable bruits or headaches.

Preoperative Management

- Admit patient.
- Standard laboratory investigations (as indicated in AVM section).
- Complete investigations including high-resolution fine cut CT and MRI to better assess the patients' injuries.
- In case of a multi-trauma, first stabilize the patient. Use ATLS protocol and address the more critical injuries.
- To treat visual loss and increased intra-ocular pressure, medications such as dexamethasone, ß-blockers and acetazolamide may be considered while optimizing the patient's condition prior to definitive treatment.

Technique

- The treatment objective is to eliminate the fistula. To this effect:
- Perform diagnostic angiography to identify the exact location and size of the fistula and its venous drainage.
- To address the high flow, an increase in the numbers of frames per second (fps) may be needed. Compared to the usual 2–4 fps, consider 7.5 fps.
- In addition to the CCF, also look for other vascular injuries/anomalies.
- Selective catheterization of both ECAs and ICAs is performed to assess the supply from these to the CCF.
- Angiography is also performed after manual compression of the CCA on the side of fistula to better assess cross flow from the contralateral side. The digital compression will attenuate the high blood flow to the fistula, enabling its visualization.
- Do not compress both carotids simultaneously.
- Also study the vertebrobasilar circulation since in a high flow fistula blood flow may be seen siphoned to the CCF.
- Perform 3D angiography if needed. In addition to studying the fistula, it will assist in the selection of appropriate working views for intervention.
- Also pay attention to the venous involvement including cavernous sinuses, superior and inferior ophthalmic veins, sphenoparietal sinus, superior and inferior petrosal sinuses and the pterygoid plexi.

- A number of treatment options are available. The following routes can be utilized for treating CCF.

  - Transarterial.
  - Transvenous via superior ophthalmic vein (if conventional routes are not available).

Transarterial Embolization of CCF

Embolic Agents

Coils

- Currently, the method of choice is transarterial coil embolization of the CCF.
- To this effect:

  - Secure arterial access using modified Seldinger technique as indicated in detail above (See 'Technique' in AVM section. Also see Chaps. 1 and 2 for detail and technique of gaining vascular access).
  - Place the guide catheter in the proximal ICA with the fistula. The tip of the catheter should be proximal to the fistula.
  - If 3D angiography is performed, select the working views from the same.
  - Prepare a microcatheter, e.g., an Excelsior SL-10 or, Excelsior 1018 microcatheter (Stryker Neurovascular, Fremont, CA), depending upon the size of coil intended to be used.
  - Select a microwire, e.g., Transend (Stryker Neurovascular, Fremont, CA) or, Synchro 2 (Stryker Neurovascular, Fremont, CA). If not pre-shaped, shape the tip of the microwire as needed.
  - Using fluoroscopy, advance the microcatheter over the microwire to the tip of the guide catheter.
  - Obtain roadmaps in the selected working views, or projections.
  - Using roadmap, advance the microcatheter over microwire and attempt to advance the microcatheter into cavernous sinus via the fistula. This may require considerable effort and manipulation.
  - Once the microwire is in the sinus, carefully advance the microcatheter over it.
  - Administer 5000 units of heparin intravenously, check ACT in 20 min. Thereafter, check the ACT hourly and administer further doses of heparin as needed to maintain ACT between 250 and 300.
  - Remove the microwire and commence deploying coils into the sinus to occlude the sinus.
  - Pay attention to the marker on the coil pusher. Once it crosses the second (proximal) marker on the catheter that indicates the coil has been completely deployed.

- Once the coil has been positioned to your satisfaction, detach it. Continue coiling until the sinus is occluded resulting in interruption of the fistula.
- To detach a GDC coil, insert the tip of an 18G needle into the patients skin in the femoral region. Attach the Black cable to the needle (for grounding). Attach the red cable to the outer tip of the coil pusher, when the coil is ready to be detached. The other end of these cables go into ports on the detacher.
- Switch the detacher on. The machine will beep when the coil is detached. Additionally, the rhythm strip on the monitor screen will become very irregular, just prior to detachment. The monitor artifact around the time of detachment has no untoward clinical implications.
- Remove the red cable from the pusher. Retract the pusher initially under direct vision, to ensure the coil has truly detached. Once detachment is confirmed, the removal is completed without fluoroscopy.
- Be careful not to lose catheter access to the cavernous sinus (CS).
- Periodically perform angiography through the guide catheter to assess the progress of intervention.
- As the fistula is occluded, less contrast will enter the CS and the previously poorly visualized ICA distal to the fistula becomes visible.
- When completely occluded, no further contrast will enter the CS.
- Perform post-embolization angiography.
- Remove the microcatheter once coiling is complete and post-intervention angiography does not reveal any complication.

Onyx

- Please refer to the AVM section above regarding technique of use.
- In case of high flow fistula, it may be advisable to initially deposit coils into the CS to slow the blood flow. This will prevent the inadvertent embolization of Onyx into the draining veins and sinuses.
- If needed, consider using the more dense Onyx 34 instead of Onyx 18.

NBCA

- Use NBCA once the flow through the CCF has been slowed in order to prevent untoward deposition in the venous sinuses.
- Be extremely vigilant about the potential for reflux into the carotid artery, which could cause a stroke. This may particularly occur when the CCF closure is near completion and the pressure gradient between the carotid artery and the cavernous sinus is lowered.

Balloons

- Balloons are no longer available in the USA for treatment of CCF.

Coil Occlusion of the Internal Carotid Artery

- The desirable treatment for CCF is the occlusion of the fistula itself, essentially resulting in ICA reconstruction. This is frequently not possible. If the CCF itself is not amenable to treatment by arterial or venous route, sacrifice of the involved ICA is an option, esp. if satisfactory supply has been confirmed from the contralateral ICA via anterior communicating (ACom) and/or supply via the posterior communicating (PCom) arteries.

Technique

- Position the Guide catheter in the proximal ICA.
- Advance a microcatheter, e.g., Excelsior 1018 (Stryker Neurovascular, Fremont, CA) over a microwire such that it is distal to the fistulous communication between the ICA and CCF but, preferably proximal to the PCom origin. It is important to occlude the ICA proximal and distal to the fistula.
- Select a coil whose circumference should be at least equal to or slightly larger than the ICA diameter. For details about deployment, refer to AVM section above. For hydrocoils, refer to transvenous coil embolization below).
- Once the coil has been positioned, observe it carefully to ensure that it will maintain its position following detachment. If the coil loops appear to be changing there position, or pulsating back and forth readily, that may indicate the deployed coil should be replaced with a larger coil.
- Detach only when satisfied that the coil is secure in its position. Otherwise, there is a risk of it embolizing into MCA or ACA and resulting in a stroke.
- After detachment of first coil, deploy and detach additional coils, such that a firm plug is created in the cavernous ICA segment.
- As the coil placement progresses, angiography will reveal flow stasis and difficulty in visualization of ICA well proximal to the coil plug. This is an anticipated angiographic finding.
- Once the embolization is complete, perform bilateral carotid angiography to confirm complete CCF occlusion.
- If there was successful sparing of the PCom origin on the involved side, there is good possibility of flow continuing through it because of retrograde ICA filling distal to coil plug.

Transvenous Embolization of CCF

- While perhaps technically somewhat more challenging and less familiar to interventionists, the transvenous approach may be ideally suited for dealing with CCF.
- Make a superficial, small skin stab incision medial to the palpable arterial pulsations.
- Using modified Seldinger technique access the femoral vein, which lies medial to the arterial pulsations.

- Dark, non-pulsating venous blood will emanate from the needle at low pressure.
- Place a sheath in the vein in the same manner as when an artery is catheterized. The sheath should be at least 6 Fr.
- Connect the sheath to a continuously running flush of heparinized saline and secure the sheath to adjacent skin using 2-0 silk suture.
- If not already present, a sheath is secured in the femoral artery and connected to a continuously running flush of heparinized saline. To prevent the likelihood of arteriovenous fistula formation, when possible the artery and vein should not be catheterized at the same femoral site.
- A diagnostic catheter connected to a continuously running flush of heparinized saline, is advanced through the sheath and over a guidewire into the uninvolved CCA for angiography and roadmap assistance. During the procedure, it will need to be repositioned on the involved side to assess the resolution of CCF.
- Advance the Guide catheter (e.g., 6 Fr Envoy) connected to a continuous heparinized saline flush into the femoral vein over wire (e.g., 0.035 Glidewire), using fluoroscopy
- Navigate upwards to the inferior vena cava.
- The course of inferior vena cava is usually to the right of aorta and will lead to right atrium.
- The Guide catheter is advanced over wire into the superior vena cava.
- Direct the guidewire to the left or superiorly, depending on which IJV needs to be catheterized.
- Unlike the arteries, valves will be encountered in the veins. Resistance will be felt if the valve is closed. Do not attempt to push through forcefully. Time the advancement and manipulation of the wire with inspiration. Then advance the catheter over the wire. Once the veins have been traversed, the valves are no longer a concern since none are present in the sinus.
- When performing road mapping to assist with navigation through the venous system, remember to wait at least 3 s after the injection, before stepping on the peddle to get the road map.
- Position the guide catheter in the IJV.
- Prepare the microcatheter and connect it to a continuously running solution of heparinized saline. The size of the microcatheter will depend upon the size of coils intended to be used, e.g.,
- Excelsior SL-10 (Boston Scientific, Fremont, CA) for GDC 10 coils, or Excelsior 1018 if use of larger caliber coils is planned.
- Advance the microcatheter over microwire to the tip of guide catheter.
- If needed, repeat the roadmap in the working view.
- Navigate the microwire through the inferior petrosal sinus (usually at junction of IJV and sigmoid sinus) or superior petrosal sinus (usually at junction of transverse sinus and SS) into the CS.
- Advance the microcatheter over the wire into the involved cavernous sinus.
- Remove the microwire.
- Administer 5000 units of heparin intravenously, check ACT in 20 min. Thereafter, check ACT hourly and giver further doses of heparin as needed to maintain ACT between 250 and 300.

- Select the appropriate sized coils.
- Set up the coil detacher, if using GDC coils.
- If needed, replace its battery to ensure proper functioning throughout the procedure.
- Stick an 18G needle into the patient's skin in the femoral region. Attach the Black cable to the needle (for grounding). The other end of this cable is inserted into the appropriate portal on the detacher.
- One end of the second cable (red in color) is inserted into the detacher. The other end of this cable is intended for the outer end of the coil pusher.
- Soften the coil by pushing it out of its sheath into a bowl of sterile, warm Ringers lactate
- Retract the coil back into is sheath and then loosen the microcatheter RHV. Advance the sheath through the RHV until it abuts the hub of the microcatheter. Tighten the RHV around the sheath.
- Advance the coil into the microcatheter until the end of the pusher is almost in the sheath.
- Loosen the RHV to retract and set aside the sheath and then retighten it around the pusher so that there is no backflow, but the pusher can be easily advanced/retracted.
- Advance the coil into the cavernous sinus under direct vision using fluoroscopy.
- Complete deployment into the cavernous sinus will be indicated when the marker on the coil pusher just crosses the marker on the catheter (proximal to the tip marker) forming a 'T'.
- Prior to detaching the coil from the pusher, ensure that the coil is stable. If the coil is pulsating, changing its shape or location, such findings are indicative of the fact that the coil may be too small. Exchange the coil for one that has a loop of larger diameter. Additionally, longer length may also be required, e.g., an 8×30 coil may be replaced by a 10×30, or larger coil depending upon the measurements.
- When the coil is ready to detach, attach the free end of the red cable to the outer end of the coil pusher.
- Switch the detacher on. The machine will beep when the coil is detached. Additionally, the rhythm strip on the monitor screen will become very irregular, just prior to detachment. These monitor findings around the time of detachment are an artifact and have no untoward clinical implications.
- Remove the red cable from the pusher and initially withdraw the pusher while visualizing it under fluoroscopy, to confirm that the coil indeed was successfully detached. Once detachment is confirmed, step off the fluoroscopy pedal and withdraw the pusher completely.
- Rarely, the coil does not detach, in which case after confirming suitable positioning, detachment is attempted again.
- Place as many coils as needed.
- Be careful not to lose catheter access to the cavernous sinus CS.
- Periodically perform angiography through the guide catheter to assess the progress of intervention.
- Once the procedure is complete, perform post-intervention angiography.

Hydrocoils

- If hydrocoils (Microvention, Aliso Viejo, CA) are used these are softened by using a steamer.
- 'Unlock' the coil by sliding off the short piece of black tubing securing the coil pusher to the sheath.
- The coil is pushed forward and held in the steam for less than a minute, until it appears soft. Then, retract the coil back into the sheath.
- It is imperative that no blood is allowed to enter the microcatheter, as this will cause the hydrocoil to expand within the microcatheter. To prevent the blood backflow, a short length of tubing with a one way stopcock is interposed between the RHV and the microcatheter. Prior to opening the RHV, the stopcock is turned so that the microcatheter is closed to the RHV, preventing backflow. Once the coil in its sheath is advanced through the RHV tighten the RHV around the sheath (just enough to still enable passage of coil through the sheath) and then open the one way stopcock to access the microcatheter.
- Advance the sheath to the hub. The rest of the deployment is the same as for GDC.
- As hydrocoils tend to expand on exposure to blood, the time available to deploy or retract is limited, usually 5 min.
- Once satisfactorily positioned, hydrocoil is detached using a handheld device (V-Grip™, Microvention, Aliso Viejo, CA). This is slid over the tip of the coil pusher.
- The light on the device will turn green indicating satisfactory connection. If this does not happen, ensure the pusher is dry (wipe the tip with a dry sponge) and that the detaching device itself is in working order.
- Once the green light is on, push the blue button on the detachment device. Some operators prefer pushing it once and letting go, while others maintain it in a depressed position until the light color changes (either is acceptable).
- The light on the detachment device will turn orange and there will be a beeping sound to indicate that the coil has detached.
- At this point using fluoroscopy, retract the pusher. When it is visually confirmed that the coil is detached, withdrawal of the pusher can be completed without further fluoroscopy.
- The rest of the procedure is the same as for GDC, or other types of coils.

Onyx/NBCA

- The technique of their usage via transvenous route remains the same as previously described.
- It is imperative that if there is any risk of venous embolization due to high flow, first slow down the flow by placing a few coils.
- In case of Onyx, remember to use a DMSO-compatible microcatheter.
- In case of NBCA, consider a flow directed, non-reinforced microcatheter.

Embolization via Superior Ophthalmic Vein

- This route is a consideration if the standard arterial or venous access is not available.
- We have not needed to utilize this route. We would recommend consulting an ophthalmic surgeon for providing access to superior ophthalmic vein, if the interventionalist is unfamiliar with this route.
- Secure a 5 Fr angiocath in the vein.
- Attach an RHV to it, which is connected to a continuously running flush of heparinized saline. Ensure the entire system is free of air bubbles or other potential emboli.
- Depending upon the type of embolic agent to be used, select and prepare the microcatheter and microwire.
- While the procedure will be undertaken similar to as if the access was from the usual peripheral locations, remember there will be some technical difficulty due to the considerable length of the microcatheters, wires, etc.
- When performing roadmap/angiogram be gentle and use less contrast as the superior ophthalmic vein leads directly to CS. In case of roadmaps, the usual 3–5 sec delay after the injection will not be necessary.

Postoperative Management and Follow-up

- Admit the patient to NSICU for at least overnight observation. Further ICU stay is dependent upon clinical condition.
- Consult or arrange follow-up with ophthalmic surgery.
- 0.9% NS + 20 meq KCl @ 150 cc/hr × 2 h, then decrease to 100 cc/hr if patient is NPO.
- Keep right/left leg (whichever side was used for procedure) straight × 2 h (in case of angioseal closure) or 6–8 h (in case manual compression was applied), with HOB elevated 15°.
- Check groins, DP's, vitals and neuro checks q 15 min × 4, q 30 min × 4, then q hr.
- Maintain mild hypotension overnight in case of a smaller AVM.
- Advance diet as tolerated.
- Review/Resume pre-procedure medications (hold oral hypoglycemics, until good PO intake established).
- Ensure arrangements for postoperative/post-discharge follow-up.
- D/C next morning after mobilizing (if no complications/other ongoing medical concerns requiring hospitalization).
- F/u on outpatient basis in 4 weeks.
- F/u angiography at 3 months.

Problems Encountered During Onyx Administration and Solutions

• Table 14.3 shows some possible problems and solutions.

Table 14.3 Problems/Solutions During Onyx Administration

Problem	Solution
DAVF incompletely occluded with persistence of CVR	If transvenous access to the DAVF is no longer possible through the standard routes, if feasible place a burr hole over the involved sinus. For accurate placement of the burr hole, do roadmapping first (with arterial injection). Additionally, may use radiopaque markers to localize the site of scalp incision and burr hole placement
Resistance encountered during Onyx injection	If transvenous access to the DAVF is no longer possible through the standard routes, if feasible place a burr hole over the involved sinus. For accurate placement of the burr hole do roadmapping first (with arterial injection). Additionally, may use radiopaque markers to localize the site of scalp incision and burr hole placement
Difficult catheter removal or catheter entrapment	• Remove any slack. Gently apply traction to the catheter for a few seconds, putting the catheter on 3–4 cm stretch. Repeat this process intermittently, until the catheter is successfully retracted and removed • If above fails, remove slack from catheter by putting a few centimeter traction on the catheter and placing it under slight tension. Firmly holding the catheter, pull it by making a snapping motion (from left to right) at the wrist, resulting in 10–15 cm displacement, to remove the catheter from the Onyx caste • If above fails, then in order to prevent a bleed from a ruptured malformation due to too much traction, the option of leaving the microcatheter in the vascular system should be considered. To do so, cut the hub of the microcatheter off • Slide the guide catheter out over the microcatheter • Clamp the microcatheter to prevent potential air embolism or bleeding • Pass the guidewire provided in the angioseal kit (or, in case of a longer sheath a standard guidewire) through the sheath (not through the microcatheter) • Slide out the sheath over the wire and microcatheter, taking care not to lose wire access • Transiently, remove the clamp from the end of microcatheter to enable completion of sheath removal • After sheath removal, place the microcatheter under stretch and clamp it with a hemostat right next to the skin • Complete the arteriotomy closure with angioseal then, maintaining the microcatheter under tension and cut it just below the skin, applying downward pressure on the skin with the hand being used for cutting. Allow the residual catheter to retract into the soft tissue • The presence of arteriotomy plug in addition to its usual function will also assist in keeping the catheter sessile enabling endothelialization • The patient will need to be on Plavix 300 mg L.D. followed by 75 mg p.o daily for 4 weeks and then discontinue • The patient should also be on ASA 81 to 650 mg (usual dose 325 mg) daily for 3 months, or indefinitely

(continued)

Table 14.3 (continued)

Problem	Solution
Onyx is not visualized as it is being injected	• After approx. 0.3 ml of Onyx has been injected to cover the volume of microcatheter, it should be visualized during fluoroscopy thereafter. Therefore, if during the procedure Onyx is no longer visualized when it previously was, stop the injection and determine the cause. Continuing to inject under pressure while none is emanating from the distal tip of the microcatheter may cause the catheter rupture.
	• Assess whether the previously deposited Onyx is preventing visualization. Consider if alternative orthogonal views need to be obtained
	• Ensure that the Onyx is thoroughly mixed with tantalum by maintaining it on the mixer (set at 8) for at least 20 min
Rupture or breakage of catheter	• This may occur consequent to injecting under pressure. Therefore, avoid doing so. Assess whether the catheter can be withdrawn in its entirety. If this is possible, retract and discard the catheter
	• If a catheter fragment is left behind, consider if it is safer to leave it in situ
	• Assess the feasibility of its removal, as well as, the possibility of migration downstream
	• Assess whether the fragment can be retrieved endovascularly using snares or merci retriever. To do so, place a rapid transit catheter (Cordis, Miami, FL) adjacent to the catheter fragment by advancing it over microguidewire (e.g., Synchro 14)
	• Remove the microguidewire and advance an alligator retrieval device (ev3, Plymouth, MN) though the microcatheter, until it reaches the tip of the microcatheter
	• Holding the microcatheter, advance the retrieval device slightly forward. This will result in opening of the jaws of the device (visualized fluoroscopically by separation of radiopaque markers). Attempt to engage the proximal tip of the fragment. Once the fragment appears to be engaged, advance the microcatheter slightly forward while holding the alligator device in position, to close the jaws of the device
	• Maintaining slight tension on the alligator device, withdraw it and the microcatheter together as a unit completely through the guide catheter and the patient's body
	• Sometimes, it may not be possible to withdraw the catheter fragment completely. Even relocating it to less critical regions (compered to intracranial vasculature) e.g., branches of ECA, or peripheral vasculature of lower extremity might be more acceptable.
	• Also, bear in mind the possibility of accidentally embolizing the fragment to an even more critical location, causing the patient greater harm
	• If it is not possible to remove it endovascularly and removal of the fragment is a strong consideration, then consider open surgery for its retrieval. Conventional surgery will carry greater risks
Vasospasm	• Vasospasm may be consequent to rough catheter/wire manipulation, navigation or, too rapid injection of DMSO
	• Ensure that the DMSO is injected very gradually. The rate should be around 0.16 ml/min and not to exceed 0.3 ml/min
	• Be meticulous and gentle during manipulation. If the vasospasm is believed to be consequent to the instrumentation and is not resolving, verapamil may be injected through the microcatheter. 5–10 mg are injected gradually as the catheter is withdrawn through the spasmodic segment. Up to 20 mg may be given into each arterial tree. Inject gradually to avoid significant drop in BP
	• In case of CCA/ICA, the vasospasm usually attenuates as the manipulation is discontinued. In case of persistent vasospasm, verapamil may be administered
	• Vasospasm of ECA or its branches usually does not warrant treatment

Problems Encountered During NBCA Administration and Solutions

• Table 14.4 shows some possible problems and solutions.

Table 14.4 Problems/solutions during NCBA administration

Problem	Solution
Visualization of NBCA entering draining vein/sinus	• Stop injecting NBCA as soon as the embolization into the venous system is visualized. Wait for a few seconds and then carefully resume injection. If any further venous embolization is noted, terminate the injection • In case of a high flow AVM or DAVF, consider preparing a high concentration NBCA • Alternatively, placing coils prior to NBCA administration may slow the blood flow and prevent inadvertent venous embolization
microcatheter tip appears stuck	• To avoid the gluing in of the catheter, avoid proximal reflux of NBCA • Use a non-reinforced microcatheter, e.g., Regatta, or Spinnaker Elite, which is easier to break off in case it becomes adherent to the glue mass • If it appears that it is not possible to break free the microcatheter, then it may need to be cut at the femoral entry point and left in the vascular system (see Onyx section above, Problem: 'Difficult catheter removal or catheter entrapment')

Problems Encountered During PVA Administration and Solutions

• Table 14.5 shows some possible problems and solutions.

Table 14.5 Problems/solutions during PVA administration

Problem	Solution
Difficulty injecting PVA through the microcatheter	• Withdraw the catheter and inspect for damage. Replace it, if necessary. Do not attempt to injection forcefully or 'clear' the microcatheter while within the patient. Such an attempt may lead to rupture of the catheter, or embolization of PVA into normal cerebral vasculature, causing stroke.

Table 14.6 Problems/solutions during coil embolization

Problem	Solution
ICA stasis, or difficulty visualization during coil occlusion of ICA	• This is an anticipated finding and not a complication. The ICA is not visualized well proximal to the coil plug because of the flow stasis
Difficulty deploying the coil	• This may be consequent to the coil having expanded within the catheter (e.g., hydrocoil), a kink in the pusher, or defect in the microcatheter. Do not use excessive force to push or pull the coil
	• Remove the coil from the catheter and examine it. If the coil is not defective, then the microcatheter may need to be changed
	• If it is not possible to remove the coil through the microcatheter, then remove the microcatheter along with the coil

Problems Encountered During Coil Embolization and Solutions

• Also refer to similar section in Chap. 12 'Treatment of Aneurysms'.
• Table 14.6 shows some possible problems and solutions.

Suggested Readings

1. Berenstein A, Lasjaunias P, Ter Brugge KG. Surg Neuroangiogr. 2004;2(2):695–735 (Heidelberg: Springer).
2. Halbach VV, Hieshima GB, Higashida RT, et al. Carotid-cavernous fistulae: indications for urgent therapy. AJNR Am J Neuroradiol. 1987;8:627–33.
3. Hurst RW, Rosenwasser RH (eds). Interventional Neuroradiology. New York: Informa. 2008:231–238; 275–303; 335–351.
4. Onyx® Liquid Embolic System, Instructions for Use. Micro Therapeutics Inc., Irvine, CA.
5. Polyvinyl Alcohol Foam Embolization Particles. Instructions for use. Cook Medical.
6. Trufill® n-BCA Liquid Embolic system. Codman Product brochure.
7. Yao TL, Eskioglu E, Ayad M, et al. Improved image interpretation with combined superselective and standard angiography (double injection technique) during embolization of arteriovenous malformations. Neurosurgery. 2008;62:140–1 (discussion 141).

Stroke

15

Indications and Case Selection

- Intravenous TPA is administered when the onset of stroke is known to be <3–4.5 h. The patient is assessed for any contraindications.
- Persistent symptoms of stroke despite adequate medical management (Fig. 15.1).
- Intra-arterial rt-PA may be indicated for patients where angiography may be performed and treatment administered within 3 and 6 h after symptom onset with an NIHSS score of greater than 4, or those with an NIHSS score of greater than 20 and the ability to be treated within 6 h.
- Posterior circulation strokes (Fig. 15.2) may be treated endovascularly for up to 24 h (due to a lesser likelihood of hemorrhagic conversion of infarct).

Contraindications

- Most contraindications are relative and have to be weighed against the risk of not intervening. These contraindications include:

  - Hemorrhagic infarct.
  - CT demonstrating hypodensity or mass effect consistent with evolving infarct of more than one-third of middle cerebral artery territory.
  - Recent major surgery.
  - Pregnancy.
  - When considering stenting, contraindication to anticoagulants and/or thrombolytics.

© Springer International Publishing AG 2017
S.H. Khan and A.J. Ringer, *Handbook of Neuroendovascular Techniques*,
DOI 10.1007/978-3-319-52936-3_15

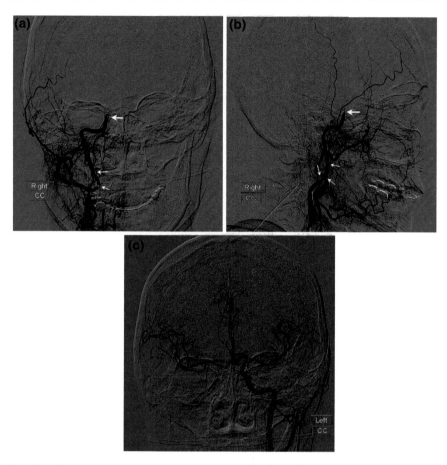

Fig. 15.1 Cerebral angiography AP (**a**) and lateral (**b**) views. Demonstrating occlusion of the distal RICA (*thick arrow*), just proximal to its bifurcation into ACA and MCA. The cerebral vasculature is not visualized. Irregularity in the lumen of the ICA is also appreciated (*thin arrows*), which probably was the source of the occlusive embolus. Clinical, CT, and MRI did not demonstrate as large a stroke as one would expect based on these images. LICA angiography (**c**) demonstrating crossflow across to the ACom to the contralateral ACA and MCA, explaining why the right cerebral infarct was not extensive

Preoperative Management

- This is usually under the supervision of a stroke neurologist. Ensure the following:
- Rapid transfer to a stroke center/facility with endovascular capabilities.
- ABC's.
- Ensure patient has two intravenous lines, preferably 18G or larger.
- Start monitoring BP, pulse oximetry, ECG, O$_2$ saturation, cardiac rate and rhythm, respiratory rate.

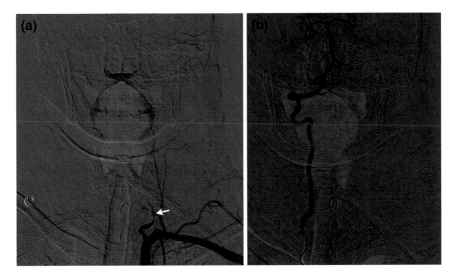

Fig. 15.2 **a** Left vertebral angiography manifesting occlusion (*arrow*). Right vertebral angiography (**b**) demonstrates adequate supply to the posterior circulation including left PICA, in the same patient. Consequently, intervention for the LVA occlusion was not required

- Insert a Foley catheter.
- Verify laboratory values including Platelet count, BUN, CR, APTT, PT/INR.
- ß-HCG for females of reproductive age group.
- Maintain MAP ≥ 90 mm Hg.
- CT scan head, CT angiography (CTA) head and neck and where available, CT perfusion (CTP). (The use of CTP is currently not included in the stroke guidelines. One of the authors uses it, the other does not, relying on the therapeutic window.)
- MRI head (select cases).
- Be cognizant of renal insufficiency, diabetes, congestive heart failure, etc., in which case consider diluted nonionic contrast agent and maintain contrast load to minimum.
- If the patient is within 3- to 6-h time window, and there are no contraindications start TPA (See below).

Chemical Recanalization

Abciximab (Reopro®, Eli Lilly and Co., Indianapolis, IN)

- To lyse clots which appear to comprise of primarily platelets (L.D. loading dose of 0.25 mg/kg IA or IV over a few minutes, followed by continuous IV infusion of 0.125 μg/kg/min (max. 10 μg/min) for 12 h, then d/c.

- Abciximab is usually administered when the arterial occlusion is consequent to a platelet plug. This may be iatrogenic, e.g., during intervention when platelet plugs may form over a wire and subsequently be shorn off when the catheter is advanced over the wire.

TPA

- 0.9 mg/kg IV (max 90 mg) with 10% of total dose administered as an initial IV bolus over 1 min, and the remainder is infused over an hour. This intravenous dose is administered within the therapeutic (3–4.5 h) window.
- The maximum intra-arterial dose is 22 mg. It is independent of any previously administered intravenous dose.
- Up to 20 mg of IA TPA can be administered with relative safety into each arterial tree.
- In case of cranial sinus thrombosis (CST), usually 2–5 mg are administered IA through the thrombus and then an infusion started at a rate of 1 mg/h, usually for 12 h. If clot burden is still there on angiography, a longer duration of administration until the clot resolves is a consideration.
- In CST, the infusion is prepared in a concentration of 1 mg/10 ml (0.1 mg/ml), for a rate of 10 ml/h.

Technique

Abciximab

- Advance a microcatheter over microwire using appropriate views and position it just proximal to the iatrogenic clot. Administer 0.25 mg/kg IA over a few minutes. Preform angiography 15–20 min later to assess the results.
- Direct the anesthesiologist/nurse to start the infusion at 0.125 µg/kg/min (max. 10 µg/min) for 12 h. This infusion may also be deferred until the arteriotomy site has been closed following completion of intervention.

TPA

- Advance a microcatheter over microwire using appropriate views and position it in the affected artery distal to the clot.
- Administer 1–2 mg TPA manually distal to the clot.
- Then administer an infusion of 0.5 mg/ml at 20 ml/h (10 mg/h).
- The infusion is prepared by mixing 10 mg of TPA in 20 ml on normal saline, resulting in a concentration of 1 mg rt-PA per 2 ml saline (or 0.5 mg/ml). Use an infusion pump for more precise administration.

- Perform angiography every 15 min (following infusion of 2.5 mg TPA) as the catheter is gradually drawn back through the clot. Re-cross the lesion after each angiogram. If the artery is still occluded, inject 1–2 mg rt-PA manually and resume the TPA infusion.
- Discontinue TPA if

  - adequate recanalization is achieved,
  - extravasation of contrast material is noted on angiography,
  - a maximum dose of 90 mg has been administered, or
  - the administered dose approaches the maximum dose without clinical or angiographic improvement.

- It may be noted, since the introduction and success of stentrievers, mechanical thrombectomy is attempted as a first approach in intervention, rather than spending time on IA thrombolysis. TPA administration is more frequently being used as 'clean-up' procedure following thrombectomy.

Mechanical Recanalization

Indications and Case Selection

- Ischemic stroke when the patient has failed IV-t-PA therapy.
- Ischemic stroke when the patient is not a candidate for IV-t-PA therapy, e.g., greater than 3–4.5 h since onset of stroke, or significant risk with TPA or heparin usage, e.g., recent major surgery.

Contraindications

- Hemorrhagic stroke, or when thrombectomy may result in significant hemorrhagic conversion of stroke.
- CT demonstrating hypodensity or mass effect consistent with evolving infarct of more than one-third of middle cerebral artery territory.
- Recent major surgery.
- Pregnancy.
- In case of stenting, contraindication to anticoagulants and/or thrombolytics.

Equipment

- Choice of devices for stroke intervention.
- Catheter wires.
- Thrombectomy devices.

- Stentrievers.
- Merci.
- Penumbra system.
- Pronto device (for CST).

Drugs

- 0.9% NS + 20 meq KCl @ 75 cc/h (adjust to higher rate if needed to maintain target MAP).
- Fentanyl 25–100 μg IV prn.
- Versed 0.5–1 mg IV prn.

Devices

- 18G Single-wall needle.
- 6-Fr short sheath (10 cm, Pinnacle; Terumo Interventional Systems, Tokyo); Use 8 Fr or 9 Fr from outset, if there is a good chance of endovascular intervention with stentrievers, Merci® or Penumbra® systems.
- Use a long sheath if the patient has tortuous vasculature.
- Guide catheter: 6-Fr Envoy® MPC guide catheter (90 cm) or,
- Merci® balloon guide catheter.
- Neuron™ 070 guide catheter.
- Diagnostic catheter: front angled catheter 5 Fr (Glidecath®; Terumo Interventional Systems, Tokyo).
- Glidewire® (Terumo Interventional Systems, Tokyo).
- Microwire (exchange length): Transcend EX 0.014 300 Floppy, or
- Transcend EX 0.014 300 ES, or Synchro2 (soft).
- For microwire thrombolysis: Excelsior™ SL 10 microcatheter.
- Stentriever systems:
- Presently, there are two products available in the US market. Both are comparable in usage and results. These are Trevo® (Stryker Neurovascular, Fremont CA) and Solitaire™ (ev3 Neurovascular, Irvine CA). One obvious difference between the two is that Trevo is visible fluoroscopically through its entire extent, while Solitaire has radiopaque markers at its proximal and distal ends with the intervening component being radiolucent.
- Here the use of Trevo is described (Solitaire usage is very similar). Trevo has a modified proximal end that enables attachment of the Abbott Vascular DOC® guidewire extension. The guidewire extension makes it possible to remove or exchange a catheter, while maintaining the retriever in position. The extension can be detached, once the catheter exchange is complete.

For Using Trevo Stentriever

- Trevo XP Provue retriever 4 × 20 (the most commonly used size).
- Trevo Pro 18 microcatheter.
- Merci Concentric balloon guide catheter.
- Torque device and insertion tool.

For Using Merci® Retrieval System

- Merci® balloon guide catheter.
- Merci® microcatheter.
- Merci® Retriever device (options: L4, L5, L6, X6, and K_{Mini}).
- See Table 15.1 for appropriate microcatheter and retriever selection.

For Penumbra System™ (Alternative to Merci® Retrieval System)

- Reperfusion catheter
- Separator
- Aspiration tubing (sterile)
- Pump canister tubing (non-sterile)
- Pump canister and lid
- Pump filter
- Use Table 15.2 and Fig. 15.3 for selection of the appropriate size.
- For angioplasty:
- Gateway™ PTA balloon catheter (Size: ≤ artery proximal and distal to the lesion).

Table 15.1 Appropriate microcatheter and retriever selection

Merci retriever	L4	L5	L6	X6	K_{Mini}
Merci microcatheter	18L	18L or 18X	18L	14X	14X
Helix loop diameter (mm)	2.0	2.5	2.7	1.5–3.0	2.1
Helix length (mm)	2.5	4.5	4.5	7.0	2.5
Filaments	Yes	Yes	Yes	No	No
Resheathable (in vivo)	Yes	Yes	Yes	No	No

Table 15.2 Catheter size

Vessel size	Reperfusion catheter + separator
<2 mm, e.g., M3	026 Reperfusion catheter/separator pair
2–3 mm, e.g., M2, P1	032 Reperfusion catheter/separator pair
>3 mm, e.g., ICA, M1, VA, BA	041 Reperfusion catheter/separator pair

Vessel Size   Separator/Reperfusion Catheter Size Selection
(mm)

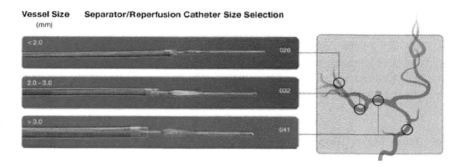

Fig. 15.3 Various sizes of penumbra aspiration catheters and separators. Note that the separators are color coded. Their recommended usage in the arterial tree is also indicated

- Inflation device with manometer.
- Stent: Wingspan™ Stent system (Size: = {or slightly oversized} the artery proximal and distal to the lesion. Length: should extend at least 2 mm beyond the proximal and distal aspect of lesion).
- Rotating hemostatic valve (RHV) and adaptor: 2.
- Syringes 60 cc, 10 cc (at least 3), 20 cc (at least 4), 3 cc (for ACT and angioplasty balloon preparation).
- Three-way stopcock: 3.
- Torque device.
- Telfa strip.
- Mandrel for shaping microwire tip.
- Angioseal™ closure device.

Technique

- Time is of the essence in stroke… work fast.
- If neuroimaging (CT/MRI) and clinical scenario indicate mechanical thrombectomy with Merci® Retriever system, start out with a large (8 Fr or 9 Fr) sheath to save time.
- In an elderly patient where there is a great likelihood of vessel tortuosity (including in the iliac region), consider a longer sheath (30–45 cm) or a shuttle sheath (90 cm; Cook Medical).
- Gain access with 18G single-wall needle (instead of micropuncture, to save time) using modified Seldinger technique.
- Insert the short sheath over J-wire (see Chap. 2, Specifics for micropuncture Technique section). Or, insert a longer sheath, e.g., shuttle sheath over a Glidewire® (Terumo®) or Bentson® (Cook Medical) wire, if the patients vascular anatomy is known to be tortuous.
- Secure sheath in position using 2-0 silk suture.

Diagnostic Angiography

Due to the frequent performance of CTA during stroke management, these days diagnostic angiography is usually unnecessary and one can directly proceed to intervention. However, if needed, the technique is as follows:

(a) *Rapid*

- Irrigate a 5-Fr pigtail catheter with heparinized saline and attach it to an RHV, which in turn is attached to a three-way stopcock connected to a continuous heparinized saline flush and a neonatal transducer, enabling a flow rate of 30 ml/h.

- Irrigate the glidewire in its containing ring and then insert it into the pigtail catheter.

- Introduce the catheter with glidewire into the sheath and once in the sheath advance the glidewire to lead the catheter.

- Under fluoroscopic guidance, with the glidewire leading, navigate to the ascending aorta.

- Remove the glidewire from the catheter and store it in heparinized saline basin.

- Center the image intensifier or detector over the patient's head, ensuring both right and left sides are in the field.

- The magnification should be decreased so that both the cervical and cerebral vasculature are in the field.

- Angiography is performed in AP view.

- Perform angiography with contrast injection at a rate of 20 ml/s for a total volume of 30 ml.

- The above method of angiography will demonstrate the cervical and cranial, as well as, anterior and posterior circulations concurrently for a rapid diagnosis of the site of lesion.

- Withdraw and remove the pigtail catheter. Disconnect it from the RHV. The RHV can then be used for the guide catheter.

(b) *Standard*

- In case the clinical symptomatology is indicative of the location of lesion, proceed with a 5-Fr front angled catheter (Glidecath; Terumo®, Tokyo,

Japan) to perform diagnostic imaging, instead of above-mentioned aortic arch injection.

- Perform angiography of the involved side, e.g., if patient has left hemiparesis, study the right carotid vasculature.
- Alternatively, diagnostic imaging may be performed with a guide catheter, e.g., Envoy (Cordis Endovascular Systems, Miami Lakes, FL), potentially eliminating the need to switch catheters at the time of intervention.
- Use at least a 6- or 7-Fr guide catheter, in anticipation of intervention. This will save the step of exchanging for a larger-sized guide catheter.
- After the diagnostic images, maintain the tip of guide catheter in the artery of interest, e.g., CCA or ICA.
- In case of ischemic stroke, usually 4-vessel angiography is not required at the outset.
- If any difficulty is encountered due to vessel tortuosity, don't waste time and quickly proceed to using a Simmons 2 or Head hunter H-1 type catheters (Terumo Interventional Systems, Tokyo) to complete the diagnostic imaging.
- After diagnostic imaging, if difficulty was encountered in vessel selection with the diagnostic catheter, use exchange length wire (260–300 cm) for replacing the diagnostic catheter with a guide catheter.
- If the patient does not have a difficult vasculature, an OTW catheter exchange is unnecessary and simply withdraws the diagnostic catheter. Using glidewire advance the guide catheter into its position in the usual manner.
- If OTW exchange is needed, it is performed as follows:

  - Activate the hydrophilic coating of EL Glidewire (Terumo®, Tokyo, Japan) or Bentson (Cook Medical Inc., Bloomington, IN) wire, by wiping its entire length with a moist Telfa.
  - In case an EL Bentson (200 cm) wire is used, be sure to shape its tip into an angle (e.g., 45°). Otherwise, considerable difficulty may be encountered in vessel navigation.
  - Loosen the knob of the RHV and introduce the wire into its hub and then advance it through the catheter.
  - Under fluoroscopic guidance, advance the tip of the wire into the target vessel, e.g., ICA (preferable, to save the steps involved in gaining ICA access later) with enough wire distal to catheter tip to maintain purchase.
  - Under fluoroscopic guidance, withdraw the diagnostic catheter while maintaining the wire tip in position. Take care that the wire is not inadvertently advanced into the intracranial ICA, or retracted resulting in loss of purchase.
  - Discontinue fluoroscopy once the diagnostic catheter is outside the patient.
  - Continue to ensure the wire does not move.

Preparation of Guide catheter

- Detach the diagnostic catheter from the RHV and replace it with a 6-Fr Envoy® or Concentric balloon guide catheter.
- Ensure that the guide catheter and the attached RHV with its saline flush system are free of any air bubbles.
- Ascertain all connections are secure and will not fall apart during procedure.
- Leave the third port of the stopcock (which is perpendicular to RHV sidearm) for contrast administration, etc.

Insertion of Guide catheter

- Introduce the tip of the guide catheter over the proximal tip of wire and insert it into the sheath.
- Using fluoroscopy, ensure that the distal tip of the wire remains in its position and is not inadvertently advanced, or retracted.
- Advance the guide catheter into the ICA and position it in the vertical cervical ICA segment, or if needed, even intracranially in the cavernous segment, if safely possible. Sometimes due to vascular tortuosity or stenosis of the ICA, the guide catheter can only be positioned in the CCA.
- Once the guide catheter is in place, remove the wire while wiping it with wet Telfa and store it in a basin with heparinized saline.
  Note: sometimes the vessels are so tortuous that it may be best to leave the Simmons 2 catheter in as the guide catheter.
- If the initial decision is to perform thrombolysis, using the microwire proceed as follows.

Preparation of Microcatheter and Microwire

- Take the sterile packaging containing the Excelsior SL 10™ (Stryker Neurovascular, Fremont, CA) microcatheter out of its packet and place on preparation table using sterile precautions. Conversely, may use Rapidtransit (Codman) or a similar catheter as well.
- Flush the protective hoop bearing the catheter with normal saline.
- Take the catheter out of its protective hoop.
- Remove the shape maintaining stylet out of its distal tip.
- Flush the catheter with normal saline by attaching a syringe to the proximal hub of the catheter.
- Attach the microcatheter to an RHV that in turn is attached to a continuous heparinized saline flush.
- Take the sterile packaging containing the 0.014″ Transcend™ wire out of its packet and place it on preparation table using sterile precautions.
- Irrigate the wire in its protective hoop, using the portal provided.

- Then gently introduce the distal tip of the microwire through the RHV into the catheter without distorting the shape of the tip. Advance the wire through the catheter until about 5 cm of it protrudes beyond the catheter tip (alternatively, the wire may be backloaded into the microcatheter by introducing the stiffer end into the catheter tip and pushing it, until the stiff end emerges from the loosened knob of the RHV at the other end.
- Grab the emergent end and pull, until only about 5 cm of wire protrudes beyond the catheter tip.
- Using the provided mandrel, shape the distal tip of the wire to enable easier navigation through the patient's cerebral vasculature.
- Ensure that there are no air bubbles in the microcatheter system.

Insertion of Microcatheter

- Loosen the knob of the RHV connected to the guide catheter.
- Introduce the distal tip of the catheter into the RHV of the guide catheter.
- Once the microcatheter is within the guide catheter, advance the microwire such that it leads the microcatheter.
- Tighten the knob of the guide catheter RHV just enough so that back bleeding is prevented, while the microcatheter and wire can be manipulated easily.
- Keep the entire system straight.
- Advance the microcatheter until the tip of the wire is just proximal to the tip of the guide catheter.

Thrombolysis

- Select working views by performing cerebral angiography through the guide catheter.
- Attach torque device to the proximal (outside) end of guidewire.
- Using roadmap guidance advance the guidewire, using the torque device to rotate the wire as needed while it is advanced.
- Then advance the microcatheter over the wire, ensuring that the wire is leading the catheter at all times.
- Continue to alternatively advance guidewire and microcatheter, until the target vessel is reached.
- Attempt to cross the clot with the guidewire and then slowly withdraw the wire while rotating it, to disrupt the clot.
- Once wire is proximal to the clot, perform angiography to assess results.
- If needed, perform additional passes with the wire to achieve clot lysis.
- Consider supplementing mechanical thrombolysis with TPA or abciximab (see 'Chemical Thrombolysis' above).
- Perform angiography alternatively with thrombolysis to assess re-establishment of blood flow.

- Consider giving the tip of the microwire a 'J' shape. This will diminish the likelihood of the tip perforating through the vessel wall (consequent to the inability to visualize the occluded vessel segment). The J tip will also diminish the likelihood of inadvertent selection of branches such as ophthalmic, or posterior communicating artery.

Note: Given the availability of effective devices such as stentrievers over the past few years, in case of stroke we recommend immediately proceeding to the same in the IR Lab. Mechanical thrombolysis (supplemented with chemical thrombolysis and aspiration through microcatheter) is a consideration when thrombectomy with stentrievers is not an option.

Thrombectomy

I. To Perform Thrombectomy Using the Trevo System

The Trevo Kit has the following components:

- Trevo XP Provue retriever 4 × 20 (the most commonly used size)
- Trevo Pro 18 microcatheter
- Torque device and insertion tool
- Merci Concentric balloon guide catheter.

Indications and Case Selection

- Patients within 8 h of experiencing ischemic symptoms
- Patients who are ineligible for IV TPA
- Patients who fail IV TPA therapy
- One can use CT perfusion study demonstrating a viable penumbra as an indication for intervention. Or, go with the above-mentioned time window.

Contraindications

- Radiologically demonstrable large ischemic infarct.
- More than 8 h since onset of stroke in anterior circulation and 12 h for posterior circulation (relative contraindication), unless CTP shows viable penumbra and the completed infarct to be less than one-third of the hemisphere (Fig. 15.4a–h).

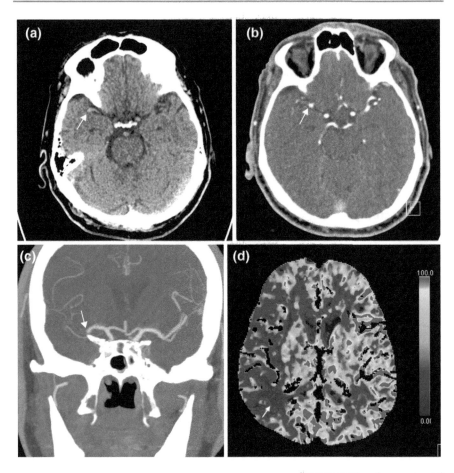

(images continued on next page)

Fig. 15.4 A 66-year-old who presented with left hemiparesis and dysarthria. At presentation, the onset of symptoms had been for more than 6 h. **a** A CT scan demonstrates the hyperdense clot (*arrow*) in right middle cerebral artery (*MCA*). The CTA **b** demonstrates the abrupt cutoff of MCA at same site (*arrow*). A clot can be appreciated ahead of the cutoff. **c** A coronal reconstruction better demonstrates the MCA cutoff (*arrow*). Also noticeable is the paucity of MCA branches when compared to the contralateral side. The CTP performed **d** demonstrates significantly attenuated cerebral blood flow of right hemisphere compared to left. The *arrow* indicates an area where there is no flow (refer to the color code bar on the right side of the image). However, the cerebral blood volume (*CBV*) is not significantly impacted other than in the previously indicated area with no flow (**e**). The mean transit time (*MTT*) in the right cerebral hemisphere is increased (**f**) when compared to the unaffected left MCA territory. There is clearly a large mismatch between CBV and MTT. These images confirm an area of large penumbra that is potentially salvageable. Angiography performed (**g**) confirms the MCA occlusion (*arrow*). Due to contrast reflux, external carotid branches are visible (*asterisk*). A Trevo stentriever was used for thrombectomy, resulting in successful clot removal on first pass (**h**)

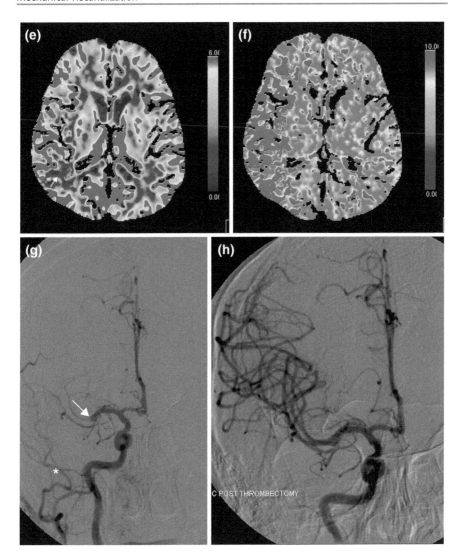

Fig. 15.4

Preparation of Balloon Guide catheter

- Take the Merci® balloon guide catheter out of its packet and place on preparation table using sterile precautions.
- If diagnostic angiography was done first, simply detach the diagnostic catheter from the RHV-saline flush system and use the flush system for the balloon guide catheter. Ensure the entire system is free of air bubbles.

- Otherwise, prepare the system as follows:

  - Attach a three-way stopcock to an RHV and attach tubing from a continuous saline flush to the three-way stopcock portal that is in line with the RHV.
  - Attach the RHV to the guide catheter.
  - Ensure that the guide catheter and the attached RHV-saline flush system are free of any air bubbles.
  - Ascertain all connections are secure and will not fall apart during procedure.
  - Leave the third port of the stopcock (which is perpendicular to RHV side-arm) for attachment of syringe to perform clot aspiration.

Insertion of guide catheter

- Introduce the tip of the guide catheter over the proximal tip of EL-wire (if one was left in place prior to diagnostic catheter removal) and insert it into the sheath.
- (If a wire is not already in position, then perform the standard guide catheter insertion over 90-cm glidewire).
- Using fluoroscopy, ensure that the distal tip of the wire remains in its position and is not inadvertently advanced, or retracted.
- Advance the balloon guide catheter into the ICA and position it in the vertical segment of cavernous ICA. Sometimes due to vascular tortuosity or stenosis of the ICA, the guide catheter can only be positioned in the CCA.
- Once the guide catheter is in place, remove the wire while wiping it with wet Telfa and store it in a basin with heparinized saline.
- Perform in vivo balloon preparation, if it was not done ex vivo, by attaching a three-way stopcock to the balloon inflation port. The inflation device is attached to the stopcock in line with the port, while a 20-cc syringe is attached to the available remaining portal of the three-way stopcock. This inflation system contains bubble-free two-third contrast and one-third saline solution. The 20-cc syringe contains 2–3 cc of the solution, with the rest being in the inflation system and intervening tubing. Close the stopcock to the inflation device. Aspirate with syringe held upright and then gently release, replacing aspirated air with contrast solution. Repeat this twice or until no further air bubbles are evacuated. Now turn the stopcock so that it is closed to the syringe.

Preparation and Insertion of Stentriever

- Flush the retriever package hoop with saline. Hydrate for a minimum of 2 min before removing retriever from hoop.
- Connect rotating hemostasis valve to microcatheter hub. The RHV is connected to a continuously running flush of heparinized saline.
- Advance the microcatheter over microwire into the neurovasculature and position the distal tip of microcatheter distal to thrombus.

- Remove the microwire from the microcatheter. Inject contrast through micro-catheter to visualize distal vasculature. Then, flush microcatheter.
- Remove insertion tool (a plastic tubing) and the preloaded stentriever within as a unit from the hoop, by pinching the tool and the stentriever at the point where the stentriever exits the tool. Do not allow the stentriever to exit the insertion tool tip or to retract further into insertion tool.
- Introduce insertion tool half way into the RHV and use the infusion line to flush it, until saline exits the proximal end of the insertion tool. Flushing of the insertion tool is important to enable smooth advance of retriever through the tool.
- Then advance the tool and retriever as a unit further into the RHV, until it is seated in the hub of microcatheter. Then tighten the RHV around the tool to secure it and prevent its movement.
- Advance the retriever through the tool into the microcatheter, until half its length has been inserted into the microcatheter. Remove the insertion tool.

Thrombectomy with Stentriever

- Advance the stentriever until the distal tip aligns with tip of microcatheter. The distal tip is within 8 cm of exiting microcatheter tip when (a) distal end of retriever shaft marker reaches the microcatheter hub, or (b) proximal end of retriever shaft marker reaches the proximal end of RHV.
- Retract the microcatheter while applying gentle forward force to stentriever to deploy shaped section of stentriever within clot. Position microcatheter tip marker just proximal to shaped section of stentriever. It is important to maintain the microcatheter tip marker just proximal to shaped section of stentriever during manipulation and withdrawal, to prevent kinking or fracture during manipulation and withdrawal.
- After deploying the stentriever, visualize the strut expansion. Wait 5 min to enable the clot to integrate into the stentriever.
- Inflate the balloon of the guide catheter to occlude the vessel and attach a 60-cc syringe to guide catheter to the free portal of the three-way stopcock on RHV of the guide catheter.
- Position and lock torque device onto stentriever at microcatheter hub.
- Slowly withdraw retriever and microcatheter together as a unit to guide catheter tip, while applying aspiration to guide catheter with the 60-cc syringe.
- Apply vigorous aspiration to guide catheter with the 60-cc syringe and with-draw retriever and microcatheter inside guide catheter.
- Continue aspirating until stentriever and microcatheter are nearly withdrawn from guide catheter.
- Deflate balloon guide catheter.

- Disconnect the RHV of balloon guide catheter and fully remove the stentriever, microcatheter, and RHV as a unit from the guide catheter.
- Attach 60-cc syringe to balloon guide catheter hub and aspirate.
- Clean the device with saline and inspect stentriever for damage. Do not use stentriever if core wire, shaped section, or platinum coil appear misshapen compared to when first removed from package.
- If not damaged, a stentriever may be used for up to three retrieval attempts. An advancement and complete withdrawal constitute one retrieval attempt (Fig. 15.5).

Problems Encountered During Stentriever Usage and Solutions

- Table 15.3 shows a problem/solution during stentriever usage.

II. To Perform Thrombectomy Using the Merci System

The Merci device has of three components:

- Merci balloon guide catheter.
- Merci microcatheter.
- Merci retriever.

Indications and Case Selection

- Patients with large clots that have proven refractory to resolution by TPA.
- Patients seen outside the therapeutic time window.
- Retrieval of foreign bodies lodged in cerebral vasculature.
- When chemical thrombolysis is contraindicated.

Contraindications

- Radiologically demonstrable large ischemic infarct.
- More than 6 h since onset of stroke in anterior circulation and 12 h for posterior circulation (relative contraindication).

Preparation of Balloon Guide catheter

- Take the Merci® balloon guide catheter out of its packet and place on preparation table using sterile precautions.

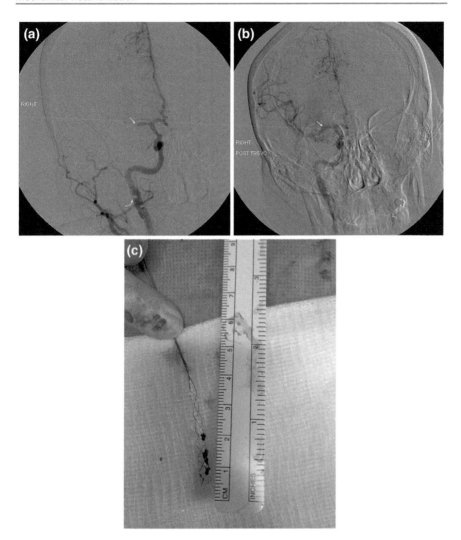

Fig. 15.5 A 39-year-old who had traumatic right internal carotid artery (*ICA*) dissection during motor vehicle accident. During resuscitation in the emergency room, she was noted to have left hemiparesis and difficulty with speech, which was found to be consequent to right MCA occlusion (**a**, *arrow*). The source of this embolic occlusion was the proximal traumatic ICA dissection (curved arrow). Successful thrombectomy was achieved with Trevo stentriever on fourth attempt (**b**) and MCA circulation re-established. The *arrow* indicates the site of previous occlusion. The clot that had caused occlusion can be seen entangled in the stentriever (**c**)

- If diagnostic angiography was done first, simply detach the diagnostic catheter from the RHV-saline flush system and use the flush system for the balloon guide catheter. Ensure the entire system is free of air bubbles.

Table 15.3 Problem/solution during stentriever usage

Problem	Solution
Withdrawal of stentriever into balloon guide catheter is difficult	• Deflate balloon of balloon guide catheter and simultaneously withdraw guide catheter, microcatheter and stentriever as a unit through sheath. Remove sheath if necessary

- Otherwise, prepare the system as follows:

  - Attach a three-way stopcock to an RHV and attach tubing from a continuous saline flush to the three-way stopcock portal that is in line with the RHV.
  - Attach the RHV to the Merci® guide catheter.
  - Ensure that the guide catheter and the attached RHV-saline flush system are free of any air bubbles.
  - Ascertain all connections are secure and will not fall apart during procedure.
  - Leave the third port of the stopcock (which is perpendicular to RHV side-arm) for attachment of syringe to perform clot aspiration.

Insertion of Guide catheter

- Introduce the tip of the guide catheter over the proximal tip of EL-wire (if one was left in place prior to diagnostic catheter removal) and insert it into the sheath.
- (If a wire is not already in position, then perform the standard guide catheter insertion over 90-cm glidewire).
- Using fluoroscopy, ensure that the distal tip of the wire remains in its position and is not inadvertently advanced, or retracted.
- Advance the balloon guide catheter into the ICA and position it in the distal ICA, but below the siphon. Sometimes due to vascular tortuosity or stenosis of the ICA, the guide catheter can only be positioned in the CCA.
- Once the guide catheter is in place, remove the wire while wiping it with wet Telfa and store it in a basin with heparinized saline.

Preparation of Microwire, Merci® Microcatheter and Retriever Device

- Take the microwire, Merci® microcatheter and retriever device out of their packets and place them on preparation table observing sterile precautions.
- Irrigate the microcatheter and guidewire in their protective hoops.
- Attach an RHV to the microcatheter.
- Then loosen the RHV and gently introduce the distal tip of the microwire into the catheter, without distorting the shape of the tip. Advance the wire through the catheter until about 5 cm of it protrudes beyond the catheter tip (alternatively, the wire may be backloaded into the microcatheter by introducing the

stiffer end into the catheter tip and pushing it, until the stiff end emerges from the other end of the catheter (through the open RHV, grab the emergent end and pull, until only about 5 cm of wire protrudes beyond the catheter tip).

- Using the provided mandrel, shape the distal tip of the wire to enable easier navigation through the patient's cerebral vasculature.
- Retract the shaped tip of the wire into the tip of the catheter.
- Ensure that there are no air bubbles in the microcatheter system and that the microcatheter remains moist at all times.
- Flush the Merci® retriever with heparinized NS in its hoop.
- Remove the retriever from its hoop and ensure that it remains moist at all times.
- Flush insertion tool and backload retriever into insertion tool.
- Retract the retriever into insertion tool so that only the tip is visible beyond the insertion tool.

Insertion of Merci microcatheter

- Loosen the knob of the RHV connected to the Merci, Envoy® or Neuron™ guide catheter.
- Introduce the distal tip of the microcatheter into the RHV of the guide catheter.
- Once the microcatheter is within the guide catheter, advance the microwire so that it leads the microcatheter.
- Tighten the knob of the guide catheter RHV just enough so that back bleeding is prevented, while the microcatheter and wire can be manipulated easily.
- Keep the entire system straight.
- Advance the microcatheter until the tip of the wire is just proximal to the tip of the guide catheter.
- Select working views by performing cerebral angiography through the guide catheter.
- Attach torque device to the proximal (outside) end of guidewire.
- Using roadmap guidance, advance the guidewire. Use the torque device to perform continuous half rotations one way then the other, as the wire is advanced.
- Advance the microcatheter over the wire, ensuring that the wire is leading the catheter at all times.
- Continue to alternatively advance guidewire and microcatheter, until the target location is reached, which is distal to the thrombus.
- Remove the guidewire, cleaning it with Telfa as it is withdrawn from the microcatheter and store it in the saline basin.
- Perform angiography through the microcatheter to visualize the occlusive thrombus and distal vasculature.
- Flush the catheter after the contrast injection.
- Introduce the insertion tool into the RHV of microcatheter and advance it into the hub of the microcatheter.

- Advance some length of the retriever through the insertion tool and then withdraw and remove the insertion tool.
- Advance the retriever until all coils are ahead of microcatheter. This will be indicated by the distal end of the retriever shaft marker reaching microcatheter hub or, proximal end of retriever shaft marker reaching proximal end of RHV.
- Position microcatheter tip marker just proximal to retriever loops. Maintain this position of microcatheter with respect to retriever loops through the procedure to diminish the likelihood of retriever fracture.
- Withdraw the retriever and microcatheter together, until the retriever loops engage the distal part of the thrombus.
- At this stage, may rotate the retriever loops to further engage the clot. Ensure that no more than five revolutions are made, to prevent retriever fracture.
- Position and lock torque device onto retriever at microcatheter hub.
- If a Merci balloon guide catheter is placed, inflate the balloon (See above 'insertion of guide catheter' page—for balloon preparation) and attach a 60-cc syringe to it.
- Withdraw retriever and microcatheter slowly and concurrently as a unit while applying aspiration to balloon guide catheter with the 60-cc syringe under fluoroscopic control.
- If the retriever loops are noted to straighten out, reduce the tension to allow the helix to reform.
- While maintaining vigorous aspiration with the 60-cc syringe, withdraw the retriever and microcatheter together as a unit into the guide catheter.
- Continue aspiration while nearly completely withdrawing the retriever–microcatheter from the guide catheter to aspirate any embolic residual.
- Disconnect the RHV from the guide catheter and fully remove the retriever, microcatheter, and RHV as a unit through the sheath. If needed, remove the sheath.
- Deflate the guide catheter balloon.
- Perform angiography to assess whether recanalization has occurred.
- May repeat procedure with Merci microcatheter and retriever, if further recanalization is needed.
- Ensure that the microcatheter and retriever device are free of clot prior to reintroduction into the guide catheter.
- Once the thrombectomy is complete, perform post-intervention angiography and then retract and remove guide catheter.
- Close femoral arteriotomy site.

Problems Encountered During Merci Device Usage and Solutions

- Table 15.4 shows problem/solution during Merci device usage.

Table 15.4 Problem/solution during Merci device usage

Problem	Solution
Merci guide catheter or retrieval system is difficult to advance or keeps getting displaced proximally	• It has been our experience that the Merci balloon Guide catheter is relatively poor in maintaining its position and the problem is compounded when the vasculature is tortuous. In such a situation, when possible we have used Envoy Guide catheter as substitute. We have also found the Neuron™ delivery catheter (Penumbra, Inc., Alameda, CA) much superior to the Merci Guide catheter in maintaining its position. Alternatively, Cello™ Balloon Guide catheter (8F, Covidien) is a comparable replacement for the Merci Guide catheter • Another alternative in tortuous vasculature is to form a coaxial system such that after positioning a Guide catheter, the microcatheter and distal access catheter (e.g., Navien™ or, DAC®) are advanced over microwire. The guide catheter is progressively advanced over these, while removing slack. The greater support results in successful navigation of cerebral vasculature

III. **To Perform Thrombectomy Using the Penumbra System**

- The Penumbra system comprises of:

  - Reperfusion catheter.

  - Separator.

  - Aspiration tubing (sterile).

  - Pump canister tubing (non-sterile).

  - Pump canister and lid.

  - Pump filter (Fig. 15.6a).

Problems Encountered During Using of Penumbra System and Solutions

Aspiration Pump Setup

- Attach filter to aspiration pump without over tightening or cross threading the filter (Fig. 15.6b).
- Secure canister lid on canister. A considerable pressure may be required to click the lid into place.
- Place the white insert into the canister well of the aspiration pump.
- Place canister with lid into the aspiration pump.

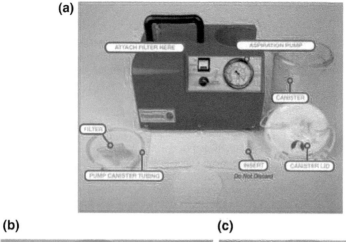

(images continued on next page)

Fig. 15.6 a Penumbra pump system with its various components including canister. **b** The system assembled. **c** The various parts of the system are highlighted including the flow switch that is used by the surgeon to turn the aspiration on and off, in the sterile field. **d** The gauge (also shown magnified), demonstrating the recommended suction range that is between 20 and 25. The recommended range is also highlighted on the gauge in *green*. **e** The canister positioned in its well in the aspiration pump must be visible to operator at all times to visualize the blood and clot dripping into the canister. *Courtesy* Penumbra, Inc., Alameda, CA

(d)   **(e)**

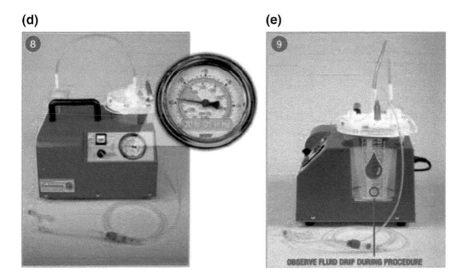

Fig. 15.6

- Connect the pump canister tubing from the center of canister lid to the filter.
- Open the sterile aspiration tubing onto the sterile field.
- Ensure flow switch is set to off.
- Attach the blue connector of the sterile aspiration tubing to the port on canister lid which is marked with blue sticker (Fig. 15.6c).
- Turn on the aspiration pump and check the gauge reads between −20 and −25 (see Fig. 15.6d).
- Ensure that all connections and canister lids are secure, all ports on the canister lids should be closed and ascertain the regulator knob is completely turned clockwise.
- Ensure that the full length of the canister is visible to you during the procedure (Fig. 15.6e).

Reperfusion Catheter and Separator Size Selection

- Select the appropriate reperfusion catheter and separator pair that will access the occluded site without occluding the vessel (see Fig. 15.3).
- As indicated above, place a 6-Fr or larger guide catheter, in the ICA or VA (depending upon location of embolic occlusion).

Reperfusion Catheter and Separator Placement

- Using a 0.014″ microguidewire, advance the reperfusion catheter to the site of occlusion, using the same technique as that for microcatheter (described above).
- Position reperfusion catheter immediately proximal to the occlusion.

- Remove the microguidewire from the reperfusion catheter.
- Introduce the matching separator (see Table 15.1) into the reperfusion catheter using the provided light blue introducer.
- Place a torque device on the proximal end of the separator
- Tighten the torque device onto the separator in a location such that when the torque device abuts against the RHV ('hubbed'), the radiopaque marker on the separator bulb distally extends approximately 4 mm past the radiopaque marker on the distal tip of reperfusion catheter (Fig. 15.7a).

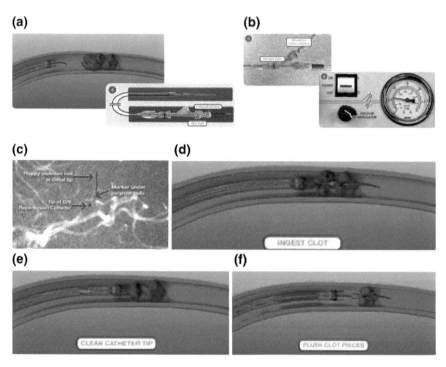

(a)

(b)

(c)

(d)

(e)

(f)

Fig. 15.7 **a** The distal aspect of penumbra aspiration catheter is proximal to the embolic clot. The bulb of the separator is within the catheter. The *inset* shows the aspiration catheter with separator. The bulb of the separator is outside the catheter, and the torque device tightened down upon the separator proximally is abutting the hub. Pulling the torque device backward will retract the separator bulb into the catheter, while pushing it forward causes the bulb to protrude out for the fixed distance. The thick band near the catheter tip is radiopaque and therefore visible during fluoroscopy. **b** The *upper plate* demonstrates sterile aspiration tubing attached to the sideport of the RHV. The torque device on the separator is abutting the RHV. The lower plate demonstrates the power switch and the suction gauge. The needle is at 24, within the recommended zone of 20–25. **c** Angiogram demonstrating an MCA branch with 'cutoff' due to embolic occlusion. A penumbra aspiration catheter and separator have been advanced into the affected vessel. A *radiopaque marker* indicates the tip of the catheter. A smaller marker identifies the bulb. The wire leading the bulb extends into the opercular segment of MCA. **d** The separator has been advanced to engage the clot by 'hubbing' the torque device. The bulb is within the clot. **e** During the course of mechanical lysis and aspiration, the bulb is seen retracted back into the catheter. A back and forth movement is performed with the separator to break up the clot and aspirate its fragments. **f** The progressive mechanical lysis and aspiration of the clot. *Courtesy Penumbra, Inc., Alameda, CA*

Preparation for Aspiration

- Connect the reperfusion catheter to sterile aspiration tubing by attaching male luer lock to side port of RHV
- Ensure that the blue female end of the aspiration tubing is attached to the port on canister with the blue sticker (as instructed above)
- Turn aspiration pump on (Fig. 15.7b).

Thrombus Removal

- Set the sterile aspiration catheter to the 'ON' or green position.
- Observe and note baseline aspiration flow rate in both the sterile aspiration tubing and dripping in the canister.
- Position the separator such that the radiopaque marker on the separator is approximately 4 mm distal to the radiopaque marker on the reperfusion catheter (Fig. 15.7c).
- Ensure that the separator movement is short (<2 cm), such that the separator's midshaft (green in color) does not exit RHV.
- Aspirate clot by advancing the reperfusion catheter until aspiration flow slows or stops in the sterile aspiration tubing and/or pump canister (Fig. 15.7d).
- Clean the catheter tip when the blood flow stops or slows, by moving the separator in and out of reperfusion catheter (Fig. 15.7e).
- Flush the clot pieces by extending the separator cone beyond the distal tip of the reperfusion catheter, to enable clot aspiration (Fig. 15.7f).
- Increased friction between the reperfusion catheter and separator may be indicative of thrombus becoming lodged in these devices. Remove and clean both devices. If the friction or fatigue persists, replace one or both devices. Figures 15.8 and 15.9 demonstrate cases treated with Penumbra system.

Reperfusion Catheter Does not Clear After Several Separator Movements

- If the reperfusion catheter continues to remain blocked and aspiration flow cannot be re-established, then retract the tip of the reperfusion catheter proximal to the thrombus to an open segment of the artery and attempt to clean it by moving the separator cone in and out of reperfusion catheter.
- Aspiration of clot from the reperfusion catheter will occur when the separator cone extends beyond the tip of the reperfusion catheter.
- If flow is still not re-established, then completely retract the separator out of the patient. Inspect the separator cone and wipe off any adherent material.
- If flow is not re-established by cleansing of the separator, then completely remove the reperfusion catheter and inspect it. Flush it on the table or, replace if it is damaged.
- Reintroduce the system into the body as described above.

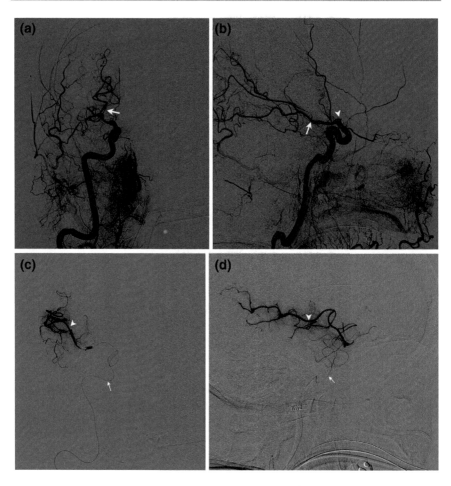

(images continued on next page)

Fig. 15.8 RICA half Towne's (**a**) and lateral (**b**) views demonstrating 'vessel cutoff' (*arrowhead*) consistent with occlusion of the ICA, just beyond origin of PCom artery (*arrow*). A filling defect at the origin of PCom is consistent with the presence of thrombus. (**c** and **d**) Following advancement of microcatheter (*arrow*) into the MCA, microangiography in AP and lateral views have been performed. One of the MCA trunks and its branches are visualized (*arrowhead*). The AP view demonstrates proximal luminal irregularity consistent with the presence of embolus. (**e** and **f**) Intervention with penumbra resulted in recanalization of the distal ICA and ACA (*arrow*). There is retrograde filling of the MCA branches (*thin arrows*) via collaterals. The embolus previously visualized at PCom origin has advanced further in the artery (*arrowhead*). (**g** and **h**) Due to the retrograde filling of MCA branches, they are visualized in a delayed fashion in the late capillary–early venous phase

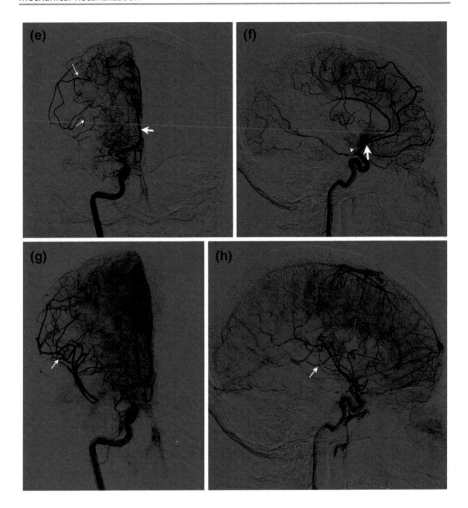

Fig. 15.8

Reperfusion Catheter Is Unable to Maintain Stable Position at Proximal Face of Clot

- Advance the reperfusion catheter to a more distal position, e.g., within the clot and commence aspirating.
- Use the separator to clear the reperfusion catheter.
- If necessary, reposition the catheter proximal to the thrombus in an open segment of the vessel to achieve better aspiration of the ingested clot.
- If readjustment of reperfusion catheter does not appear to solve the problem, consider if the guide catheter can be advanced further up to provide better support.

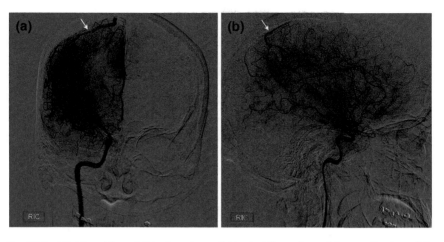

Fig. 15.9 AP (**a**) and lateral (**b**) views in another case where successful recanalization of the MCA has been performed using Penumbra system. Note the early draining vein (*arrow*)

Combining Stentriever and Penumbra Systems for Clot Extraction

- Aspiration of thrombus usually takes time (mean 45 min).
- Fibrin rich or highly adherent clots, e.g., from atrial fibrillation and CHF generally require longer time and effort.
- Blood loss up to 500 cc or more may occur by aspiration during thrombus removal
- Ensure there is no proximal flow limiting stenosis. If it exists perform intervention to rectify it prior to undertaking thrombus aspiration using the Penumbra system.
- Perform post-procedure cerebral angiography.
- If procedure is complete, retract and remove guide catheter.
- Close femoral arteriotomy site.

IV. **Combining Stentriever and Penumbra System for Clot Extraction**

- Another effective alternative is to combine the two techniques described above.

- In this case, a 7-Fr shuttle sheath is positioned in artery of interest.

- Through this, a 5 Fr penumbraACE™ 60 aspiration catheter is advanced.

- A 3 Max microcatheter is advanced through the ACE 60 to the target vessel. Finally, a stentriever is advanced through the microcatheter. When the stentriever is being retracted, the aspiration is turned on.

V. Angioplasty and Rescue Angioplasty

Indications

- Mechanical disruption of an occlusive thrombus using balloon angioplasty, which may fragment the thrombus and present a greater surface area for thrombolytic agent binding and may improve the efficacy of chemical thrombolysis.
- Focal symptomatic intracranial stenosis in an accessible location, i.e., proximal to A2, M2, and P2 persistent vessel occlusion or stenosis because of ineffective chemical or mechanical thrombolysis re-occlusion of reopened arteries consequent to thrombosis or vasospasm. In such cases, rescue angioplasty with or without stenting may prevent re-occlusion in a stenotic artery and permit distal infusion of thrombolytic agents.
- Concomitant stenting is performed in case of vessel dissection at site of stenosis, or if the vessel is unlikely to remain patent with chemical thrombolysis and angioplasty alone.
- Goal:

  - Dilatation of the stenosis to 75–80% of the normal vessel caliber proximal and distal to stenosis. Do not attempt to achieve normal diameter or overdilatation, which may result in dissection or vessel rupture.

- In case of angioplasty for embolic occlusion, the goal is re-establishment of blood flow through the occluded vasculature.

Technique
Preparation of Inflation Device

- Fill a 20-cc syringe with 15 cc contrast and 5-cc heparinized NS (2/3:1/3 concentration).
- Attach a three-way stopcock to the inflation device and connect the 30-cc syringe containing contrast medium to the sideport of the stopcock.
- Aspirate the contrast into the inflation device, leaving only 1–2 cc within the syringe.
- Purge any air out of the barrel and tubing of the inflation device, all the way to the distal portal of the stopcock.
- Leave inflation device on table, until needed.

Preparation of PTA Balloon Catheter for Angioplasty

- Two sterilely draped tables lying side to side and free of clutter are used to support the length of the interventional devices.
- Place the balloon catheter on the preparation table using sterile precautions.

- Lubricate the balloon catheter system in its protective hoop using heparinized 0.9% NS
- Remove the balloon catheter from its protective hoop and place it on the table using sterile folded towels on it if necessary, to keep it secure and extended along its length.
- Remove the stylet from the distal tip of the catheter.
- Attach a syringe with heparinized NS to the hub of the catheter and flush the catheter, until NS drops are noted at the distal tip of the catheter.
- Place a 0.014″ Transcend™ or Synchro2™ wire on the preparation table using sterile precautions.
- Irrigate the wire in its protective hoop, using the portal provided.
- Backload the stiff end of the wire into the distal tip of the angioplasty catheter, until it emerges from the hub of the catheter.
- Now gently grasp the stiff end of the wire at the hub and pull it out of the hoop until only a few cm of wire extends beyond the distal tip of catheter.
- Using a mandrel, shape the distal tip of the microwire to enable easy navigation to the stenosis.
- Withdraw the tip of the wire into the distal tip of the catheter, such that there is no wire extending beyond the catheter tip.
- Ensure the wire does not get kinked during manipulation.
- Remove the balloon protector from the distal tip of the angioplasty catheter by sliding it off.
- We prefer a negative pressure preparation after the balloon is positioned across the lesion by aspirating the inflation lumen with a large syringe held upright, containing 2–3 ml of the dilute contrast solution and then slowly releasing the negative pressure created. With the syringe held upright, the air from the inflation lumen will rise as bubbles in the syringe and then be refilled with the contrast solution.
- Alternatively, the balloon catheter can be prepared as described below. However, the smooth contour of the undilated balloon may be lost, which will cause difficulty negotiating the site of lesion. Therefore, we do not employ this method.
- Alternative balloon preparation technique: Take a 3-cc syringe containing contrast and
- Heparinized NS in 2/3 and 1/3 concentration and attach it to a three-way stopcock.
- Attach the stopcock to the balloon port (the side arm of the angioplasty catheter).
- Hold the syringe with the nozzle pointing down and aspirate for 5 s to remove air from the balloon and then release the plunger.
- Close the stopcock to the balloon and disconnect the syringe and evacuate air from the syringe.
- Reconnect the syringe to stopcock and open the stopcock to the balloon.
- Re-aspirate and release plunger, until bubbles no longer appear.
- If bubbles persist, do not use the system.

- Detach the syringe after air purgation is complete.
- Lubricate the balloon catheter shaft to activate the hydrophilic coating.

Deployment of PTA Balloon Catheter for Angioplasty

- Gain arterial access and position a guide catheter in pertinent artery (e.g., ICA or VA) as described above.
- Attach the hub of the balloon catheter to an RHV such that the proximal tip of the microwire in the catheter extends out from the hub of the RHV.
- Ensure the balloon catheter is continuously flushed with heparinized NS via the sideport of the RHV attached to a three-way stopcock, which connects to the tubing of the flush system.
- Ensure there are no air bubbles in the balloon catheter and that NS is dripping continuously from its distal tip.
- Ensure the distal tip of the microwire is not extending beyond the tip of balloon catheter.
- Loosen the knob of the RHV attached to the guide catheter and carefully insert the balloon catheter through it.
- Tighten the knob of RHV again, so that a seal is created around the balloon catheter, but it can still be advanced through the guide catheter without any difficulties.
- Once the distal aspect of balloon catheter is within the lumen of guide catheter, advance the microwire so that it leads the balloon catheter.
- Continue to advance the balloon catheter and wire assembly until the proximal markings on the balloon catheter align with the hub of the guide catheter. This alignment indicates that the balloon catheter tip has reached the distal tip of the guide catheter.
- Perform fluoroscopy to confirm location of the microcatheter, wire, and guide catheter.
- Perform angiography to visualize the lesion using the free port of the stopcock connected in the guide catheter system and select the appropriate working views for treating the lesion.
- Attach a torque device to the guidewire.
- Using road map guidance, advance the wire with constant half rotatory motion to cross the lesion.
- Ensure there is adequate length of wire distal to the lesion.
- Advance the balloon catheter over the wire using road map guidance.
- The two marker bands on the distal aspect of the balloon catheter tip, which indicate the proximal and distal ends of the angioplasty balloon, are positioned across the lesion.
- Confirm appropriate positioning by visualizing the marker for the tip of the balloon catheter, followed by the two marker bands indicating either end of the angioplasty balloon. For better visualization of markers also use native imaging and magnification, as necessary.

- Perform angiography to ascertain appropriate positioning of the balloon relative to the stenosis.
- Repeat angiography every time the position of the balloons is adjusted, until completely satisfied with the position of the balloon.
- Recover the inflation device from the table.
- Use the distal free port of the stopcock attached to the inflation device (which is in line with the inflation device) to make a wet (meniscus to meniscus) connection to the balloon port of the balloon catheter.
- Ensure that this connection is secure so that it will not disconnect during angioplasty.
- Close the stopcock to the inflation device.
- Aspirate the syringe (with nozzle pointing down) attached to the sideport of the stopcock to purge air out of the balloon angioplasty system.
- Slowly release the plunger of the syringe, so that the air is replaced with the contrast left in syringe for purpose. Repeat this step once, or twice.
- Close the stopcock to syringe.
- Reconfirm balloon position fluoroscopically.
- Using the chart provided with the balloon catheter slowly begin inflating the angioplasty balloon using the balloon inflation device, e.g., to perform an angioplasty to 1.57 mm using a 1.5-mm balloon, slowly inflate to 9.0 atm.
- Inflate slowly by turning the screw provided on the inflation device at a rate ≤ 1 atm/15 s (to 'stretch' not 'crack' the vessel).
- Step on fluoroscopy pedal frequently to visualize progression of angioplasty.
- During inflation, the balloon may acquire a 'waist' due to the stenosis. This resolves with the progression of angioplasty.
- Once the goal pressure is reached deflate the device.
- Confirm complete balloon deflation fluoroscopically.
- In order to achieve complete deflation, one may need to open the stopcock to the syringe and vigorously aspirate. Close the stopcock to syringe while aspiration is fully applied.
- Confirm complete balloon deflation fluoroscopically.
- Document the balloon inflation time from commencement of balloon inflation to deflation. The timer provided on the angiography unit may be used for this purpose.
- Perform f/u angiography to evaluate results of angioplasty.
- If needed, repeat the angioplasty.

Removal of PTA Balloon Catheter

- Confirm complete balloon deflation by visualizing it fluoroscopically.
- Ensure wire access across lesion is not lost during catheter removal.
- Loosen the knob of the RHV attached to the Guide catheter.

- Under continuous fluoroscopy, begin catheter withdrawal while the microwire remains in position across the lesion.
- This is a two-person maneuver: One operator controls the balloon catheter at the hub of the RHV and the second operator withdraws the balloon catheter over the wire while constantly observing the tip of the wire on the monitor to ensure it is not withdrawn inadvertently.
- The first operator is responsible for stepping on the fluoroscopy pedal, until the catheter successfully exits the RHV of the Guide catheter.
- The entire assembly is kept straight to ensure adequate control and maneuverability.
- The second operator progressively steps away from the first while withdrawing the catheter over wire to keep the system straight.
- Be vigilant to ensure the wire or catheter is not contaminated during the process by coming into contact with unsterile surfaces.
- As soon as the distal tip of the balloon catheter exits the hub of RHV, the first operator grabs the wire and secures it by forming a loop and holding it just next to the hub. The RHV knob is tightened around the wire. Then, the first operator uses a moist Telfa™ strip to wipe off the extraneous wire proximal to distally as the second operator completes the removal of the catheter of the wire.
- Wipe off the balloon catheter with heparinized NS and store in a saline bowl, in case it may be required for reuse.
- Maintain wire access across lesion esp. if the intention is to place a stent following angioplasty.

Selection of Appropriate Wingspan™ Stent

- Study the angiogram to select the appropriate size of stent.
- Measure the diameter of the vessel where its caliber in normal, or relatively so
- Select a stent by the size of the vessel. If needed, select a slightly oversized stent. However, don't undersize the stent since, that will risk its dislodgement and distal migration.
- The length of the stent should be such that at least 2 mm of the stent extends proximal and distal to the lesion, e.g., for a vessel with a diameter of 4.4 mm and a lesion length of 4 mm, use a 4.5-mm stent (which expands to 4.9 mm) with a 9-mm length (see Table 11.3, Chap. 11 Intracranial Angioplasty and Stenting for sizing guidelines).

Preparation of Wingspan™ Stent

- Open the pouch and transfer the packaging tray to preparation table using sterile precautions.
- Examine the system to rule out any damage.
- Using a 15-cc syringe, flush the dispenser hoop with saline.

- Carefully pull out the proximal hub aspect of the system from the tray.
- Locate the RHV of the outer body and tighten it onto the inner body of the stent system.
- Now transfer entire system out onto the table from the tray and dispenser hoop.
- Inspect the stent delivery system for any damage or flaws.
- Inspect to ensure that the stent is preloaded into the distal tip of the system.
- Locate the hub of the inner body, which is the most proximal aspect of the system and attach an RHV to it.
- Flush the lumen of the inner body with heparinized saline.
- Loosen the previously tightened RHV of the outer body and flush the lumen of the outer body with heparinized saline to purge air from the system.
- Gently advance the pusher of the inner body of the system until the proximal radiopaque markerband bumper is just proximal to the stent.
- Retighten the RHV of outer body to lock onto the inner body, so that the entire system will move as a single unit.
- There is an option of connecting heparinized saline flush to the side ports of the RHVs of the outer and inner bodies.

Deployment of Wingspan™ Stent

- Fluoroscopically ascertain that the guidewire is still across the lesion.
- Perform angiogram in working view.
- Backload the stent system onto the guidewire.
- Loosen the hub of the RHV of the guide catheter and advance the stent system into it.
- When the stent system is just short of the tip of the guide catheter, obtain a roadmap to assist in navigation.
- Advance the stent system over the guidewire until the stent is at the site of intended deployment, with the distal marker bands on the stent just distal to this locus.
- At this point, ascertain the positions of the following: distal tip of the guidewire, distal marker bands on the distal tip of the stent, proximal marker band on the stent pusher/bumper.
- The distal tip of the guidewire should be crossing the lesion and well distal to the distal marker bands on the stent.
- The distal marker bands on the stent should be just distal to the site of the lesion.
- The proximal marker band should be proximal to the lesion.
- Perform angiography and adjust position of stent if needed, until satisfied with position.
- Repeat angiography after each adjustment.
- Loosen the RHV of the outer body and slightly withdraw the hub of the outer body until the stent is directly aligned with the lesion.

- Tighten the RHV and if needed pull back on the system to ensure that all slack has been removed and the system is completely straight.
- Perform angiography to ascertain satisfactory final position.
- Ensure that the vessel distal to the lesion is visualized.
- Loosen the RHV of the outer body.
- Now deploy stent under continuous fluoroscopy as follows:
- Keep the inner body hub stationary with the one hand.
- Continue to withdraw the hub of the outer body with the other hand.
- Visualize the markerband at the distal end spread out into multiple smaller markers, indicating the opening of the stent.
- Continue deployment in a smooth motion until the stent is completely deployed.
- Do not attempt to move the stent or advance the outer body once the deployment is underway. After completion of deployment, retighten the RHV of the outer body and gently withdraw the entire system maintaining wire access across the lesion.
- Once system is out of the Guide catheter RHV, secure the wire, stop fluoroscopy, and remove the system off the wire. This is a two-person maneuver.
- Perform angiography to ascertain satisfactory result before giving up wire access and only then, withdraw the guidewire.
- Perform standard AP lateral cerebral angiography to document results and to rule out any new vessel cutoff or change in comparison with pre-procedure angiogram.
- Retract the guide catheter to the femoral artery and perform femoral angiogram in $\approx 45°$ ipsilateral oblique view.
- If the arteriotomy is proximal to femoral bifurcation and the vessel size is ≥ 4.9 mm, perform closure with angioseal.
- Clean and dress site.
- Break sterile field.

Postoperative Management and Follow-up

- Admit patient to NSICU for at least overnight observation. Further ICU stay will depend upon extent of stroke and clinical condition.
- 0.9% NS + 20 meq KCl @ 150 cc/h $\times$ 2 h, then decrease to 100 cc/h if patient is NPO.
- Keep right/left leg (whichever side was used for procedure) straight $\times$ 2 h, with HOB elevated 15°.
- Check groins, DP's, vitals and neurochecks q 15 min $\times$ 4, q 30 min $\times$ 4, then q h.
- Plavix 300 mg LD then, 75 mg PO daily $\times$ 4 weeks, if stent was placed.
- ASA 81–325 mg PO daily.
- Advance diet as tolerated.

- Perform baseline TCDs on POD 1, or within first few days of procedure prior to patients' discharge.
- Review/resume pre-procedure medications (except oral hypoglycemics that are resumed once PO intake is established).
- Ensure that the patient is being followed by (preferably, admitted under the auspices of) a stroke neurologist and that there is post-discharge follow-up by him/her.
- Transfer to stroke ward/step down unit after mobilizing (if no complications/other ongoing medical concerns requiring ICU hospitalization).
- D/C home or rehab after acute issues related to stroke addressed.
- F/u on outpatient basis in 4 weeks.
- F/u angiography at 3 months.

Problems Encountered During Angioplasty and Stenting and Solutions

- Cerebral artery rupture during procedure.
- See Chap. 19 'Complications, Avoidance and Management'.

Pronto Device (for Cranial Sinus Thrombosis)

Indications

- Acute CST, not responding to other management and where there are no contraindications to endovascular intervention (Figs. 15.10 and 15.11).
- It may be noted that Pronto™ or similar aspiration catheters are not FDA approved for use in venous or cranial sinus system.

Contraindications

- Vessel size less than 2 mm.
- Chronic or atherosclerotic clot, e.g., an infarct involving more than one-third of the cerebral hemisphere which could be converted to a hemorrhagic infarct.

Femoral Venous Access

- If CST was already diagnosed or suspected based on neuroimaging and clinical symptomatology, prepare vascular access to femoral artery and vein.
- When feasible, access the femoral artery and vein on separate limbs since accessing adjacent vessels on the same limb runs a small risk of arteriovenous fistula formation.

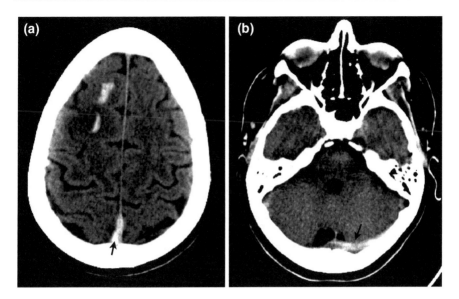

Fig. 15.10 CT scan axial section, without contrast, in a 35-year-old female with CST. The *arrow* points to an acute clot in the superior sagittal sinus (SSS; **a**) and left transverse sinus (**b**). There is a venous hemorrhagic infarct of the right frontal lobe (**a**) (*permission to reprint courtesy of Marshfield Clinic. From Khan et al.* [2]. *Copyright 2009 Marshfield Clinic. All rights reserved*)

- Access the femoral artery in the standard fashion described above.
- Advance a 5-Fr front angled catheter (Terumo™) with continuously running heparinized saline flush solution over a glidewire into the CCA.
- Perform diagnostic angiography. Ensure that angiography continues well into the venous phase and that the cranial sinuses are within the imaging field.
- Once CST is diagnosed/confirmed, gain access to the femoral vein using modified Seldinger technique, as described above for femoral artery and place a 7-Fr short sheath and secure the sheath in place with 2-0 silk suture.
- The femoral vein lies medial to the femoral arterial pulse.
- Attach a syringe to the micropuncture needle and apply gentle aspiration pressure enabling venous blood to enter the syringe and confirm venous access. Unlike the artery, venous blood does not emanate out pulsating briskly when the vein is accessed.
- Attach a 6-Fr Envoy™ guide catheter to a continuously running solution of heparinized saline, ensuring the system is free of air bubbles.
- Introduce the Envoy™ guide catheter into the sheath within the femoral vein.
- Advance it through the inferior vena cava over glidewire™, with the glidewire leading.
- With the glidewire leading and continuing with live fluoroscopy, advance into the right ventricle and then superior vena cava.
- Select the appropriate subclavian vein and then the jugular vein.
- To assist jugular access, roadmapping is performed.

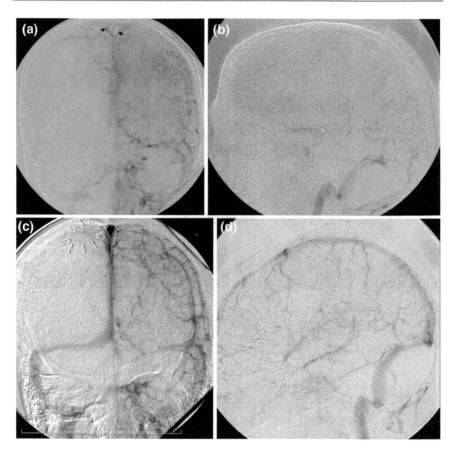

Fig. 15.11 Cerebral angiography AP (**a**) and lateral (**b**) views performed prior to intervention demonstrate the absence of major cranial sinuses. The arrows in (**a**) point to a thin rim of contrast enhancement surrounding the clot in the lumen of SSS. A microcatheter was placed in the SSS and TPA administered overnight. The following day, the clot was successfully aspirated with Pronto V3 thrombectomy catheter, resulting in successful reconstitution of cranial sinuses (**c** and **d**). The surgical clip artifact (**c**) is because of a craniotomy performed for evacuation of the expanding right frontal hematoma. (*permission to reprint courtesy of Marshfield Clinic. From Khan et al.* [2]. *Copyright 2009 Marshfield Clinic. All rights reserved*)

- To perform the roadmap of the venous system, fluoroscopy is performed in a delayed fashion with at least a 3-s delay from the time of contrast injection to stepping on the fluoroscopy pedal. The arterial and capillary phases are bypassed in this manner.
- Some difficulty may be encountered entering the jugular vein. This is because unlike the arterial system, valves are encountered in the veins. May need to time the advancement through venous valve with the patient's inspiration.
- Advance and position the Envoy catheter in the IJV or sigmoid sinus.

- If Penumbra system is selected, its' technique remains as indicated above. Another option is pronto catheter.

Pronto™ Aspiration Catheter Preparation

- Prepare a 5-French Pronto V3™ thrombectomy catheter (Vascular Solutions, Inc. Minneapolis, MN), which is a direct aspiration catheter usually used for dialysis fistula thrombectomy. Pronto V3 is a 140-cm rapid exchange catheter, with a 30-ml locking aspiration syringe. It has a luer adapter at its proximal end for connecting to the aspiration syringe.
- (Another similar aspiration catheter may also be used, e.g., Fetch®, Possis Medical, Minneapolis, MN. However, we do not have any personal experience with it).
- Open the pouch and transfer the tray containing pronto V3 to operating table using sterile technique.
- Attach a 10-ml syringe filled with heparinized saline to the flushing luer of the carrier tube and completely flush to activate the hydrophilic coating.
- Remove the catheter from the carrier tube and inspect for any bends, kinks, or other damage.
- Remove the wire stylet from the wire lumen.
- Flush the catheter and wire lumen with heparinized saline.
- Draw 5 ml of heparinized saline into the 30-ml syringe.
- Connect the syringe to the stopcock and connect the attached extension line to the catheter.
- Flush the entire connection to remove all air from the catheter, extension line, stopcock, and syringe. Then, turn the stopcock to the 'Off' position.
- With the stopcock in the 'Off' position, pull back the plunger on the 30-ml syringe to the desired amount of extraction volume. Twist the plunger to lock the syringe in the vacuum position.

Deployment

- If a microwire is not already in place, insert a 0.014 microwire (e.g., Transend EX 0.014, introduce the proximal end of wire into the distal tip of the catheter. The introduced end of wire will exit from the provided exit notch further proximally.
- Retract the wire until its distal tip is just within the distal tip of catheter.
- Advance the pronto catheter and guidewire as a unit into the guide catheter loosening the RHV to enable advancement of the catheter-wire complex, but not so loose as to allow bleeding via the RHV.
- Once the pronto catheter is within the guide catheter, advance some wire ahead of it, so that the wire is leading the pronto catheter.

- When the catheter-wire unit reaches the tip of the guide catheter, perform road mapping, remembering to step on fluoroscopy pedal in a delayed fashion, to enable visualization of the venous system.
- Advance the pronto catheter over the wire into the thrombus.
- Once appropriately positioned, completely withdraw the wire.
- Turn the stopcock to 'ON' position.
- Gradually retract the catheter to enable clot aspiration.
- Once proximal to the clot and out of cranial system, the catheter may be retracted more expeditiously. Close the RHV of the guide catheter after removing the pronto catheter.
- Ensure that it is free of blood and if necessary, flush it to make it so.
- Evacuate the clot out of the pronto catheter system onto the provided filter system by pushing forward on the plunger of the syringe. This will enable assessment of the amount of clot extracted.
- Clean the Pronto™ catheter off any clot residuals. If needed, make additional passes with Pronto™ catheter to remove additional clot from the acutely occluded sinus.
- Following completion of clot extraction, perform cerebral angiography for documentation of results.
- Remove the diagnostic and guide catheters.
- If the requirement of vascular access is not anticipated in the near future, the femoral artery sheath is exchanged for an angioseal closure device over wire and the arteriotomy is plugged.
- Remove the sheath from the femoral vein and apply manual pressure upon the venous puncture site for 5–10 min.
- Clean and dress puncture sites.
- Break the sterile operating field.

Postoperative Management and Follow-up

- Admit to NSICU. Duration of ICU stay will depend upon extent of stroke and clinical condition.
- 0.9% NS + 20 meq KCl @ 150 cc/h till further orders.
- NPO.
- Keep right/left leg (whichever side was used for procedure) straight × 2 h, with HOB elevated 15°.
- If patient on heparin or Reopro drip, continue postoperatively for 12 h.
- Check groins, DP's, vitals and neurochecks q 15 min × 4, q 30 min × 4, then q h.
- ASA 81–325 mg PO daily.
- Advance diet as tolerated.
- Review/resume pre-procedure medications (except oral hypoglycemics that are resumed 48 h after intervention and once oral intake is established).

Table 15.5 Problems and solutions

Problem	Solution
Difficulty in navigating and positioning the Pronto™ catheter at desired location	• Negotiating the jugular-sigmoid system may prove difficult esp. as the size of the catheter increases. Using a 'buddy wire' may help in advancing the pronto catheter—microguidewire unit
Inability to aspirate clot due to apparent plugging or occlusion of the catheter	• Advance or slightly retract the catheter to see whether the aspiration can be re-established. If not, completely withdraw the catheter out of the body and then clean it. Do not attempt to evacuate clot out of the pronto catheter while it is still in the vascular system

- F/u CT head postoperative day 1 and as needed during hospitalization.
- Ensure patient is followed by (and preferably admitted under the auspices of) stroke neurologist and that there is post-discharge follow-up by him/her.
- F/u on outpatient basis in 4 weeks, 3 months, 6 months, 1 year and then as necessary.
- Conversely, if the patient is being treated in conjunction with a stroke neurologist, and there are no active issues requiring neurosurgical attention, the patient may be followed by neurologist alone after the initial postoperative follow-up.

Problems Encountered During Pronto Device Usage and Solutions

- Table 15.5 shows some problems and solutions.

Suggested Readings

1. Khan SH, Ringer A. The technique of angioplasty and stent placement in acute ischemic stroke. J Neurol Res 2011;I(3):81–9.
2. Khan SH, Adeoye O, Abruzzo TA, Shutter LA, Ringer AJ. Intracranial dural sinus thrombosis: novel use of a mechanical thrombectomy catheter and review of Management strategies. Clin Med Res. 2009;7(4):157–65.
3. Pearse M. Interventional and endovascular therapy of the nervous system. A practical guide. New York: Springer-Verlag; 2001. p. 269–89.
4. Ringer A, Nichols C, Khan SH, Pyne-Geithman G, Abruzzo T. Angioplasty and stenting for management of intracranial arterial stenosis. In: Bendok B, Batjer H, Naidech A, Walker A, editors. Hemorrhagic and ischemic stroke. Thieme Medical Publishers; 2011.
5. Merci User Guide.
6. Penumbra System™ User Guide.
7. Wingspan User Guide.

Kyphoplasty

16

Indications and Case Selection

- Pathological fractures due to:

  - Osteoporosis.
  - Malignancy including multiple myeloma; metastasis, e.g., from breast CA, lung CA, lymphoma.
  - Benign osteolytic lesions, e.g., hemangioma, giant cell tumor.

Contraindications

- Infection of skin or soft tissue that will be traversed during procedure.
- Osteomyelitis.
- Bleeding disorders.
- Retropulsion of bone fragment or tumor mass into spinal canal.

Preoperative Management

- Verify lab values including platelet count, BUN, CR, APTT, PT/INR, and ß-HCG (in pre-menopausal females).
- Liquids only on morning of procedure.
- NPO (for ≈6 h) when procedure performed under GA (almost always done under local anesthesia with mild-to-moderate sedation).
- Continue prescribed medications, e.g., antihypertensives. However, NSAIDs and ASA to be discontinued a week prior to procedure.
- Obtain informed consent for kyphoplasty of affected levels.
- Ensure two IV lines inserted (18G & 20G).

© Springer International Publishing AG 2017
S.H. Khan and A.J. Ringer, *Handbook of Neuroendovascular Techniques*,
DOI 10.1007/978-3-319-52936-3_16

- Position patient prone on neuroangiography table.
- Attach patient to pulse oximetry and ECG leads for monitoring O$_2$ saturation, HR, cardiac rhythm, respiratory rate, and BP.

Equipment

- Betadine or Chloraprep™ scrub.
- Methyl methacrylate, e.g., KyphX® HV-R™ Bone Cement (which has barium sulfate pre-added on a 30% w/w basis).
- Syringes 5 cc (2).
- Needle 18G (for drawing lidocaine from bottle).
- Needle 22G (for local infiltration of lidocaine).
- Spinal needle 18G.
- 11-gauge Jamshidi needle.
- K-wire (one for each treatment site).
- Graduated cannula.
- Biopsy syringe.
- Balloon with manometer.
- Cannula with stylet (for cement insertion).
- Cement mixer, e.g., Kyphon® Mixer.
- Pre-assembled kits are available. We preferentially use Kyphon®.
- Drugs

    - 1% Lidocaine for local infiltration.
    - Fentanyl 25–50 µg IV prn.
    - Versed 0.5–1.0 mg IV prn.

Technique

- Position the patient prone on the neuroangiography table.
- The head should be turned to a side as comfortably as possible, on a pillow.
- Arms are drawn up and positioned outside the irradiation field.
- Perform fluoroscopy to demarcate the vertebra of interest using a towel holder and skin marker.
- Ensure the lesion is visualized in a true lateral and AP position by ascertaining that the endplates are aligned esp. in the region of interest.
- The positions of working AP and lateral positions are selected and saved.
- Identify and demarcate the vertebra of interest.
- Select and demarcate the point of entry (see below) on the skin.
- There are some technical differences in performing this depending upon the spine level. These are as follows.

Lumbar

Point of Entry

- Identify and demarcate the center of each pedicle at level of interest by AP fluoroscopy.
- Also demarcate the spinous process.
- Join the demarcated pedicle points by a straight line.
- The point of entry is at the level of this bipedicular line as follows:

  - L1, L2: 8 cm lateral to midline.
  - L4, L5: 12 cm lateral to midline.

- Infiltrate the point of entry with local anesthesia.
- Make a small stab incision (about 5 mm) at the anesthetized site.
- Introduce a spinal needle into the incision at a 60° angle to the vertical plane.
- Advance the spinal needle along the bipedicular line on AP fluoroscopy, anterior to the transverse process, to the junction of the ipsilateral pedicle and the posterior vertebral body at their lateral walls (Fig. 16.1).

Thoracic

Point of Entry

- Demarcate the top of the pedicle on AP fluoroscopy.
- Also demarcate the spinous process.
- Join the demarcated pedicle points.
- The point of entry is at the level of this bipedicular line.
- Measure the distance from the spinous process to the pedicle. The skin entry point is approximately $1.5\times$ the spinous-pedicle distance, lateral to the pedicle.
- Infiltrate the point of entry with local anesthesia.
- When bone is encountered, it may also be infiltrated with local anesthesia through the spinal needle.
- The needle course is via the potential space between the rib head, transverse process, and pedicle. To this effect, advance the needle obliquely until the rib head is felt. Follow the posterior wall of the rib and advance the instrument anterior to the transverse process. The trajectory is relatively fixed once between the rib and transverse process and is confirmed on lateral fluoroscopy.

Entry into Vertebral Body

- Withdraw the spinal needle.
- Insert an 11-gauge Jamshidi needle through the stab wound and advance it along the same trajectory as the spinal needle, using fluoroscopy.

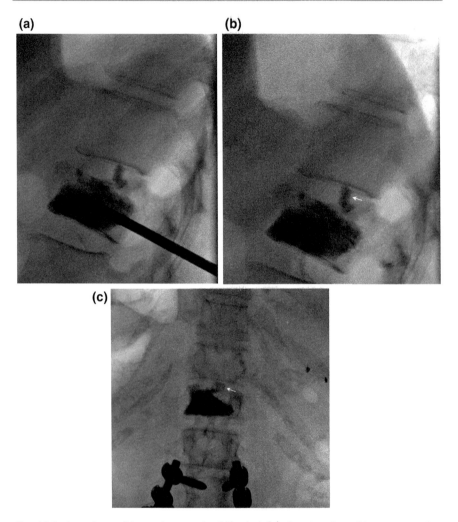

Fig. 16.1 A patient with persistent pain following L1 fracture that did not respond to conservative management. Extrapedicular kyphoplasty was performed. An extrapedicular approach was undertaken and methyl methacrylate injected into the vertebral body through the inserted cannula (**a**). The procedure was discontinued when cement was noted to extend into the disk space (*arrow*, **b**). The anteroposterior view (**c**) demonstrates the considerable amount of cement that can be deposited into the vertebral body by the extrapedicular approach. Again noted is some cement extravasation into the disk space

- Once the junction of the ipsilateral pedicle and the posterior vertebral body is reached (and felt), use a mallet to advance it obliquely toward the plane of the contralateral pedicle on AP view.
- The Jamshidi should be just through the cortex of the VB at the level of pedicle.
- Readjust trajectory as necessary during advancement.
- On lateral view, the Jamshidi reaches the anterior 1/3 of the vertebral body.

- Keep in mind the curvilinear shape of the anterior border of vertebral body on the axial view. Therefore, the anterior cortical margin between the pedicles on AP view extends further anterior than the cortical margins lateral to the pedicles. The more posterior cortical margin cannot be appreciated on lateral fluoroscopy. Therefore, to prevent an instrument from extending anterior to the vertebral body, even though it may appear to be within the vertebral body on both AP and lateral images, avoid advancing any instrument more anteriorly than ¾ of the vertebral bodies AP dimension (on lateral view) unless it is nearly centered between the pedicles on AP view.
- Take care not to dislodge instruments during manipulation, as reinsertion may prove difficult.
- Remove the stylet from the Jamshidi and insert a K-wire.
- Using a mallet, advance the k-wire maintaining trajectory and ensuring not to go beyond ¾ of the vertebral body on AP dimension and lateral views.
- Remove the Jamshidi and advance a graduated cannula over the K-wire, using mallet as necessary under fluoroscopy.
- Remove the K-wire.
- Advance a biopsy needle with attached syringe through the cannula into the vertebral body.
- Aspirate with the syringe to obtain a biopsy sample.
- Remove the biopsy needle and pushing the syringe plunger, transfer the core biopsy specimen into a sterile jar with saline, maintaining sterility.
- Advance balloon with manometer (select psi on manometer) through the cannula under fluoroscopy.
- Inflate the balloon approximately 40 psi at a time, checking progress under fluoroscopy.
- The balloon may be inflated up to 400 psi.
- Deflate and remove the balloon.
- Insert a cannula filled with cement, ensuring the distal tip of the cannula is within vertebral body.
- Deliver the cement into the vertebral body under fluoroscopy using the pusher provided. Use a rotating motion on the pusher.
- Prior to withdrawal of cement cannula, use a rotating motion so that the cement is not deposited in the tract extravertebrally. Additionally, ensure the pusher is completely extended to the distal tip of the cement cannula.
- Use as much cement as necessary to treat the vertebral body
- Use constant fluoroscopy while depositing cement to ensure it does not break though into the disk space; extravertebrally, into the neural canal, or embolise into veins.
- If there appears to be beginning of errant deposition, wait a few minutes to allow the deposited cement to firm up and then continue injection, ensuring the cement remains within the vertebral body. Alternatively, change the depth of cement cannula in the vertebral body and continue cement deposition.
- Confirm final result by AP + lat fluoroscopy and then withdraw all instruments

- Withdraw the graduated cannula over the cement cannula and pusher to ensure there is no deposition of cement along the track in soft tissues. Usually, 3–11 cc of methyl methacrylate may be easily deposited.
- Take single-shot X-rays for future reference.

Postoperative Orders

- Flat in bed for one hour with HOB 15°.
- Sit up for one hour.
- Then mobilize.
- Resume diet.
- Resume preoperative medications.
- Discharge after 2 h of observation, if remains stable and not hospitalized for ongoing treatment.

Suggested Reading

Ringer AJ, Bhamidipaty SV. Percutaneous access to the vertebral bodies: a video and fluoroscopic overview of access techniques for trans-, extra-, and infrapedicular approaches. World Neurosurg. 2013;80(3–4):428–35.

WADA Test

Indications

- To determine hemispheric dominance for speech.
- Test injection prior to embolization of a vessel feeding an AVM when the functional significance of a vessel or pedicle in question is unclear, e.g., due to inadequate angiographic visualization or embolization of a region with high risks (such as spinal cord or in the brain).
- When suppression of both neuronal and axonal activity is desired, amytal injection is followed by 40 mg lidocaine injection (e.g., in spinal AVMs).

Preoperative Orders

- Fluids only for breakfast.
- Continue prescribed medications (including ASA and antihypertensives) except antiseizure drugs, which would have been withheld by neurologist.
- Labs: CBC, APTT, INR, electrolytes, BUN, CR.
- ß-HCG for females of reproductive age group.
- Insert IV and commence 0.9% N.S. at 75 cc/hr.
- Consent the patient.

Equipment

Micropuncture Kit

- 5 Fr short sheath (10 cm).
- 5-Fr front angled catheter (Terumo®).

© Springer International Publishing AG 2017
S.H. Khan and A.J. Ringer, *Handbook of Neuroendovascular Techniques*,
DOI 10.1007/978-3-319-52936-3_17

- Glide wire (Terumo®).
- Three-way stopcock.
- Touhy connector.
- Flush system with heparinized saline (6000 units heparin per 1000 ml saline).
- Three 10-cc syringes (for contrast injection).
- One 10-cc syringe (for local anesthesia). Label the syringe.
- Three 20-cc syringes (for Flushing catheter/lines).
- Three 5-cc syringes (for Sodium Amytal).

Angiopack that Includes

- Mandrel.
- Sharps holder.
- Towels.
- 4 × 4 Gauze sponges.
- A pair of scissors, one needle driver, one mosquito forceps.
- Plastic basin (for holding catheter and wires).
- Two small plastic cups, one colored and the other transparent (for contrast or drugs, if needed).
- Plastic clamps for securing tubing to drape sheet.
- Drape sheet.

Drugs

- Fentanyl 25–100 μg IV q hr prn.
- Versed 0.5–1 mg IV prn.
- 1% Lidocaine (for local anesthesia prior to arteriotomy).

Sodium Amytal

- Dilute 500 mg in 10 cc 0.9% NS to yield a concentration of 50 mg/cc.
- Transfer this to a sterile plastic cup on procedure table and label the cup.
- Add additional 10 cc 0.9% NS to plastic cup and mix, to yield a concentration of 25 mg/cc of Sodium Amytal.

Procedure

- Position the patient supine on angiography table.
- Palpate pulse at both femoral regions.
- Palpate both DP's. Use Doppler USG if needed.

- Prep and drape patient in a sterile fashion.
- Gain arterial access using modified Seldinger technique and secure a short sheath in position using 2-0 silk suture.
- Attach the sheath to continuous running flush of heparinized saline.
- Use 5-Fr front angled catheter with guidewire attached to a continuous flush system for angiography.
- Access the carotid artery on the side of suspected pathology first.
- Perform standard AP and lateral cervical angiography.
- Then select the ICA. For this purpose, may use the acquired angiography run as 'Fluoro Fade.'
- Perform standard AP and lateral cerebral angiograms.
- Allow the neurologist to commence their testing.
- When directed, inject 100 mg of Sodium Amytal (4 cc of the preparation described above) through the catheter into the ICA. May need to give additional boluses of 25 mg (1 cc) or modify the original bolus, per neurologist's request.
- If the test is negative (unchanged neurological exam), rule out a false negative, e.g., amytal did not go into the vessel being tested (the vessel being tested must be seen on an angiogram). Additionally, if there is a high-flow lesion present, then amytal may have passed through the high-flow vessels, instead of the vessels of interest. In such a situation while the WADA test may appear negative, the actual occlusion of vessel of interest may lead to neurological deficits.
- If the test is positive (neurological symptoms), then treatment such as embolization may be contraindicated from that position. Catheterization further distally with repeat WADA testing should be performed to assess whether more selective catheterization and embolization are feasible. Bear in mind repeat amytal injections in itself may cause the patient to become confused, sleepy, and uncooperative.
- Following completion of testing for the side, retract the diagnostic catheter into the arch and access the contralateral carotid.
- Perform standard AP and lateral cervical angiography.
- Select the ICA, and use the previously acquired run as 'Fluoro Fade,' if needed.
- Perform standard AP and lateral cerebral angiograms.
- Allow the neurologist to continue with their testing.
- When directed, inject 100 mg of Sodium Amytal (4 cc of the preparation described above) through the catheter into the ICA. May need to give additional boluses of 25 mg (1 cc) or modify the original bolus per neurologist's request.
- May retract the catheter back into the aortic arch or descending aorta when the testing is well underway, and no further amytal injections will be required.
- Once the neurological examination is complete, retract the catheter into the femoral region.
- Obtain an ipsilateral oblique ($\approx$33–45°) view of the femoral region at the site of arteriotomy, centering on the femoral head and neck region.
- If the femoral angiography confirms the arteriotomy to be proximal to femoral bifurcation and the size of vessel at arteriotomy ≥ 4 mm, then perform angio-seal closure (see Chap. 3).

- Following completion of procedure, palpate both DP's
- If above requirements are not met, perform manual compression (see Chap. 3).

Postoperative Orders

- Patient to remain flat in bed for 2 h with HOB 15°, with the leg with arteriotomy to remain straight.
- Neurological, groin, and DP checks q 15 min X 4, then q 30 min X 4.
- 0.9% NS at 125 cc/hr for 2 h.
- Advance diet.
- Resume preoperative medications.
- Discharge after 2 h of observation, if patient remains stable, return to baseline ambulation and voiding

Suggested Reading

Technical aspects of surgical neuroangiography. In: Berenstein A, Lasjaunias P, Ter Brugge KG, eds. Surgical Neuroangiography. Heidelberg:Springer-Verlag. 2004;2.2:926–29.

Pharmacological Agents

Additional Contributor: Kiranpal S. Sangha

18

Heparin

Mechanism

- A glycosaminoglycan, with immediate anticoagulant effects, that indirectly inhibits thrombin by modulating antithrombin III (AT III) activity.
- It also indirectly neutralizes and inactivates factors IXa, Xa, XIa, and XIIa and restores electronegativity of endothelial surfaces.
- Prevents thrombin-platelet? Aggregation and inhibits von Willebrand factor.
- The half-life of IV heparin is approximately 1.5 h.

Indications and Case Selection

- Prevention of procedure related thromboembolic complications during cerebral angiography (used in flush solutions) or neuroendovascular procedures (therapeutic doses).

Side Effects

- Idiosyncratic immunologically mediated thrombocytopenia

Dose

Use for Flush System

- 6000 IU per litre of 0.9% normal saline (6 IU per cc) for flush systems used in the neuroendovascular operative suite.

© Springer International Publishing AG 2017
S.H. Khan and A.J. Ringer, *Handbook of Neuroendovascular Techniques*,
DOI 10.1007/978-3-319-52936-3_18

- 2500 IU per litre of 0.9% normal saline (2.5 IU per cc) in the operating room. The lower dosage is a precaution against excessive bleeding from operative sites, e.g., during craniotomy.

During Endovascular Intervention

- In coil embolization of intracranial aneurysms, the goal ACT is between 250 and 300 sec.
- In stenting, the goal ACT is between 300 and 350 sec.
- After securing vascular access, administer 3000–5000 IU heparin. In case of ruptured aneurysms, heparin may be deferred until the framing coil is placed.
- Obtain ACT 20 min after the first heparin dose and then hourly. Administer intermittent boluses of IV heparin depending upon the value of ACT.
- See Table 18.1 for goal ACT in various endovascular procedures.
- Consider short-term postoperative anticoagulation after endovascular intervention. According to our weight-based protocol, the patient is administered 900 IU if the weight is <70 kg and 1300 IU for >70 kg for 12 h following intervention.

Heparin Dosing for Post-Coiling Neurosurgery Patients

- Suggested protocol: Weight 75 kg or less—900 units/h, no bolus doses, for 12 h.
- Weight above 75 kg—1300 units/h, no bolus doses, for 12 h.
- Labs: no ACT or other laboratory draws required.
- *Alternative*: The most commonly used heparin weight-based protocol uses bolus dose of 80 u/kg/h followed by a maintenance IV infusion rate of 18 units/kg/hour.
- Infusion rate 900–1300 units/h

Table 18.1 Goal ACT in various endovascular procedures. Reprinted with permission from [1], with permission from Wolters Kluwer Health, Inc.

ACT (s)	Indications
High (300–350)	Procedures involving deep arterial injury, e.g., percutaneous transluminal angioplasty with/without stenting
	Procedures with significant stasis of blood flow e.g., balloon occlusion of parent vessels
Moderate (250–300)	Procedures in which above mentioned thrombogenic elements are absent, e.g., embolization of an aneurysm, coiling of ruptured aneurysm, arteriovenous malformations

Pt weight	Dose in units/kg/h
50 kg	18
60 kg	15
70 kg	13
75 kg	12
80 kg	16
90 kg	14
100 kg	13
110 kg	12
120 kg or higher	11

Major Complications

- Hemorrhage.
- Conversion of ischemic stroke to hemorrhagic stroke.
- Heparin-induced thrombocytopenia (HIT): a potential life-threatening complication seen in up to 5–30% of patients exposed to unfractionated heparin. Due to the potential of significant HIT-induced thromboembolic complications, clinical, and laboratory surveillance of those receiving high-dose or long-term heparin (1 week or greater) is recommended.

Contraindications

- Some practitioners consider systemic heparinization during endovascular intervention for an acutely ruptured aneurysm or AVM a contraindication. A majority do not. In case of an acutely ruptured aneurysm, we have found heparinization to be safe, when initiated after placement of the first coil. In unruptured aneurysms, heparinization may be initiated as soon as arterial access is secured.
- Severe thrombocytopenia.
- Heparin-induced thrombocytopenia.
- An uncontrolled active bleeding site.

Reversal

- Heparin is reversed by intravenous administration of protamine sulfate at 1 mg per 100 units of circulating heparin (not to exceed 50 mg total).
- A preloaded syringe of 50 mg should remain available at all times during most endovascular procedures, to enable rapid bolus administration in case of an emergency.

- While normally protamine is administered as an IV infusion over 10–30 min to prevent idiosyncratic hypotension and anaphylactoid symptoms, in case of endovascular emergencies (e.g., vessel perforation or intracranial aneurysm perforation), anticoagulation must be immediately reversed by rapid IV bolus of protamine (10 mg over 1–3 min).

Abciximab (ReoPro®)

Mechanism

- Antibodies that prevent binding of fibrinogen to platelet GP IIb/IIIa receptors.

Indications and Case Selection

- Acute management of endoarterial thrombus associated with a neurointerventional device.
- Acute arterial occlusion complicating a procedure.
- Dissection with thrombus adherent to an intimal flap.
- Prophylaxis for extracranial or intracranial stent implantation for atherosclerosis.

Dose

- Loading Dose: 0.25 mg/kg followed by continuous IV infusion of 0.125 µg/kg/min (max 10 µg/min) for 12 h, then d/c.

Side Effects

- Major bleeding: Older patients and those with lower body weight may be at increased risk. To minimize this risk, use lower doses, local trans-catheter rather than systemic infusions, shorter courses of the drug and avoid concomitant heparin therapy.
- Thrombocytopenia.
- Pseudo-thrombocytopenia.
- Utricaria, diarrhea, and elevated serum amino-transferase levels.

Major Complications

- Major bleeding.
- Hemorrhagic conversion of infarct.

Contraindications

- Active internal bleeding.
- Recent (within 6 weeks) gastrointestinal (GI) or genitourinary (GU) bleeding of clinical significance.
- History of cerebrovascular accident (CVA) within 2 years, or CVA with a significant residual neurological deficit.
- Bleeding diathesis.
- Thrombocytopenia (<100,000 cells/μL).
- Recent (within 6 weeks) major surgery or trauma.
- Severe uncontrolled hypertension.
- Presumed or documented history of vasculitis.

Reversal

- Discontinue drug infusion.
- Allow 10–30 min for clearance of the drug from plasma, then

  - Administer Platelets transfusion.

- Surgical intervention should be delayed for 12–24 h after discontinuation of abciximab infusion.

Aspirin (ASA)

Mechanism

- A cyclo-oxygenase inhibitor that prevents formation of prostaglandins from arachidonic acid.

Indications and Case Selection

- Prophylaxis of intra- (short-term) and post-procedural (short+ and long-term) thromboembolic events during endovascular procedures, e.g.,

  - diagnostic cerebral angiography,
  - coil embolization of aneurysms,
  - stent implantation (typically with a second antiplatelet agent),
  - balloon test occlusions,
  - therapeutic occlusion of large arteries.
  - Occasionally administered in conjunction with a second antiplatelet agent.

- Subacute management of procedural complications, e.g.,

  - parent artery coil herniations,
  - thrombus or clot on coil phenomena,
  - in-stent thrombus (alone or in combination with a second agent).

Dose

- 325–1300 mg orally, daily.
- Uncoated ASA achieves peak plasma concentrations within 30–40 min.
- Enteric-coated ASA achieves peak plasma concentrations in up to 6 h.
- 60% of the population is resistant to the antiplatelet effect of low-dose (81 mg) ASA.
- 30% of the population is resistant to the antiplatelet effect of 325 mg/day regimen.

Side Effects

- GI erosions.
- Renal Insufficiency.
- Headaches.
- High-dose (unlike low-dose) regimens impede BP management by interacting with agents such as angiotensin-converting enzyme (ACE) inhibitors, or furosemide.
- Unpredictability of individual response (ASA resistance).

Major Complications

- Major bleeding including of GI system.

Contraindications

- Uncontrolled hypertension.

Reversal

- Reversal may be achieved by platelet transfusion.

Clopidogrel (Plavix™)

Mechanism

- Platelet ADP receptor antagonist.

Indications and Case Selection

- Prevention of intraprocedural and short-term post-procedural (4–12 weeks) thromboembolic events related to endovascular procedures. These include:

  - Coil embolization of wide-neck cerebral aneurysms where stent will be used.
  - Stent implantation (with a second antiplatelet agent).
  - Therapeutic occlusion of large arteries (often with a second antiplatelet agent).

- Subacute management of procedural complications (alone or in combination with a second agent), e.g.,

  - Parent artery coil herniations.
  - Thrombus or clot on coil phenomena.
  - In-stent thrombus (may be more effective than other agents).

Dose

- 75 mg PO daily, start 5 days prior to the actual procedure because there is a 3- to 7-day latency period to full therapeutic effect.
- LD: 300 mg PO, if there was no time to achieve therapeutic effect over a course of days. A therapeutic effect can usually be achieved within 2–3 h of LD.

Side Effects

- Bone marrow suppression (less risk than Ticlid™; perform CBC blood test every 2 weeks for the first 3 months).
- Neutropenia (risk similar to ASA at 0.2–0.5%).
- TTP.
- GI events: abdominal pain, dyspepsia, gastritis, diarrhea, constipation rash and other skin disorders.

Major Complications

- Major bleeding.

Contraindications

- Hypersensitivity to the drug.
- Active bleeding.

Reversal

- Platelet transfusion.

Ticlopidine

Mechanism

- Platelet ADP receptor antagonist

Indications and Case Selection

- As an alternative, in case of ASA intolerance or failure. Slightly more effective than ASA, but it has a more concerning side effect profile.

Dose

- 500 mg PO daily.

Side Effects

- Bone marrow suppression. Requires a CBC blood test every 2 weeks for the first 3 months.
- Aplastic anemia.
- Severe neutropenia (absolute neutrophil count below $450/mm^3$).
- Major hemorrhage.
- Bone marrow related complications do not appear to be common when ticlopidine is used for periods shorter than 1 month.

Major Complications

- Major bleeding.
- Bone marrow suppression.
- Severe Neutropenia.
- TTP.

Contraindications

- Hypersensitivity to the drug.
- Active bleeding.

Reversal

- Platelet transfusion along with methylprednisolone 20 mg IV.

Tissue Plasminogen Activator (TPA)

Mechanism

- Converts plasminogen to plasmin, fibrin specific.

Indications and Case Selection

- Patients with acute ischemic stroke who are:

  - 18 years of age, or older.
  - Clinical diagnosis of ischemic stroke with measurable neurologic deficit.
  - Symptom onset less than 3 h (or less than 4.5 h in some cases) prior to initiation of treatment.
  - Symptom onset >3 h but less than 6 h in case of intra-arterial administration. This time window may be increased up to 24 h for posterior circulation (which has less likelihood of hemorrhagic conversion of infarct).

- *Exclusion criteria* apply (see contraindications).

Dose

- *Intravenous*: 0.9 mg/kg (max. 90 mg). The first 10% of the calculated dose is given as an IV bolus over 1 min, and the remainder is infused over an hour for patients within the 3- to 4.5-h window.
- *Intra-arterial*: The maximum intra-arterial dose is 22 mg. It is independent of any previously administered intravenous dose.
- 1–2 mg TPA is administered manually distal to the clot.
- Then administer an infusion of 0.5 mg/mL at 20 mL/h (10 mg/h).
- The infusion is prepared by mixing 10 mg of TPA in 20 mL on normal saline, resulting in a concentration of 1 mg TPA per 2 mL saline (or 0.5 mg/mL). Use an infusion pump for more precise administration.

- Angiography is performed every 15 min (following infusion of 2.5 mg rt-PA) as the catheter is gradually drawn back through the clot.

    - The lesion is re-crossed after each angiogram.

- If the artery is still occluded, inject 1–2 mg TPA manually and resume the TPA infusion.
- Discontinue TPA if

    - adequate recanalization is achieved,
    - extravasation of contrast material is noted on angiography,
    - a maximum dose has been administered, or
    - the administered dose approaches the maximum dose without clinical or angiographic improvement.

- In case of cranial sinus thrombosis (CST), usually 2–5 mg is administered IA through the thrombus and then an infusion is started at a rate of 1 mg/h, usually for 12 h. If clot burden is still there on angiography, a longer duration of administration until the clot resolves is a consideration.
- In CST, the infusion is prepared in a concentration of 1 mg/10 ml (0.1 mg/ml), for a rate of 10 ml/h.

Side Effects

- Bleeding including ICH and systemic bleeding, easy bruising, hematemesis, hematuria, and bleeding gums.
- Antiplatelet agents, anticoagulants and invasive procedure such as CVL insertion or NG tube insertion should be avoided for 24 h.
- If not already inserted, avoid placing a urinary catheter for at least 30 min post-infusion.

Major Complications

- Intracranial hemorrhage.

Contraindications

- The following should not receive TPA treatment:

    - Brain CT scan demonstrating ICH prior to treatment.
    - Only minor or rapidly improving symptoms of stroke.
    - Clinical presentation suggestive of SAH, even with a normal CT.
    - Active internal bleeding.

- Known bleeding diathesis including platelet count $<100 \times 10^3/mm^3$.
- Heparin within 48 h with an elevated APTT.
- Current oral anticoagulation use, e.g., warfarin, or recent use with an elevated PT (>15 s) or INR (>1.7).
- Intracranial surgery, severe TBI, or previous stroke within 3 months.
- Suspected aortic dissection associated with stroke.
- Suspected subacute bacterial endocarditis or vasculitis.
- History of GI or urinary tract hemorrhage within 21 days.
- Major surgery or serious trauma within 14 days.
- Recent arterial puncture at a non-compressible site.
- Lumbar puncture within 7 days.
- History of ICH.
- Known AVM or aneurysm.
- Witnessed seizure at the same time as onset of symptoms of stroke.
- Recent acute MI.
- SBP > 185 mm Hg or DBP > 110 mm Hg at time of treatment, or patient requires aggressive treatment to reduce BP within these limits.

Reversal

- FFP transfusion.

Coumadin

Mechanism

- Inhibits formation of vitamin K-dependent clotting factors (Factors II, VII, IX, and X).

Indications and Case Selection

- Thromboembolic events, e.g., stroke.
- Prophylaxis and/or treatment of the thromboembolic complications associated with atrial fibrillation and/or cardiac valve replacement.
- DVT.
- PE.
- CST.

Dose

- A total of 5–15 mg orally, daily, maintaining an INR 2–3× control values. The anticoagulant effects of warfarin manifest when the normal clotting factors are cleared from the circulation, which may take up to 72–96 h. Therefore, heparin coverage should be provided during this time. We prefer to commence with 5 mg daily allowing the INR to reach a therapeutic level over 2–3 days, in order to avoid bleeding complications. This is particularly important in underweight elderly patients.

Side Effects

- Bleeding.
- Hypersensitivity and adverse drug interactions with medications, such as phenytoin, prednisone, and phenobarbital.

Major Complications

- ICH or other major bleeding.

Contraindications

- Pregnancy.
- Recent craniotomy or spinal surgery, ophthalmic surgery, or major trauma surgery.
- ICH.
- Bleeding from GI, GU or respiratory tracts.
- Dissecting aorta.
- Percarditis or Pericardial effusions.

Reversal

- Phytonadione (Vitamin K) 1–2.5 mg IV and transfusion of FFP.
- Rate of vitamin K administration must not exceed 1 mg/kg due to risk of allergic reaction. Intravenous vitamin K administration also carries the risk of anaphylaxis.

Verapamil

Mechanism

- Nondihydropyridine calcium channel blocker, a phenylalkylamine that reduces the influx of calcium through the L-type calcium channels in smooth-muscle cells, enabling vasodilation. Its half-life is about 3–7 h.

Indications and Case Selection

- Before balloon angioplasty: The chemical vasodilatation prior to mechanical vasodilatation may enable a smoother and safer angioplasty.
- Mild vasospasm that does not warrant angioplasty.
- Moderate vasospasm that cannot be safely treated with angioplasty.

Dose

- 1–5 mg intra-arterially. It is slowly infiltrated (over 2–10 min) into the vasospastic vessel via a microcatheter into the intracranial vessel, and via diagnostic or guide catheter into larger vessels, e.g., ICA or, VA.

Side Effects

- Bradycardia.
- Hypotension.

Major Complications

- Hypotension.
- Bradycardia.

Contraindications

- Acute MI.
- Severe CHF.
- Cardiogenic shock.
- Severe hypotension.
- Second- or third-degree AV block.
- Sick sinus syndrome.
- Marked bradycardia.
- Hypersensitivity to the drug.
- Wolff–Parkinson–White syndrome.
- Lown–Ganong–Levine syndrome.

Papaverine

Mechanism

- It is a benzylisoquinolone alkaloid that vasodilates by inhibition of cAMP and cGMP phosphodiesterases in smooth muscle, leading to increased intracellular levels of cAMP and cGMP. Papaverine may also inhibit the release of calcium from the intracellular space by blocking calcium ion channels in the cell membrane. It is a short acting, with half-life of less than 1 h.

Indications and Case Selection

- Cerebral vasospasm. However, due to its short duration of action necessitating repeated treatments, other agents, e.g., verapamil, are preferred.
- Angioplasty pre-treatment: To enable placement of balloon catheter by causing vasodilatation.

Dose

- Available in 3% concentration (30 mg/ml) at pH 3.3.
- To obtain a 0.3% concentration, 300 mg of papaverine is diluted in 100 ml of normal saline. It is administered intra-arterially through the microcatheter, which is positioned just proximal to the affected vascular segment.
- The 300-mg dose is administered at a rate of 3 ml/min.
- Do not mix papaverine with contrast agents or heparin, which may result in precipitation of crystals.

Side Effects

- Hypotension.
- Increased ICP.
- Cerebral steal, i.e., redistribution of blood flow away from the ischemic region.
- Microembolization of papaverine crystals.
- Neurotoxicity from the preservative (chlorobutanol).
- Paradoxical vasoconstriction.
- Worsening neurological status.
- Discontinue infusion immediately if these changes occur. In most cases, there is a resolution of the untoward effects with discontinuation of papaverine.

Major Complications

- Rapid increase in ICP.
- Thrombocytopenia.
- Hypotension.
- Seizures.
- Transient neurological deficits (mydriasis and brainstem depression).
- Monocular blindness.
- Precipitation of papaverine crystal emboli during infusion.
- Paradoxical worsening of vasospasm leading to cerebral infarction.

Contraindications

- Increased ICP.
- Glaucoma.
- Hypersensitivity to papaverine.
- Atrioventricular block.
- Acute myocardial infarction.
- Recent stroke.
- Liver function disorders.

Nicardipine

Mechanism

- A calcium channel antagonist with more selective effects on vascular smooth muscle than on cardiac muscle. It attenuates the influx of calcium through the L-type calcium channels in smooth-muscle cells. The half-life is approximately 8 h.

Indications and Case Selection

- Symptomatic and TCD-confirmed vasospasm.

Dose

- Nicardipine is diluted with physiological saline to a concentration of 0.1 mg/ml and administered in 1-ml aliquots to a maximum dose of 5 mg per vessel.
- It is administered by positioning the microcatheter in the cerebral vessel requiring treatment.

Side Effects

- Transient tachycardia.
- Hypotension.
- Increased ICP.

Major Complications

- Refractory intracranial hypertension.

Contraindications

- Hypersensitivity to the drug.
- Aortic stenosis.

Nitroglycerine

Mechanism

- Potent and immediate vasodilator. Vasodilatation is caused by stimulation of cGMP, which results in vascular smooth muscle relaxation.

Indications and Case Selection

- Vessel spasm during catheterization.

Dose

- 100–300 µg through the catheter.

Side Effects

- Headache.
- Orthostatic hypotension.
- Tachycardia.

Major Complications

- Severe hypotension.
- Paradoxical bradycardia.
- Anaphylactoid reactions.

Contraindications

- Hypersensitivity to drug.
- Severe anemia.
- Increased ICP.
- Sildenafil, tadalafil, vardenafil use: These have a synergistic effect with NTG, which may result in profound hypotension and cardiovascular collapse.
- Methemoglobinemia.

Fresh Frozen Plasma (FFP)

Mechanism

- Comprises of coagulation factors including labile factors V and VIII.

Indications and Case Selection

- Coagulopathy (PT or a PTT more than 1.5 times control).
- Replacement of single coagulation factor deficiencies, where a specific or combined factor concentrate is unavailable.
- Significant bleeding during endovascular procedure.
- Immediate reversal of oral anticoagulants if Prothrombin complex concentrate is not available.
- Acute disseminated intravascular coagulation.
- Thrombotic thrombocytopenic purpura.

Dose

- 10–15 ml/kg, but further doses may be required.

Side Effects

- Allergic reaction and anaphylaxis.
- Complications associated with leukocyte depletion.
- Infection.
- Graft versus host disease.
- Venous thromboembolism.

Major Complications

- Transfusion-related acute lung injury.
- Major anaphylactic reaction.

Contraindications

- FFP is contraindicated for volume expansion.
- DIC.

Platelets

Mechanism

- Platelets supply the phospholipid needed for the interaction of factors V and Xa in the intrinsic pathway of coagulation.
- Maintain the integrity of capillary endothelium.
- Adhere almost instantaneously to injured vessel wall initiating the formation of hemostatic plug.

Indications and Case Selection

- Thrombocytopenia or an abnormality of platelet function, or both.
- Multiple transfusions.

Dose

Random Donor Platelets (RDP): 1 unit per 10 kg of body weight.

- Stable patients who are not refractory to platelet transfusions can be expected to have a platelet count increase between 5000 and 7000 per unit.
- A single unit RDP contains a minimum of 5.5×10^{10} platelets suspended in 50 mL of plasma.

Single Donor Platelets (SDP): 1 apheresis unit per transfusion episode, which is equivalent to 6–8 units of pooled RDP.

- SDP are collected by apheresis and contain a minimum of 3.0×10^{11} platelets suspended in 200–600 mL of plasma.
- Platelet products may be stored for 5 days with continuous agitation. Once pooled, platelets outdate in 4 h. Unused platelets must be returned to the blood bank within 30 min of issue.

Side Effects

- Allergic reaction and anaphylaxis.
- Febrile non-hemolytic transfusion reaction.
- Infection.
- Alloimmunization.

Major Complications

- Bacterial sepsis.
- Acute lung injury.
- Graft vs host disease.

Contraindications

- Thrombotic thrombocytopenic purpura.
- Post-transfusion purpura.
- Hemolytic uremic syndrome: Platelet transfusions have been associated with rapid deterioration and death.
- Heparin-induced thrombocytopenia.
- Platelet count >100,000/mL without evidence of platelet dysfunction.
- Idiopathic thrombocytopenic purpura, unless bleeding is life threatening.

Sodium Amytal

Mechanism

- A barbiturate derivative that activates $GABA_A$ receptors.
- During Wada test when a carotid injection of sodium amytal is administered, it temporarily anesthetizes the perfused region, resulting in isolation of the contralateral hemisphere in performing cortical functions of language and memory.
- It also blocks neuronal activity, and in conjunction with lidocaine which blocks axonal activity, it is administered as a test injection in procedures such as spinal AVM embolization, or embolization of spinal tumors, prior to the injection of the embolic agent.

Indications and Case Selection

- Wada Test.
- Test injection prior to embolization of feeder vessel of AVM. In order to suppress both neuronal and axonal activity, amytal injection is followed by xylocaine injection.

Dose

- Approximately 50–100 mg per test injection via catheter.
- It is prepared for administration as follows:

- Dilute 500 mg in 20 cc 0.9% NS to yield a concentration of 25 mg/cc of sodium amytal.
- During Wada test, after catheterization of vessel of interest, 100 mg of Sodium Amytal (4 cc of the preparation described above) are injected through the catheter. Additional boluses of 25 mg (1 cc) or modification of the original bolus may be required, per neurologist's request.

Side Effects

- High doses during recirculation may suppress the contralateral hemisphere, possibly complicating the interpretation of the Wada test.
- Confusion.
- Decrease in or loss of reflexes.
- Drowsiness.
- Fever.
- Irritability.
- Hypothermia.
- Difficulty breathing.
- Bradycardia.
- May decrease effects of hormonal contraception.

Major Complications

- Death from overdose.

Contraindications

- Porphyria.
- Hypersensitivity to barbiturates.
- Significant liver impairment or respiratory disease.

Xylocaine

Mechanism

- It blocks the fast voltage gated Na^+ Channels in neuronal cell membranes. There may be inhibition of postsynaptic neurons and consequently, action potentials.

Indications and Case Selection

- Most common usage is as local anesthetic prior to arteriotomy where preparations with or without epinephrine are used.
- Cardiac xylocaine is used to test axonal function. For this purpose it may be used alone or in conjunction with amobarbital.

- It is used in functional testing in case of spinal vascular disorders.
- Provocative functional testing in cerebral AVMs.

Dose

- 10–40 mg IA of cardiac lidocaine for neurophysiological testing.
- Usually around 5 ml of 2% lidocaine for local anesthesia (max. 4 mg/ml to 280 mg; 14 ml).

Side Effects

- Headache.
- Dizziness.
- Drowsiness.
- Visual disturbances.
- Confusion.
- Parasthesias.
- Tremor.
- Tinnitus.
- Hypotension.
- Bradycardia.
- Arrhythmias.

Major Complications

- Cardiac arrest.
- Seizures.
- Coma.
- Respiratory arrest.

Contraindications

- Second- or third-degree heart block without pacemaker.
- Allergy to amide local anesthetics.
- Concurrent treatment with class I antiarrhythmic agents (e.g., flecainide, quinidine, disopyramide, procainamide).
- Hypotension not due to arrhythmia.
- Bradycardia.
- Accelerated idioventricular rhythm.
- Porphyria.

Reversal

- In case of lidocaine overdose: intravenous bolus of 20% lipid Emulsion
  1.5 ml/kg over 1 min and start IV infusion at 15 ml/kg/h. The bolus may be
  repeated twice at 5 min intervals if cardiovascular instability is not restored.
  Additionally, the infusion may be doubled to 30 ml/kg/h if instability persists
  after 5 min. Lipid emulsion is continued until cardiovascular instability is
  restored or maximum dose administered. Do not exceed the maximum cumu-
  lative dose of 12 ml/kg.
- Concurrent supportive care including following ACLS protocols is imperative,
  e.g., securing airway and hemodynamic support.
- It may be noted that the authors have not encountered cardiovascular collapse or
  CNS toxicity due to xylocaine administration during interventional procedures.
- Additionally, propofol is not a substitute for lipid emulsion in such cases. This is
  because propofol has only 10% lipids, which is too low to be of benefit in such
  cases. Furthermore, the cardio-depressant properties of propofol may be coun-
  terproductive in such situations.
- Table 18.2 shows the mechanism of action, dosage and reversal of some drugs
  commonly used in endovascualar surgery.

Table 18.2 Mechanism of action, dosage, and reversal of some drugs commonly used in
endovascular surgery

Agent	Mechanism of action	Dose	Reversal
Antiplatelet			
Aspirin	Cyclo-oxygenase inhibitor, prevents formation of prostaglandins from arachidonic acid	325–1300 mg p.o. daily	Platelet transfusion
Ticlopidine	Platelet ADP receptor antagonist	500 mg p.o. daily	Platelet transfusion + methylprednisolone 20 mg IV
Clopidogrel	Platelet ADP receptor antagonist	75 mg p.o. daily	Platelet transfusion
Abciximab	GP IIb/IIIa receptor antagonist. Antibodies that prevent binding of fibrinogen to platelet GP IIb/IIIa receptors	Abciximab bolus 0.25 mg/kg, then infusion 0.125 μg/kg/min (max 10 μg/kg/min) for 12 h	Platelet transfusion

(continued)

Table 18.2 (continued)

Agent	Mechanism of action	Dose	Reversal
Anticoagulants			
Heparin	Glycosaminoglycan; activates and modulates AT III activity, that neutralizes and inactivates factors IXa, Xa, XIa, and XIIa	70–100 U/kg IV bolus, followed by repeated boluses to keep ACT between 200 and 350. ACT monitored hourly APTT 1.5–2.5× normal values, monitored every 6 h	Protamine sulfate: 1 mg per 100 units of circulating heparin (not to exceed 50 mg total)
Enoxaparin - Low molecular weight heparin (LMWH)	Inactivates factor Xa and thereby inhibits thrombosis	Enoxaparin: 1 mg/kg twice daily s.c.	Protamine sulfate: 1 mg per 100 units of circulating LMWH (not to exceed 50 mg total). Protamine is not fully effective against LMWH and some heparin activity may return after 3 h
Warfarin	Inhibits formation of vitamin K-dependent clotting factors (Factors II, VII, IX, and X)	5–15 mg orally, daily, maintaining an INR 2–3× control values	Vitamin K 1–2.5 mg IV (rate not to exceed 1 mg/min) and FFP transfusion
Thrombolytics			
Tissue plasminogen activator	Converts plasminogen to plasmin, fibrin specific	0.9 mg/kg (max. 90 mg). First 10% of the dose given as an IV bolus and the rest is infused over an hour IA dose: up to 22 mg in each arterial tree; given in boluses of 1–2 mg. *In stroke*: Infusion at a rate of 10 mg/h, with angiography every q 15 min *In CST:* Infusion at a rate of 1 mg/h	FFP transfusion

Suggested Readings

1. Khan SH, Abruzzo T, Sangha KS, Ringer A. Use of anti-platelet, anticoagulant and thrombolytic agents in endovascular procedures. Contemp Neurosurg. 2007;29(18):1–7.
2. Mustard JF, Kinlough-Rathbone RL, Packham MA. History of platelets. In: Gresele P, Page C, Fuster V, Vermylen J, editors. Platelets in thrombotic and nonthrombotic disorders. UK: Cambridge University Press; 2002. p. 3–24.
3. Joshi S, Meyers PM, Ornstein E. Intracarotid delivery of drugs. The potential and the pitfalls. Anesthesiology. 2008;109:543–6.

4. Fitzsimmons BF, Marshall RS, Pile-Spellman J, Lazar RM. Neurobehavioral differences in superselective Wada testing with amobarbital versus lidocaine. AJNR Am J Neuroradiol. 2003;24:1456–60.
5. Khan SH, Abruzzo T, Sangha KS, Ringer A. Use of anti-platelet, anticoagulant and thrombolytic agents in endovascular procedures. Contemp Neurosurg. 2007;29(18):1–7.
6. Sayama CM, Liu JK, Couldwell WT. Update on endovascular therapies for cerebral vasospasm induced by aneurysmal subarachnoid hemorrhage. Neurosurgical Focus. 2006;21(3).
7. Winkler SR. Stroke. In: Chisholm-Burns MA, Wells BG, Schwinghammer TL, Malone PM, Kolesar JM, Rotschafer JC, Dipiro JT, editors. Pharmacotherapy principles & practice. USA: The McGraw-Hill Companies, Inc.; 2008. p. 161–74.

Complications, Avoidance and Management

19

Cerebral Artery Rupture During Procedure

Prevention

- Always be aware of location of wire tip during intervention. Excessive manipulation may cause the tip to jump forward resulting in vessel rupture (Fig. 19.1).
- Ensure there is not too much energy in the wire or catheter. If needed, gently pull the wire or catheter back, to remove any redundancy or slack. When the slack is adequately removed, the loop just proximal to the tip will be seen to pulsate and only a fraction more retraction will be required to straighten out the system with the tip withdrawing only slightly. If done carefully, access will not be lost.

What to Do Once It Has Occurred

- An awake patient will complain of sudden, severe, and persistent headache, possibly with stiff neck. While cerebral angioplasty in an awake patient may cause pain, it is transient and dissipates when the balloon is deflated. Persistence of pain is indicative of rupture. Depending upon the severity of rupture, there may be a decline in the level of consciousness. In an anesthetized (or awake) patient, the monitors may show a sudden increase in blood pressure due to the rise in ICP. There may be concomitant bradycardia.
- ABC's first. Ensure the patient has a protected airway and remains well oxygenated. Use an ambu bag if needed. Have the patient intubated, if the airway is unprotected.

© Springer International Publishing AG 2017
S.H. Khan and A.J. Ringer, *Handbook of Neuroendovascular Techniques*,
DOI 10.1007/978-3-319-52936-3_19

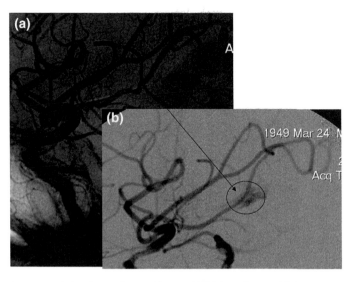

Fig. 19.1 Guidewire tip has been advanced into an MCA branch to enable ICA stenting. During manipulation, perforation of MCA occurred. In panel (**a**) the tip appears to be within the vessel. However, after the wire was retracted, contrast extravasation was noted on angiography, indicative of vessel perforation (**b**). The area of interest, where the wire tip had been, is *encircled*

- Stop and reverse therapeutic heparinization, including administration of protamine 1 mg per 100 units of heparin (maximum 50 mg). Usually, protamine is administered over 10–30 min to prevent idiosyncratic hypotension and anaphylactoid symptoms. However, in endovascular emergencies such as this one, anticoagulation must be immediately reversed by rapid IV bolus of protamine (10 mg over 1–3 min). A preloaded syringe of 50 mg should remain available at all times during most endovascular procedures, to enable rapid bolus administration in case of an emergency.
- Consider:

  - NovoSeven™ 90 µg/kg IV bolus over 2–5 min.
  - FFP.

- Immediate steps to control ICP.
- If EVD in place, open to drain CSF.
- Ensure head midline and venous return is not compromised.
- Consider anti-Trendelenberg position.
- Mannitol 1 gm/kg infused rapidly within 20 min.
- May need to direct others to perform these maneuvers while you take steps to address the complication.
- Endovascular maneuvers.

- Maintain wire (0.014″) access to the injured vessel. If access is lost, attempt to rapidly re-access the perforated vessel with wire. If successful, consider:
- Placement of a covered stent, to exclude the site of perforation. If the rupture occurred following deployment of a stent, place a second stent overlapping with the first to cover the perforation site.
- If the perforation was caused at site of balloon angioplasty during procedure, exchange for a balloon 1 mm smaller in size and inflate.
- If necessary, sacrifice the involved vessel using coils. With this approach, e.g., in the M2 segment of MCA as in Fig. 19.1, the complication of stroke is accepted with the aim of saving the patient's life.

- Neurosurgical maneuvers.

- Decompressive craniotomy, and if feasible, evacuation of the clot.

Displacement/Embolization of Detached Coil from Aneurysm

- This may occur if the coil:

- Is smaller than the circumference of the aneurysmal sac in which case, it may embolize out with the arterial pulsations.
- Is displaced by the repositioning or retraction of microcatheter.
- Was still partially in the microcatheter when detached.
- Was partially deployed and then retrieval attempted due to unsatisfactory deployment. If the coil inadvertently entangled with previously detached coils, it may pull out coil/coil mass from the aneurysm.

Prevention

- Select a coil with circumference equal to or slightly greater than the aneurysm circumference for the framing coil. Downsize gradually, as needed, for additional coils.
- Before detachment, observe the coil using live fluoroscopy. If it visibly pulsates, the chances of it being displaced out of the aneurysm are significant. Consider removing it and replacing it with a larger size coil.
- Pay particular attention to ensure that the marker on the coil has crossed the proximal marker of the microcatheter to form a 'T' before detaching it.

What to Do Once It Has Occurred

- If the coil has not displaced yet, but is threatening to do so, consider rapidly deploying additional coils to trap the offensive coil within the aneurysm.
- If the coil has already displaced out of the aneurysm then the options are as follows:

  - Assess if the coil can be retrieved endovascularly using snares or merci retriever. To do so, place a rapid transit catheter (Cordis, Miami, FL) adjacent to the coil by advancing it over microguidewire (e.g., Synchro 14).
  - Remove the microguidewire and advance an alligator retrieval device (ev3, Plymouth, MN) through the microcatheter, until it reaches the tip of the microcatheter.
  - Holding the microcatheter, advance the retrieval device slightly forward. This will result in opening of the jaws of the device (visualized fluoroscopically by separation of radiopaque markers). Attempt to engage the proximal tip of the coil. Once the coil appears to be engaged, advance the microcatheter slightly forward while holding the alligator device in position, to close the jaws of the device.
  - Maintaining slight tension on the alligator device, withdraw it and the microcatheter together as a unit completely through the guide catheter and the patient's body.
  - Sometimes, it may not be possible to withdraw the coil fragment completely. Even relocating it to less critical regions compared to intracranial vasculature, e.g., branches of ECA or peripheral vasculature of lower extremity may be more acceptable.
  - Also, bear in mind the possibility of accidentally embolizing the coil to an even more critical location, causing the patient greater harm (Fig. 19.2a–g).
  - If it is not possible to endovascularly remove the coil, a strong consideration should be given to trapping it against the wall of the vessel by using a stent as follows:

    Prowler Select Plus (0.021″ inner diameter, 5 cm distal length) (Cordis Neurovascular, Miami, FL).
    Transend microwire (0.014, or 0.010).
    Enterprise Vascular Reconstruction Device and Delivery System (Cordis Neurovascular, Miami, FL).
    The unconstrained diameter of Enterprise stent is 4.5 mm. The available lengths (in mm) are 14, 22, 28, and 37, respectively.

Technique

- The guide catheter should be positioned as close to the site of stenting as safely possible to ensure stability of the system during deployment. However, it should be at least a cm (usually more) away from the site of stent placement to enable smooth deployment.

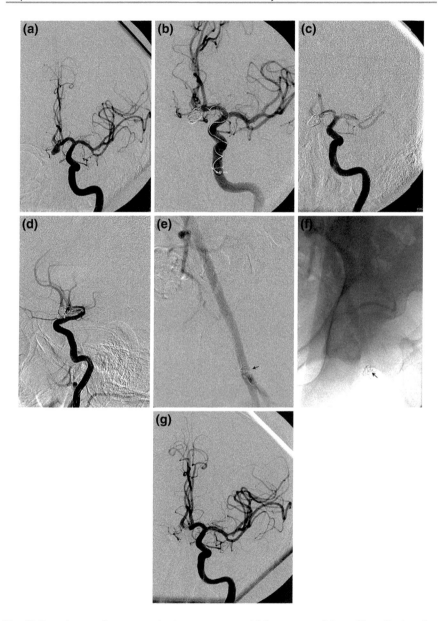

Fig. 19.2 **a** An anterior communicating aneurysm, which was treated by coiling. During the intervention, one of the coils detached prematurely resulting in a considerable length remaining outside the aneurysm and extending down into the ICA (**b**). An alligator snare was used in an attempt to grab and retrieve the errant coil. Initially, the result was rostral displacement of the coil (**c** and **d**). Eventually, the coil was successfully ensnared and retracted. However, control of the coil was lost in the femoral artery (**e**, *arrow*). The coil is better seen just inferior to femoral head on fluoroscopy image (**f**, *arrow*). The patient did not manifest any lower extremity deficit consequent to the inadvertent coil deposition. Post-intervention cerebral angiography demonstrated complete occlusion of the Acom aneurysm (**g**). There was no filling defect, vessel cutoff, or any other abnormality consequent to the earlier misadventure with the coil. After completion of intervention, vascular surgery was consulted and the errant coil was removed from the femoral artery surgically

- Our preferred stent is Enterprise stent, which is deployed as follows:
- Prepare a Prowler Select Plus microcatheter by attaching it to an RHV and removing the shaping wire from its distal tip.
- Connect the RHV to a three-way stopcock that is connected to a continuously running flush of heparinized saline.
- Ensure the microcatheter (and all catheters introduced into the patient) are free of air bubbles.
- Using fluoroscopy and roadmapping, advance a Prowler Select Plus microcatheter over a microwire and cross the site of stent deployment.
- Select the appropriate Enterprise stent and inspect the package to rule out any damage or breakage in sterility.
- Using sterile precautions, remove the dispenser hoop from the package and place it on the sterile equipment table.
- Free the delivery wire from the clip on the dispenser hoop.
- Grasp the introducer and the delivery wire at the point where it exits from the dispenser hoop. This will prevent stent movement.
- While holding the introducer and delivery wire, remove the system from the dispenser hoop. Make sure the stent is not partially deployed.
- Ensure that the wire is not kinked and the introducer is undamaged.
- Do not attempt to shape the distal end of the delivery wire.
- Loosen the RHV of the microcatheter.
- Insert the distal end of the introducer partially into the RHV.
- Tighten the RHV around the introducer.
- Press the wings of the pediatric transducer on the tubing leading to the microcatheter, which will result in increased flow. Confirm that the fluid is exiting from the proximal end of the introducer. Purge the device until the saline flush has evacuated out any air from the system.
- Slightly loosen the RHV and grasping the introducer and wire together, advance the introducer until it completely engages the hub of the microcatheter.
- Advance the delivery wire to transfer the stent from the introducer into the microcatheter. Do not torque the wire at any point.
- Continue to advance the wire until the marker at 150 cm (from the distal wire tip) enters the RHV.
- Loosen the RHV and remove the introducer off the wire.
- Using fluoroscopy, observe the stent as it is advanced toward the microcatheter tip.
- Align the stent positioning marker on the wire across the coil.
- Once positioned, confirm the following markers are visible on fluoroscopy in the following sequence distal to proximal:

  i.   Distal tip of catheter.
  ii. Distal marker on delivery wire.
  iii. Distal stent markers (appear as a single marker, until stent is deployed).
  iv. Stent positioning marker on delivery wire (this is in the mid-region of the stent.

v. Small marker indicating the extent to which the stent can be partially deployed and still recaptured (manufacturer recommends that recapture be performed only once).

vi. Proximal stent markers (appear as a single marker, until stent is deployed).

vii. Proximal marker on delivery wire.

viii. Proximal marker on the catheter (the position of this marker is not crucial provided the above are positioned adequately).

- Also ensure the distal tip of the guide catheter is visible and the catheter is stable, so it will not inadvertently collapse during stent deployment.
- Remove all slack from the system.
- Ensure the microcatheter RHV has been loosened.
- Slowly retract the microcatheter under live fluoro while holding the delivery wire stable, so that it does not move. The marker on the tip of the microcatheter will be noted to move proximally toward the markers on the delivery wire.
- As the microcatheter is retracted further, the distal stent markers will separate indicating the deployment of distal stent.
- Continue to retract the microcatheter as it passes over the stent positioning marker.
- When the catheter reaches the small marker proximal to the positioning marker, the stent can still be re-sheathed by advancing the microcatheter over the wire. However, once the microcatheter is pulled proximal to this marker, the stent can no longer be recaptured.
- Up to this point, if stent needs to be repositioned, re-sheath the stent by maintaining tension on the wire and gently advancing the microcatheter over the stent. The distal stent markers will be seen to collapse into a single marker, as before. If any resistance is encountered during microcatheter advancement, do not continue to push the catheter. Gently, retract the catheter slightly (without crossing the 'recapture limit' marker) and then re-advance.
- Retract the microcatheter over the proximal stent markers, which will result in the separation of the marker into four distinct markers, indicating the complete deployment of the stent.
- Once the microcatheter is well proximal to the stent, if needed re-advance it over the delivery wire. This will cause the microcatheter to advance within the stent and the catheter tip may be positioned distal to the stent, to maintain vascular access.
- Retract and discard the delivery wire.
- Perform angiography to confirm the vessel lumen is patent and the coil suitably trapped between the stent and vessel wall (Fig. 19.3a–i).
- If the coil herniation was consequent to a wide aneurysm neck, consideration may be given to covering the neck of the aneurysm with a stent, as well. Depending upon the location of the herniated coil from the aneurysm, this could be done by the same stent or a second stent may be deployed.
- If the aneurysm still requires further coiling, an exchange length wire may be used to exchange microcatheters and then, the microwire, e.g., Transend 0.010

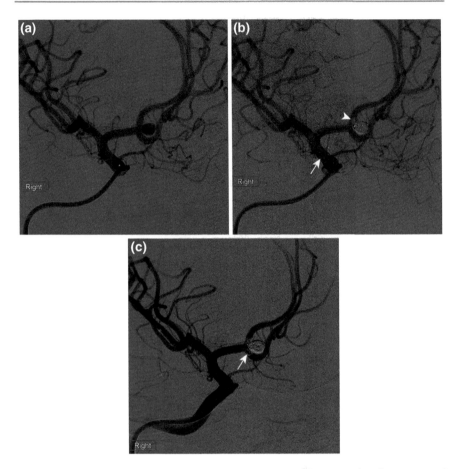

(images continued on next page)

Fig. 19.3 A ruptured anterior communicating aneurysm (**a**). Coil embolization was performed (**b**). Toward completion of the coiling, a filling defect was noted in the *right* pericallosal artery (*arrowhead*) suggestive of thrombus. In this image the final coil has been placed and the position marker on the pusher (*arrow*) is just across the proximal marker on the microcatheter, indicating the coil is ready for detachment. Following detachment, the coil herniated out of the aneurysm (**c**, *arrow*). The filling defect of *right* pericallosal was noted to worsen. The errant coil advanced up *left* pericallosal artery (**d**, *arrow*), and the affected artery was no longer visualized (compare **d** and **e**). A decision was made to trap the errant coil using an enterprise stent. To this effect, a prowler select plus catheter was advanced into the *left* pericallosal artery over a microwire (**e**). A stent was positioned in the segment with the errant coil. The guidewire is positioned beyond the coil area (*arrow*). The markings on the microcatheter, stent, and the positioning marker on the wire are appreciated further proximally. **f** The stent has been successfully deployed, resulting in reconstitution of the left pericallosal artery. The markings on either end of the stent (*arrows*) demonstrate that the segment affected by the coil is well covered. The microwire tip remains in position (*arrowhead*) in the re-apparent vessel. The coil-like structure parallel to the trapped coil is actually the positioning marker on the guidewire that indicates the *mid*-region of an undeployed stent. **g** Demonstrates satisfactory recanalization of the *left* pericallosal artery. The Prowler Select Plus catheter is appreciated in the ICA (*arrow*). The filling defect in the proximal *right* pericallosal artery persisted despite administration of Reopro. A second enterprise stent was deployed to address the filling defect in the proximal *right* pericallosal artery. The maneuver resulted in satisfactory resolution of the filling defect (**h**). Angiography performed a year later demonstrated the errant coil well trapped between the vessel wall and the stent (**i**). The filling defect in the *right* pericallosal artery is completely resolved. Both pericallosal arteries have uniform caliber and the markings on the ends of the two stents are readily appreciated

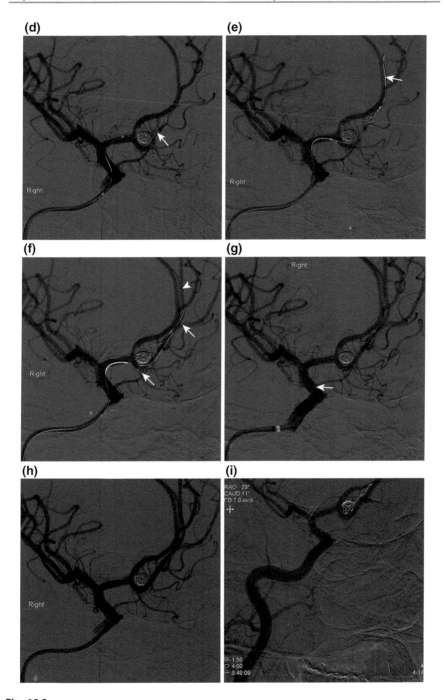

Fig. 19.3

and 0.014 used to redirect the microcatheter through the stent tines into aneurysm. Or, another consideration is to perform further coiling once the stent has endothelialized, provided most of the aneurysm has been coiled in case of ruptured aneurysms.

- In elective cases, our preference is to perform the stent placement and coil embolization in a staged fashion. Therefore, after stent placement we wait a month, with the patient on ASA + Plavix. Allowing the stent to endothelialize, decreases the likelihood of stent dislodgment during manipulation. In case of an unplanned stenting, remember to administer the patient a LD of Plavix (300 mg). Conversely, in an unruptured aneurysm, initiate Reopro, 25 mg/kg LD followed by 0.125 µgm/kg/min for 12 h. The LD of Plavix need not be administered, if Reopro is initiated.
- If the herniated coil is in a location unsuitable for stent placement, e.g., it is too distal or the vessel is too small, then consider open surgery for its retrieval. Such retrieval will carry greater risks, and these should be weighed against leaving the coil in situ and accepting a potential stroke.

Aneurysm Rupture

- This may happen during coiling of an aneurysm.
- It may also happen while performing angiography using a pressure injector in case of ruptured aneurysm, when the tip of the catheter is close to the aneurysm (Fig. 19.4a).

Prevention

- Be meticulous in technique.
- Choose a coil of the same size as the diameter of the aneurysm. Sometimes deploying a slightly larger coil is necessary to ensure stability, but too large a coil may lead to aneurysm rupture.
- Keep all wires and catheters straight, so that these devices do not build up any undue torque.
- Ensure there is no undue tension buildup in the catheters, by removing all slack. This is done by gently pulling back the microcatheter, until the proximal marker on the microcatheter is seen to pulsate.
- Watch the guidewire tip and the microcatheter tip at all times during navigation.
- Navigate while utilizing both planes. The road map used for the purpose must be without motion artifact and done with enough magnification to ensure accurate visualization. Otherwise, the guidewire or microcatheter may penetrate the aneurysm wall due to miscalculation.
- When the microcatheter tip has been placed into the aneurysm, carefully, advance and retract the microwire mimicking the action of coil deployment to

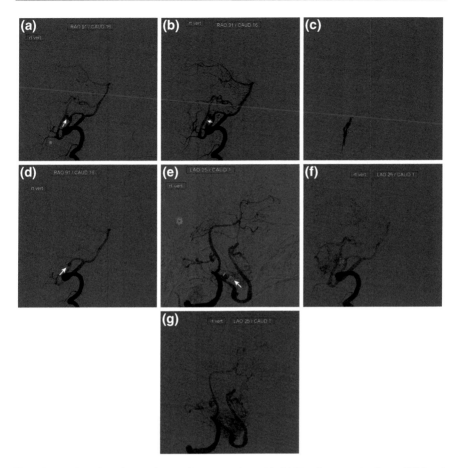

Fig. 19.4 A lateral angiogram in a patient presenting with SAH and a posterior fossa AVM and multiple PICA aneurysms (**a**). A microcatheter has been advanced into the largest and irregular shaped aneurysm. The tip of the microcatheter is much too close to the aneurysm wall (*arrow*). **b** Repeat angiography demonstrated contrast extravasation, consistent with aneurysm perforation (*arrow*). Angiography through the microcatheter also confirms the perforation **c**. Coils were rapidly deployed, allowing loops to deposit outside the aneurysm in the subarachnoid space (*arrow*, **d** and **e**). The microcatheter was gradually retracted as the coil was deployed, resulting in the coil being within and outside the aneurysm. Note there is no longer any contrast extravasation, indicating a cessation of subarachnoid hemorrhage. Complete coil occlusion of the aneurysm was achieved (**f** and **g**)

ensure that the microcatheter will not 'harpoon' forward during coil deployment and detachment.

- In a multi-lobulated aneurysm, do not attempt to advance a microcatheter tip into a region of aneurysm that is at an acute angle to the neck. The microwire may be positioned in such a location, but the microcatheter tip while being advanced will straighten the wire and most likely the microwire and catheter will perforate the aneurysm wall.

- Ensure that too stiff a coil is not placed into a ruptured aneurysm, e.g., while GDC 18 may be suitable for a large unruptured aneurysm, GDC 10 is usually a more suitable option for a similar aneurysm that presents with a rupture.
- Do not attempt to overpack the aneurysm with coils. Generally, when the aneurysm is completely filled and our catheter tip is displaced out or the smaller and softest coil does not completely deploy within the aneurysm, we consider the embolization complete.

What to Do Once Rupture Has Occurred

- Do not panic, especially if the heart rate, BP, ICP, and other parameters remain unchanged.
- Continue to coil the aneurysm to exclude it expeditiously from the cerebrovascular circulation.
- If the catheter tip is outside the aneurysm in the subarachnoid space, do not reflexively pull it back. Continue to deposit coils in the subarachnoid space as the catheter is gradually pulled back into the aneurysm. The goal is to coil outside the aneurysm, through the perforation and then within the aneurysm (Fig. 19.4b–g).
- If the patient has an external ventricular drain, open it to drain (if not done already) to prevent intracranial hypertension. By no means overdrain. Setting the drain height at 25 cm H_2O may prevent the same.
- In case of hemodynamic instability, the cause may be increased ICP. In case of posterior circulation aneurysms, the patient may not manifest increased BP in response to intracranial hypertension. There may be a paradoxical hypotension and difficulty maintaining BP due to brainstem insult.
- If an EVD is in place, ensure it is open to drain.
- In case an EVD is not in place and the patient's neurological examination deteriorates, or in a patient under GA, the monitored parameters (e.g., BP, HR, cerebral oxygenation) are indicative of deterioration, insert an EVD emergently, or have one inserted. In such a situation, the presence or absence of EVD may make a difference between life and death.

Femoral Pseudoaneurysm

Prevention

- Be meticulous with femoral artery closure.
- If an angioseal or similar device is used, deploy it attentively in order to avoid device failure.
- In case of manual compression, apply adequate pressure to initially obliterate pulse superior to puncture site for at least 15–20 min. Gradually, decrease the force of compression every 5–10 min, to ensure satisfactory closure of puncture site.

- Avoid double punctures and multiple sticks.
- Monitor pulse, BP at least every 15 min, immediately after sheath removal.

What to Do Once It Has Occurred

- Perform ultrasound to assess the pseudoaneurysm. Compression of the pseudoaneurysm with the ultrasound probe frequently also proves therapeutic.
- If ultrasound is non-diagnostic and the suspicion of pseudoaneurysm remains strong, perform an abdominal-pelvic CT (Fig. 19.5).
- Resuscitate patient with fluids and blood products as necessary.
- Consult peripheral vascular surgery for possible open surgical repair, if above steps are unsuccessful.

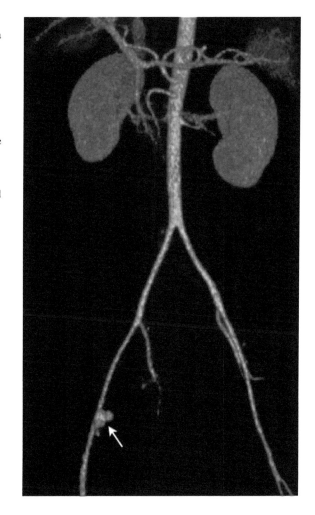

Fig. 19.5 A CT reconstruction performed in a patient who underwent a diagnostic procedure 3 days prior to presentation. The femoral arteriotomy was closed using an angioseal. While bearing down during defecation, the patient had a sensation of 'give way' in the groin. She subsequently became light headed and diaphoretic. A femoral pseudoaneurysm was detected (*arrow*). The patient responded to supportive care including saline and blood transfusions. She did not require surgical intervention

Thromboembolic Complications

Prevention

- Practice meticulous catheter hygiene. Do not allow blood to stagnate in a catheter
- Catheters should almost always be connected to continuously running flush of heparinized saline. The flush is interrupted only transiently, e.g., when injecting contrast for angiography.
- When the wire is within the catheter during navigation causing flush to be interrupted, do not persist with catheterization for longer than 3 min. Retract the wire, back bleed the catheter for at least its' total volume, and then flush forward with heparinized saline to free the catheter of any blood. Then, the wire may be re-inserted and navigation resumed.
- When manipulating wire, ensure the tip is continuously being rotated so that it does not inadvertently cause scraping of embolic material from the vessel wall.
- Do not advance catheter tip without the wire leading.
- In an interventional case, heparinize patient.
- Never ever attempt to overcome a resistance felt in the catheter, by injecting with greater force. The resistance may be due to blockage from a blood clot in the catheter. Back bleed the catheter for its volume and then flush. If no back bleeding occurs despite pulling the catheter slightly back, remove the catheter completely and investigate the cause of blockage on the side table. If the catheter is noted to have significant clot burden, replace it with a new one.

What to Do Once It Has Occurred

- It is diagnosed by a luminal filling defect or a vessel cutoff downstream (Fig. 19.6a).
- The following options can be used separately or in combination:
- If in an accessible location and a guide catheter is in position, advance a microcatheter over a microwire such that the microcatheter tip is adjacent to the clot. Remove the microwire. Disconnect the microcatheter hub from the heparinized saline flush system and attach a 3-ml syringe to the hub. Gently pull back syringe plunger in an attempt to aspirate the clot. Retract the microcatheter while maintaining aspiration (Fig. 19.6b).
- Once the microcatheter is out of the guide catheter, discharge its contents on a gauze piece and inspect for any aspirated clot.
- Perform angiography to assess whether or not the clot has been removed.
- Administer Reopro (L.D. loading dose of 0.25 mg/kg followed by continuous IV infusion of 0.125 μg/kg/min (maximum 10 μg/min) for 12 h, then discontinue. Usually, this will suffice.

(a)   **(b)**

(c)   **(d)**

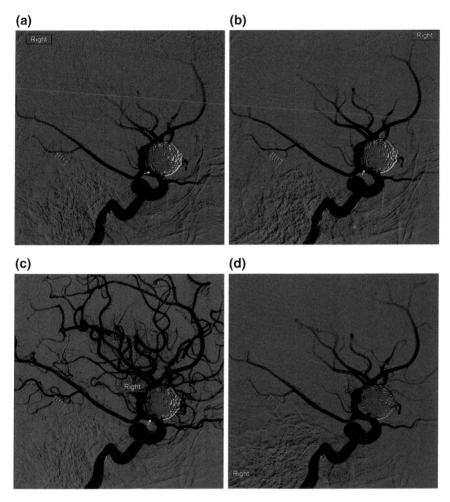

Fig. 19.6 At culmination of coil embolization of a right ophthalmic aneurysm, a luminal defect in the adjacent ICA was noted (**a**, *arrow*). The microcatheter already in position for coiling was used to aspirate the clot. However, this proved unsuccessful (**b**, *arrow*). Reopro was administered adjacent to the clot, through a microcatheter. It resulted in attenuation of the luminal defect (**c**, *arrow*). Repeat angiography demonstrated complete resolution of the clot and restoration of normal ICA lumen (**d**)

- If a microcatheter is in position, the loading dose can be administered via the microcatheter into the clot and adjacent artery, prior to the first attempt at aspiration as described above (Fig. 19.6c, d).
- Check for resolution of luminal defect by performing angiography after each remedial maneuver, e.g., following administration of Reopro, following aspiration.

- Consider using Penumbra System to attempt removing the clot. This is not an option in distal or terminal vessel cutoff. If Penumbra or similar interventional devices are used, patient should be placed on heparin prophylaxis for approximately 12 h (900 IU/h for 12 h for patients less than 70 kg, and 1300 IU/h for 12 h for patients >70 kg). This postoperative heparinization is not necessary, if Reopro is used.
- If angiographic abnormality persists, e.g., luminal defect, then depending upon extent of defect, consider deploying a stent across the site to restore the luminal caliber. If a stent is deployed and was preceded by Reopro, start the patient on ASA 325 mg daily, indefinitely and Plavix 75 mg daily the following day, for 1 month. A loading dose of Plavix is not necessary as the Reopro will persist in the patient's system for around 72 h.

Dissection

- It may happen consequent to significant device manipulation.

Prevention

- Practice meticulous technique. Advance catheters over wire. Do not forcefully push wires. Continue to half-rotate wire back and forth as it is being advanced.
- Provide adequate sheath/guide catheter support in case of tortuous vasculature, e.g., consider using a longer than the usual 10–11 cm sheath, or even a shuttle sheath.
- Maintain the guide catheter as close to the site of intervention as safely possible. However, do not force the guide catheter up if resistance is encountered and do not place a large, stiff catheter in a vessel segment unsuitable for it.

What to Do Once It Has Occurred

- Assess the extent of dissection. If it is minor, innocuous appearing and without a raised intimal flap, no intervention may be necessary. The site of dissection could be re-examined after an interval to verify resolution. If managed conservatively, place the patient on aspirin, with or without Plavix.
- If the dissection is significant, place a suitable stent across the affected segment (see chapter on intracranial and extracranial stenting, as the case may be) and commence patient on ASA and Plavix.
- Plavix 75 mg PO daily is usually administered for a month. ASA is usually continued indefinitely.

ICH

- This may occur because of factors such as: Performing an invasive procedure and the patient is commenced on anticoagulants soon thereafter, e.g., a ventriculostomy is done with a consequent unrecognized active bleeding. The patient then undergoes a planned intervention with usage of heparin (Fig. 19.7a–h).
- Uncontrolled high blood pressure in the presence of antiplatelet/anticoagulants/, thrombolytic agents and manipulation during intervention may be contributory.

Prevention

- Refrain from performing unnecessary procedures while patient is/will be on heparin.
- Keep a low threshold of suspicion and aggressively investigate in case of any untoward change in the patient's neurological status.
- Perform CT head early in part of workup for declined level of consciousness. Bear in mind the artifact from coils, metal in bolts, humming birds, etc., may make the identification of early ICH challenging. Therefore, the CT scan should be reviewed carefully.

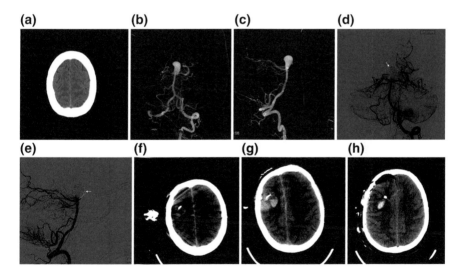

Fig. 19.7 A patient presenting with posterior fossa SAH consequent to ruptured aneurysm. A ventriculostomy was placed due to declined level of consciousness and enlarged ventricles. An upper cut of a CT scan prior to any intervention is largely unremarkable **a**. The basilar tip aneurysm (**b** and **c**) was coiled uneventfully (**d** and **e**, *arrow*). Per protocol, the patient was placed on IV heparin postoperatively. The patient initially did well, but subsequently complained of a headache. A CT scan was obtained which revealed an ICH (**f**). Heparin was stopped. However, the hematoma continued to expand (**g**), with a progressive decline in level of consciousness, requiring a craniotomy for evacuation of hematoma (**h**)

What to Do Once It Has Occurred

- Stop the heparin, and if required, reverse it using protamine.
- Assess whether decompressive craniotomy/craniectomy is required.

Retroperitoneal Hematoma

- This may occur because of unrecognized bleeding from femoral access site, especially if patient is on anticoagulants or antiplatelet agents.

Prevention

- The patient should undergo groin checks, pulse checks, and vital sign monitoring every 15 min for an hour, then every 30 min for an hour, and then at least every hour for 12 h, or until the patient is in hospital in case of overnight procedure.
- In case the vital signs, patient diaphoresis, thready pulse, etc., are indicative of blood loss, fully investigate the potential causes including, obtaining an abdominal-pelvic CT scan and femoral ultrasound.

What to Do Once it Has Occurred

- Supportive care including IV fluids and if need be PRBC.
- If bleeding from the access site is suspected, perform USG to confirm. The USG probe may also be used therapeutically to apply pressure and stop the bleeding.
- Reverse anticoagulants.
- Vascular surgery consultation.
- Consider discontinuing antiplatelet agents. This may be very problematic if the patient has had a recent stent insertion, as it creates the risk of in-stent thrombosis. In such a situation, decision has to be made on a case by case basis taking into account the risks of continuing or discontinuing antiplatelets. Sometimes a compromise can be made, e.g., Plavix is discontinued while continuing ASA.
- Retroperitoneal hematoma, unless significant, is managed with conservative, supportive care.

Radial Artery Thrombosis

Prevention

- Perform arteriotomy as atraumatically as possible.
- Ensure the ulnar artery is patent (do modified Allen's test).
- Use the smallest caliber of sheath/catheter needed for the procedure.
- Continue heparinized saline flush.
- Do not maintain sheath any longer than necessary. Remove sheath after procedure while the patient is still anticoagulated.

What to Do Once It Has Occurred

- Usually, it is clinically asymptomatic or symptoms are self-limiting.
- If symptomatic, do a Doppler study to confirm diagnosis.
- Obtain vascular surgery consultation.
- Consider LMWH.

Device Failure

Stretched Coil

- This is a mechanical failure or unraveling of the coil.
- The considerations are similar to those for errant coil, described above.
- If irretrievable, immobilize it against the wall of the vessel by placing a stent that will trap the coil between it and vessel wall (Fig. 19.2).

Stent Deployment Failure

- If the stent is still within the microcatheter, remove the Microcatheter/sheath along with contained stent.
- If the stent is partially deployed, attempt to retrieve it back into the microcatheter. If this is not possible, then retract the entire system along with the stent outside the patient or, if complete retraction is not possible, retract to deploy the stent in a more neutral location, e.g., ECA or its branches.

Errant Placement of Stent

- Consider if it is feasible to leave the stent as is because that may be the safer option.
- If not then, introduce a microcatheter (e.g., Excelsior SL 10 or Prowler Select Plus) over the wire.
- Use the microcatheter to introduce an alligator snare or a similar retrieval device. Grab the stent and pull to the tip of the catheter. If possible, withdraw the stent and microcatheter into the guide catheter. Once within the guide catheter, remove the entire system. If the stent cannot be retracted into the guide catheter, maintain it at the tip of the catheter and pull out system. Maintain wire access, whenever possible.
- Again, if the stent cannot be retrieved or repositioned with reasonable risk, the better option may be to accept the malposition.

Merci Device Fracture

- To prevent device fracture, position the microcatheter tip marker just proximal to retriever loops. This position of microcatheter with respect to retriever loops should be maintained through the procedure, to diminish the likelihood of retriever fracture.
- The manufacturer recommends that no more than five revolutions be made with the retriever to prevent its fracture.

What to Do Once It Has Occurred

- Attempt to retrieve it by advancing alligator snare or similar device through the microcatheter and grasping the fractured retriever.

Index

© Springer International Publishing AG 2017
S.H. Khan and A.J. Ringer, *Handbook of Neuroendovascular Techniques*,
DOI 10.1007/978-3-319-52936-3